Nutrition: An Approach to Good Health and Disease Management

Edited by

Esperanza J. Carcache de Blanco and Jay Mirtallo

The Ohio State University
Columbus, OH
USA

DEDICATION

Dr. Esperanza Carcache de Blanco dedicates this edition to her students, teaching assistants, and post-docs as they are the main source of inspiration in her day-to-day journey. She also would like to express her sincere appreciation to her teachers as they transmitted valuable knowledge, ethical principles, and advice. Finally, she wishes to express her thanks and gratitude to her family for providing love, affection, encouragement, and support.

Esperanza J. Carcache de Blanco
The Ohio State University
USA

CONTENTS

FOREWORD

The Center for Disease Control and Prevention is reporting staggeringly high overweight and obesity statistics in the United States and the percentages continue to climb year after year. Complications from obesity and worsening of diseases associated with obesity are putting a financial burden on individuals, families and the nation. Increased costs are associated both directly with higher medical health consumption and expenditures and indirectly with associated sick time and absenteeism. Because of this escalation in obesity, including pediatric obesity, life expectancy for the younger generation is now lower than that of their parents, a phenomenon that has never before been reported. Analogous to obesity, the percentages of individuals struggling with eating disorders are also climbing. Unhealthy eating behaviors for the sake of weight loss including starvation, purging and laxative abuse are placing individuals at risk for osteoporosis, esophagitis, gastric rupture and cardiovascular and endocrine system complications, as well as death.

A basic understanding of the fundamentals of nutrition and the importance of healthy nutrition has never been more critical than it is now. The responsibility for understanding and teaching the value of healthy nutrition can no longer be expected only from a dietitian. It is imperative that all healthcare providers be able to converse with their patients about healthy nutritional behaviors and preventive steps to incorporate into their daily lives to reduce disease complications and/or prevent disease altogether. A review of the patient's diet and nutritional behaviors should be incorporated into every patient visit and all healthcare providers should be assuring that patients have an understanding of proper nutritional habits.

The authors have presented up-to-date, evidence-based, clinically relevant material at a level appropriate for a healthcare provider. The chapters span from the necessary foundational knowledge of macronutrients to the nutritional role of micronutrients and phytochemicals. An appreciation for food regulation, socio-economic factors and cultural issues which must be considered when evaluating the patient's diet and recommending necessary changes, are also discussed. Lastly, and of great importance, managing the patient with respect to co-diseases is reviewed.

Drs. Carcache de Blanco and Mirtallo have shown remarkable thought and skill in compiling a comprehensive, well-organized text providing necessary nutritional information to health care providers. They are to be commended for identifying a void in the healthcare literature and taking the necessary steps to rectify the problem. This book is of great value and will enhance any nutrition course and curriculum.

Jane Gervasio
Butler University College of Pharmacy and Health Science
4600 Sunset Avenue
Indianapolis, IN 46208-3485
USA
E-mail: jgervasi@butler.edu

PREFACE

Healthy lifestyles and dietary changes have become a major global custom and represent in business a trillion-dollar-plus market. Regrettably, this tendency is related to a dramatic global rise in lifestyle related ailments. Nutrition; therefore, plays an important role in human health, and education on the role of nutrition healthy life and disease management should be an integral part of healthcare professional programs. The level and type of nutrition are influenced by multiple factors including cultural background, education, environmental conditions, and socio-economic status. Other factors include physical activity, food habits, and disrupted biological clocks. The impact of these elements has been linked to risk of developing chronic diseases. Concomitantly, adequate nutrition and the application of pharmaconutrition concepts could optimally manage these diseases.

The focus of this book is to cover nutrition concepts important for health promotion and disease prevention supported by applications using real-life scenarios to put these principles to use immediately and have a foundation to adapt to newer concepts of nutrition that would improve their individual health as well as their relatives, friends and patients. The content of this book also provides concepts that can be used for the integration of a nutrition-based therapeutic plan into the daily assessment of patients for disease prevention and treatment. Chapters of this book include content on macronutrients, micronutrients and their main sources; dietary guidelines and major components of a healthy diet; impact of socio-economic and cultural factors in diet, nutrition, and disease risk; malnutrition; the influence of disease on nutrient metabolism; the role of inflammation in response to nutritional interventions and specific nutrition principles applied to cardiac, gastrointestinal, diabetes and dyslipidemia diseases. To reflect on the content, the authors have included applications of nutritional requirements and patient cases as a way to facilitate the use of nutrition concepts in healthcare by healthcare professionals.

The final goal of the book is to provide information on the possible role of a balanced and integrated diet to maintain good health; to prevent, manage, and treat diseases; and to describe how factors such as education, status, environmental conditions, and cultural background influence nutritional choices and health-related risks. All the topics are discussed with a rational, scientific approach. The individual that successfully integrates the knowledge in this book and completes the exercises correctly should be able to assess an individual's diet, make suggestions for lifestyle and dietary changes that promote health, educate the public on a healthy diet as well as recognize individuals at risk of malnutrition.

Esperanza Carcache de Blanco and Jay Mirtallo
The Ohio State University
Columbus, OH
USA

CONTRIBUTORS

Carcache de Blanco, EJ	College of Pharmacy, The Ohio State University, Columbus, OH 43210, USA
Eggers, NA	College of Pharmacy, The Ohio State University, Columbus, OH 43210, USA
Forestrania, RC	College of Pharmacy, The Ohio State University, Columbus, OH 43210, USA
Lee, K	Food Science and Technology, The Ohio State University, Columbus, OH 43210, USA
Manwill, P	College of Pharmacy, The Ohio State University, Columbus, OH 43210, USA
Mirtallo, J	College of Pharmacy, The Ohio State University, Columbus, OH 43210, USA
Ogavalgual, M	College of Pharmacy, The Ohio State University, Columbus, OH 43210, USA
Pascall, MA	Food Science and Technology, The Ohio State University, Columbus, OH 43210, USA

Nutrition: An Approach to Good Health and Disease Management

Professor Jay Mirtallo dedicates this book to those individuals who believe that all health professionals should have a basic knowledge of nutrition along with skills necessary to apply this knowledge in their professional practice. Professor Mirtallo would like to express his sincere appreciation and gratefulness to Mr. Peter J. Blanco Carcache for designing the book cover.

Jay M. Mirtallo
The Ohio State University
USA

CHAPTER 1

Background: Nutrition in Health and Disease

Esperanza J. Carcache de Blanco* and Jay Mirtallo*

College of Pharmacy, The Ohio State University, Columbus, Ohio, USA

Abstract: Nutrition is a key player in the well-being of healthy individuals. Nutritional models have been designed over decades in an attempt to improve dietary patterns. In the last decades the government has been involved in the monitoring of the guidelines. Particularly, USDA has participated in the revision of nutritional models based on better understanding of nutritional needs. Hence, this chapter provides an overview on nutritional models and its correlation and impact on nutrition in health and disease management.

Keywords: Basic four, basic seven, cardiovascular, daily food, diabetes, dietary goals, food guides, hypertension, ill, myplate, pharmaconutrition, protective foods, pyramids, USDA, wheel.

INTRODUCTION

The human body is a complex system and requires a diet rich in multiple components in order to be healthy and prevent or fight disease. Nutrition involves multiple "processes by which the human organism ingests, digests, absorbs, transports, and eliminates food substances" (Wardlaw and Smith, 2011). As such, nutrients in the diet are assimilated into the body and are essential in promoting normal metabolism as well as cellular and organ function. According to Wardlaw and Smith, "Nutrition is the science that links food to health and disease" (Wardlaw and Smith, 2011). With the advancement in science, nutrition has been applied to different fields. Pharmaconutrition, by Dr. of Pharmacy Paul Clayton, is defined as follows: "With the right diet and lifestyle, the body has fantastic power to both heal and repair injured functions. I call this new science "Pharmaco-Nutrition" (Clayton, 2014). From the Greek, pharmakon means drug and threpsi means nutrition, nourishment. Pharmaconutrition is a new paradigm, according to Dr. Daren Heyland from the Society of Critical Care Medicine. During the past decade, significant advances have made possible the understanding of the role of key nutrients and

***Corresponding authors Esperanza J. Carcache de Blanco and Jay Mirtallo:** College of Pharmacy, The Ohio State University, Columbus, OH 43210, USA; E-mails: carcache-de-blan.1@osu.edu; mirtallo.1@osu.edu

nutrition in general, specially, in the management of severely sick individuals (Heyland, 2007). Lately, Pharmaconutrition has evolved to cover a wider area. According to Dr. Paul Clayton,

> "Pharmaco-Nutrition is based on what we eat and premise that, with the help of scientific and documented knowledge from pharmacology, biochemistry and epidemiology, we can develop new diets and varied micro nutritional programmes, with no negative side effects, which can re-create the balance in the body's complex metabolic systems. Pharmaco-Nutrition starts by mapping out the many metabolic discrepancies in the body which, for instance, may be the cause of cardiovascular diseases and degenerative joint conditions. The results are compared with the knowledge we have already gathered from pharmacology and nutrition. This forms the basis for extensive micro nutritional programs which can contribute to restoring the metabolic balance of the body. Pharmaco-Nutrition teaches us that physical breakdown of the body, which usually develops in parallel to increasing age, can be avoided. This depends on an alteration in our way of thinking, so that illnesses and the symptoms of aging can be prevented and treated" (Clayton, 2014).

IMPORTANCE OF NUTRITION IN HUMAN HEALTH

There are different factors associated to human health and disease states. Lifestyle is an important factor; it is key to developing and maintaining an optimal state of health. According to published data, 72% men and 64% women have been reported to be either overweight or obese (Kenney *et al.*, 1999; Ryan, 2010). Reports also state that poor diet and physical inactivity directly correlates with morbidity and mortality. Disease states that have been correlated to nutrition and lifestyle factors include cardiovascular diseases with 37% (81.1 million), osteoporosis with 50% women and 25% men (50 y/o or older) having an osteoporosis-related fracture in their lifetime, and cancer with 41% to be diagnosed during their lifetime due to dietary factors associated with cancer risk (USDA and DHHS, 2010). This relationship has also been observed for conditions believed to predispose to hypertension and diabetes; pre-hypertension with 34%, hypertension with 34% (74.5 millions), pre-diabetes with 35% (78 million), and diabetes with 11% (24 million) (USDA and DHHS, 2010). These associations suggest nutrition to be important for the maintenance of health as well as disease prevention, management and treatment.

HISTORY OF FOOD GUIDES

Over the years, there have been different models in the United States created to promote a healthy diet. A healthy diet promotes health and minimizes risk of developing disease. The models (Fig. **1**) have been improved based on increased understanding of nutritional concepts (USDA, 2011). A brief description of several different models used by the USDA is presented below (Welsh *et al*., 1992).

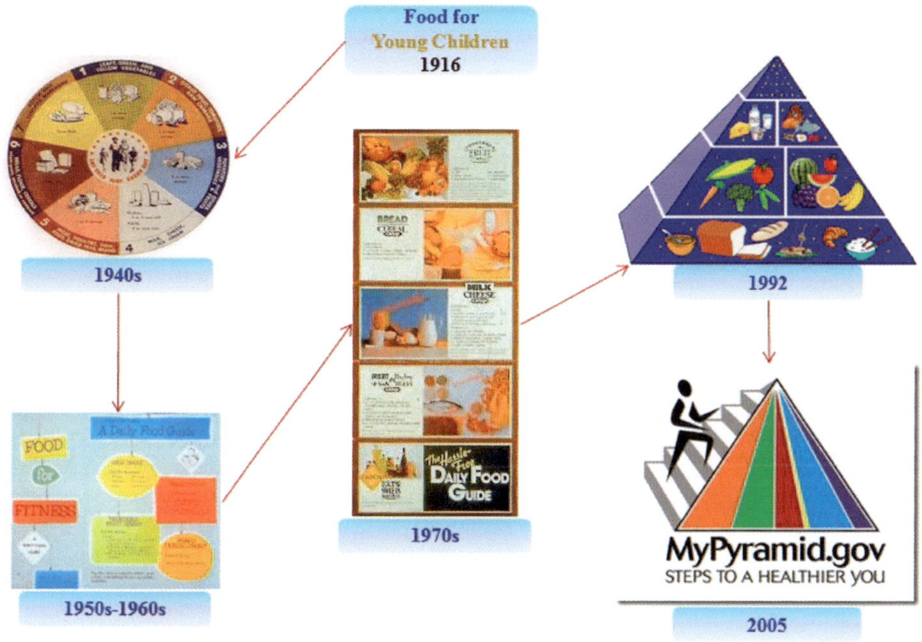

Fig. (1). History of food guides. (USDA, 2011).

Between 1916 and 1930s: The Food Guide "Food for Young Children" and "How to Select Food"

- This model established direction founded on five food groups (milk and meat, cereals, vegetables and fruits, fats and fatty foods, and sugars and sugary foods) and household measures

- The focus of this model remained on "protective foods"

In the 1940s: There was "A Guide to Good Eating (Basic Seven Groups)"

- President Roosevelt called for a National Nutrition Conference to define Recommended Daily Allowances (RDA's). The conference also focused on the potential of public education on nutrition and endorsed ten characteristics of an effective program (Table **1**) (Davis and Saltos, 1999; FSA, 1941).

- These characteristics are still recommended today.

- The foundation of the diet in this model was for nutrient appropriateness.

- The model included the number of servings per day necessary from each food group.

- The RDA provided specific suggested intakes for calories and included nine essential types of nutrients such as protein, iron, calcium, vitamins A and D, thiamin, riboflavin, niacin, and ascorbic acid (vitamin C).

- The model, however, lacked specific serving sizes and expected that individuals would include additional types of foods than that the guide suggested to fulfill the needs for calories and nutrients.

- Overall, the model was considered complex.

Table 1. Features of an effective program for public nutrition education. (Davis and Saltos, 1999; Federal Security Agency, 1941).

Public Nutrition Education Program*
• Reach out to all groups, races, sexes, creeds, ages.
• Recognize intentions for action and embrace recommendations on what to do and how to do it.
• Help advance proficient leadership.
• Drive home constantly similar ideas and through different mechanisms.
• Use every appropriate education tool available.
• Adjust tools to different groups and employ them with intelligence and proficiently.
• Include all stages of individual, family, and group situations that have an influence upon the ability to produce, buy, prepare, conserve, and consume food.
• Provide and support opportunity for involvement in making, putting into effect, and assessing local nutrition programs.
• Procure fullest participation through the use of all possible channels to reach the heart of the community.
• Be properly financed.

*Original sentences have been modified.

Between 1956 to 1970s: A new food guide "Food for Fitness, A Daily Food Guide (Basic Four groups)"

- The foundation of the model was to achieve goals for nutrient adequacy.
- It had specified amounts from four food groups (fruits, meat, milk and vegetables, and grain products).
- It was focused on providing sufficient nutrients and was widely used for about twenty years.
- It did not contain guidance on proper fats, sugars, and calorie consumption.

In 1979: A modified guide "Hassle-Free Daily Food Guide"

- The model was developed once the 1977 Dietary Goals for the United States were released.
- As a result of this model, the United States Department of Agriculture (USDA) began addressing the role of certain dietary components such as fats, sugars, and sodium in the risks of certain chronic diseases, in its 1979 publication, Food.
- The model was grounded on the Basic Four, but it also comprised a fifth group to highlight the need for moderate consumption of fats, sweets, and alcohol.

In 1984: A new food guide "Food Wheel: A Pattern for Daily Food Choices"

- The food guide model was represented by a food wheel for the first time.
- The model was first presented for a Red Cross nutrition course as a food wheel.
- The total dietary approach incorporated goals for both nutrient appropriateness and moderation.
- The use of five food groups and quantities formed the foundation for the Food Guide Pyramid later.

- The model listed amounts of food for daily intake that were given at three calorie levels.

- Since the development of this model, dietary guidelines for Americans are revised every 5 years.

In 1992: Food Guide Pyramid

- The Food Guide Graphic was, for the first time, presented as a Pyramid.

- The total dietary approach included goals for both nutrient appropriateness and moderation.

- The model was developed based on consumer research, to acknowledge new food arrangements.

- The illustration for the consumer focused on concepts of diversity, moderation, and amount.

- The model also included visualization features to represent added fats and sugars throughout five different food groups and moderation was symbolized by the small tip of the pyramid.

- The model included a range for daily quantities of food across three calorie levels.

- In 1995, these guidelines were mandated to be revised by decree, with the 1990 National Nutrition Monitoring and Related Research Act.

- Although there were many flaws in the Food Pyramid Guide, it was not revised until 2005. Issues with the 1992 Pyramid addressed in the 2005 Revision (My Pyramid – see below) are summarized as follows:

  - All fats are bad for health.
  - All carbohydrates are good dietary components.
  - Protein sources (animal or plant sources) are interchangeable.
  - Eat your potatoes.

In 2005: The guide "MyPyramid Food Guidance System"

Improvements to the original Food Guide Pyramid introduced in the MyPyramid website included the benefits of unsaturated fats, recognition of the health benefits of whole grains and an emphasis on the importance of controlling your weight. A key positive advance of My Pyramid was the inclusion of exercise and physical activity (life-style) as a part of a healthy eating strategy.

- This model was presented along with updating the Food Guide Pyramid patterns for the *2005 Dietary Guidelines for Americans* (US-DHHS and USDA, 2005), that included amounts of food for daily consumption for 12 levels of calorie.
- The model continued the "pyramid" concept, based on consumer research, but using simplified graphics.
- Detailed information of the model was made available through the website "MyPyramid.gov".
- The model added a strip for oils and the concept of physical activity as an integral part of good nutrition and health.
- The illustration in this model could also be used to describe concepts of diversity, moderation, and quantities.

Comparison of "Pyramids"

Several pyramids have been put to test as a result of this model (Fig. **2**). However, the "Mediterranean Diet Food Pyramid" has been used for comparison with other food guides.

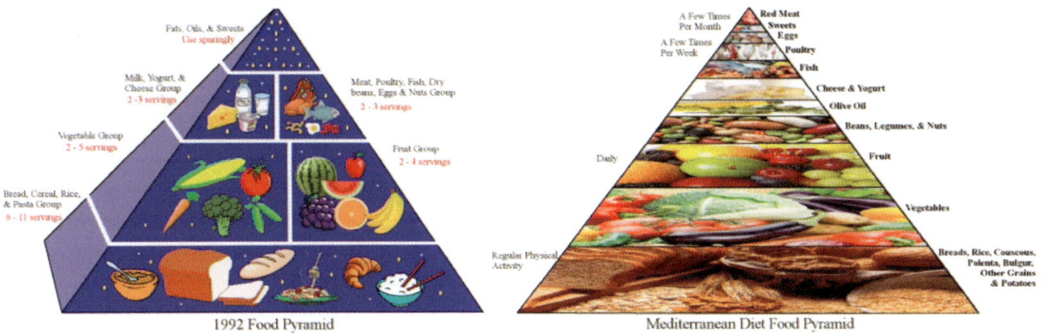

Fig. (2). Comparison of two pyramids (USDA, 2011).

Comparative data of Fig. 2.

1992 USDA Guidelines

- Six broad food groups (*e.g.* Dry beans, Eggs, Fish, Meat, Poultry & Nuts group).
- Portions based off of serving sizes (*e.g.* 2 – 4).
- No recommendation for physical exercise.
- Shows relative distribution of natural fats & sugars throughout the pyramid.
- Grains, Vegetables, & Fruits compose the base of the pyramid.

Mediterranean Diet

- Eleven specific food groups (*e.g.* Fish Group, Legume Group, Red Meat Group).
- Portions based off of relative group size in pyramid.
- Recommends regular physical exercise.
- Does not show presence of fats & sugars in other portions of the pyramid.
- Grains, Vegetables, & Fruits compose the base of the pyramid.

In 2011: My Plate

- This model was introduced along with the new USDA food patterns for the *2010 Dietary Guidelines for Americans*.
- The model has different graphics to help attract consumers' attention with a new visual cue.
- The model has an icon that reminds consumer of healthy eating, not intended to deliver specific messages.
- The visual is associated to food and is a familiar mealtime representation in consumers' minds, as identified through studies.

- The word "My" in this model carries on the personalization approach from MyPyramid.

History of Pharmaconutrition

Over 40 years ago, artificial nutrition began to be used as a supportive care. It managed metabolic support while the patient recuperated from the primary ailment. Nutrition support teams identified patients with nutritional issues (*e.g.*, malnourished or catabolic patients), performed measurements and calculations, and provided artificial nutrition in order to reduce the loss of calories, proteins, and micronutrients (to prevent or treat inflammatory disorders). Time passed and very few large-scale trials published patterns used in this practice. However, energy requirements or protein loss were object of discussion. Recently, the use of large randomized clinical trials with application of meta-analysis has correlated this practice to stronger signals of therapeutic effect. Nutritional strategies seemed to be making an impact on patient outcomes. What were most illuminating to the clinical practice guidelines were the clinically important outcomes of the largest treatment effects from studies of particular nutrients (antioxidants, arginine, fish oils, and glutamine). Thus, the concept of pharmaconutrition developed (Jones and Heyland, 2008). This new treatment model comprised valued nutrients and the application of nutritional strategies that can have significant effects on critically ill patients, particularly on immunological, inflammatory, metabolic, and other pathophysiological disorders. The focus of the study was on understanding the effect of specific nutrients on the causal disease process and on the clinical consequences. The study moved from understanding nitrogen balance or energy requirements of supported to the modulation of disease response and improvement of chances of survival (Jones and Heyland, 2008).

In summary, pharmaconutrition has been used to improve the care in ICU of critically ill patients. It has progressed from being considered as immune enhancing diet to immune modulating diet. Specialized diets are not generalized to critically ill patients because some of these diets can be even harmful to some patients. An example of a clinical application includes modulation of cytokine expression to help patients overcome a particular health related issue. Another example includes looking for a particular nutrient effect to modulate the immune system of ill patients. However, recent guidelines have suggested that parenteral nutrition therapy may be harmful to critically ill patients when not managed properly (such as inducing hyperglycemia). Thus, pharmaconutrition should be used with caution in critically ill patients. On the other hand, parenteral nutrients can be more helpful if used appropriately (Wischmeyer, 2008). Inflammatory response using parental nutrients may have positive results when compared to the use of macronutrients such as proteins using parenteral nutrition (Heyland *et al.*, 2008). Outcomes of parenteral nutrition may be improved if contemporary practices are routinely adapted in the clinical setting (Mirtallo, 2013).

Nutrients

The primary focus of nutrition in health and disease is to ingest a diet that is complete, balanced, and in an amount that promotes normal body functions. By complete, the intent is that the diet includes all the nutrients necessary for life in amounts that prevent a deficiency or symptoms from continual excessive ingestion. Nutrients are substances obtained from food that are vital for growth and maintenance of a healthy body throughout life. They function to build or repair tissues, support metabolism and organ function and provide a source of energy. The intent of a balanced diet is for the nutrients to work together for health. The statement: 'Too much of a good thing is bad" applies specifically to the human diet. Also, the absence of an essential nutrient could have devastating consequences. For example, we learned from manufacturer shortages of parenteral vitamins that adequate amounts of thiamine are required to avoid life-threatening deficiencies (Centers for Disease Control and Prevention, 1997). Lactic acidosis caused by thiamine deficiency became a clinical dilemma in patients that required parenteral nutrition (Fig. **3**) (Centers for Disease Control and Prevention, 1997). Thiamine dcficiency causes an improper functioning of α-ketoglutarate dehydrogenase. Glycolysis then shifts to an anaerobic pathway which produces lactate and subsequently, lactic acidosis.

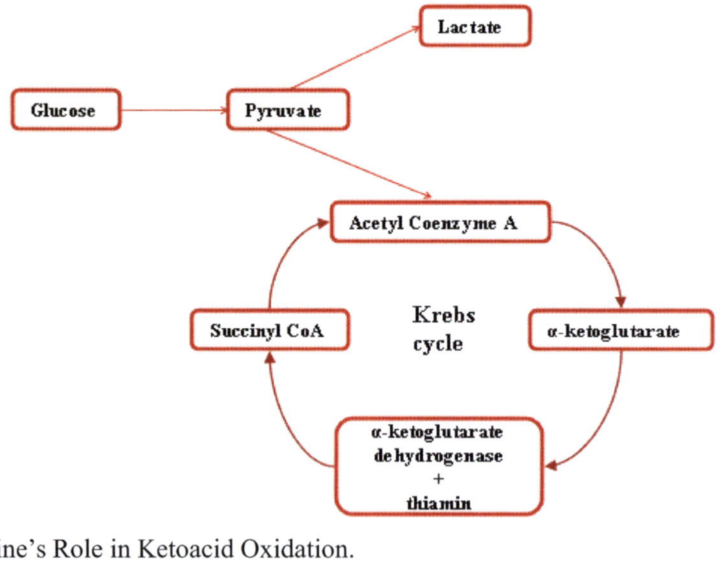

Fig. (3). Thiamine's Role in Ketoacid Oxidation.

Thiamine is an essential nutrient. An essential nutrient may be defined as a substance derived from the diet necessary for body functioning and promotion of health. Essential nutrients must be provided by the diet because they are either not synthesized by the body or not synthesized in sufficient amounts to prevent deficiency. Essential nutrients have some common characteristics. They must have at least one specific biologic function in the body. Also, omission of an essential nutrient from the diet results in a decline in biologic function. Finally, replacement of the nutrient prior to permanent damage will restore normal biologic function. Nutrients function in different ways such as the 3 specific categories described below:

1. Provide calories to meet energy needs

2. Support growth, development and maintenance

3. Sustain body (cellular) function

Classes of Nutrients

More detailed, specific content related to nutrients will be provided in subsequent chapters of this book. The intention of this section is to provide an overview and introduction to nutrients. Nutrients are divided into several classes dependent on function in the body. The major classes of nutrients are carbohydrates, lipids (fats and oil), and proteins; and other nutrients include vitamins, minerals, water, and phytochemicals.

Caloric (energy) sources are carbohydrate, lipids and proteins. Carbohydrates (Fig. **4**) are either simple or complex depending on the number of carbohydrates included in the nutrient. They are a source of glucose, a basic elementary source of cellular energy that has a specific caloric density. Fiber is a component of some carbohydrates that is a substance in food that is not digested by the processes that take place in the stomach or small intestine. Fiber functions to provide bulk to the stool facilitating normal bowel function. Dietary fiber must be distinguished from other sources of fiber not useful to human health.

Lipids are the other source of non-protein calories. They are the main form of energy in the body. Lipids' primary characteristic is their solubility in solvents rather than water. Important to human health is their source: animal (butter, lard) or plant (corn, safflower or olive oil). Essential fats regulate blood pressure and support synthesis and repair of vital cells. Lipids are also described based on their form at room temperature; fats are solid and oils are liquid. There are several types of lipids. Fatty acids are either saturated (no double bonds) or unsaturated (presence of one or more double bonds). The essential fatty acids provide fundamental biologic functions that become impaired during deficiency. Other types of lipids are triglycerides, cholesterol and *trans* fats. Triglycerides and cholesterol provide essential functions in the body but are associated with development of specific diseases at elevated levels in the body. *Trans* fats are not commonly found in nature. Most *trans* fats are created when lipids are transformed from a liquid to a solid state to facilitate storage, shipment, and shelf-life of this energy source.

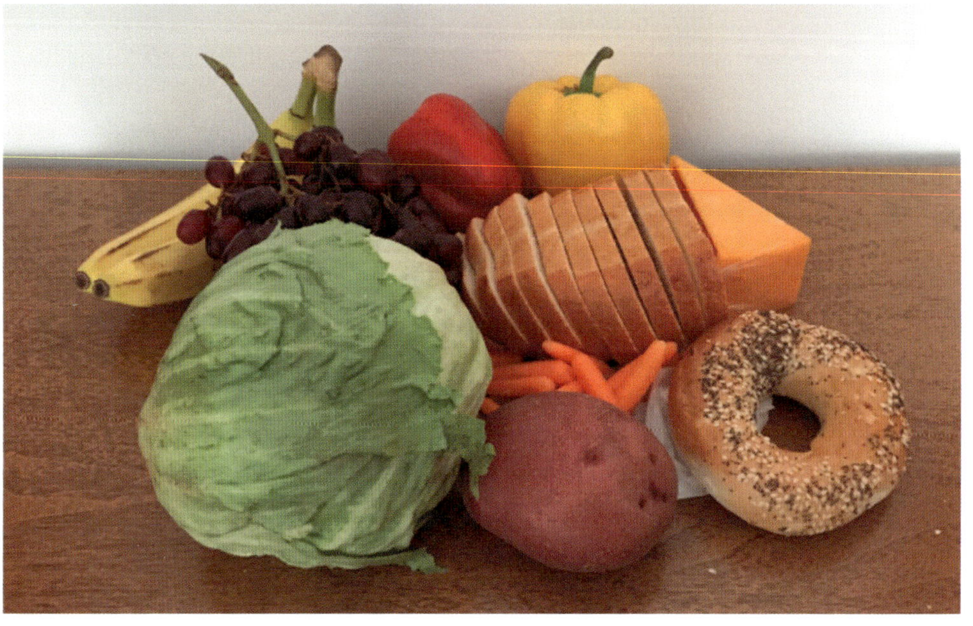

Fig. (4). Examples of sources of carbohydrates.

The next source of energy or calories for the body is protein. Protein is not often considered an energy source because of its important other functions in the body. It is the source of structural material for bone, muscle, blood, cells, enzymes, and immune cells and chemicals. Nutritionally, a primary focus is to assure protein is adequately incorporated into the body as well as functions optimally. Protein comes from animal (including dairy) as well as vegetable sources (Fig. **5**). Similar to lipids, there are several types of proteins from the diet; amino acids (essential, non-essential and conditionally essential), di and tri-peptides as well as whole proteins.

The sources of calories are also considered macronutrients because they exist in large quantities in the body (grams *vs.* milligrams or micrograms). Contrarily, micronutrients are present in the body in smaller quantities (milligrams or micrograms). These may be further classified as vitamins, minerals and the micronutrients; trace elements.

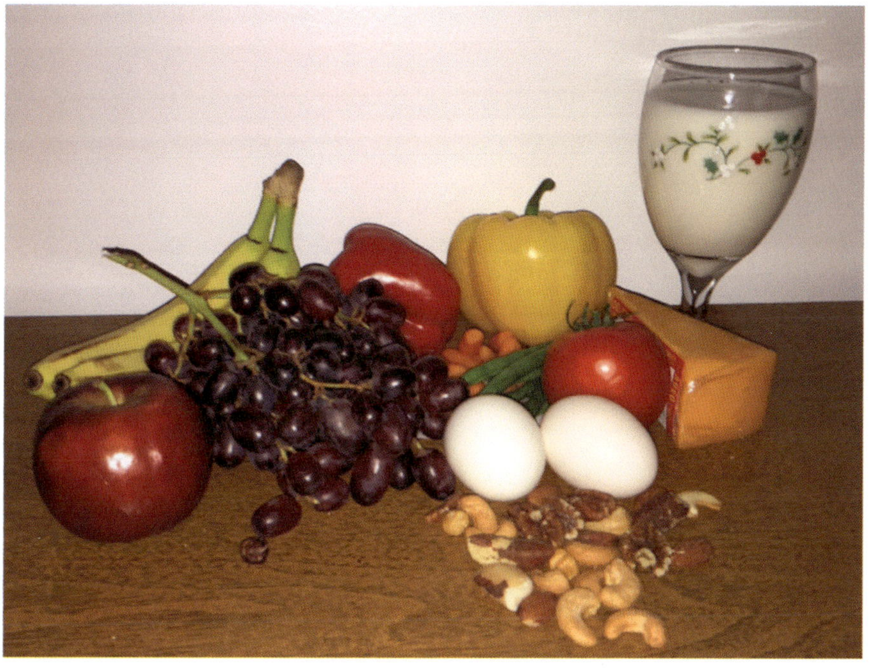

Fig. (5). Sources of protein.

Vitamins are organic compounds that are not carbohydrate, protein or lipid. They regulate or act as coenzymes in the metabolism of energy yielding nutrients. Vitamins also coordinate the growth and maintenance of tissues as well as assist in storage and utilization of energy. Vitamins are not synthesized by the body so must be provided by the diet. Classification of vitamins are either as fat-soluble (vitamins A, D, E and K) or water-soluble (thiamine (B-1), riboflavin (B-2), niacin/nicotinic acid (NI, B-5), pantothenic acid (PA), pyridoxine (B-6), biotin (Bi), cyanocobalamin (B-12) and ascorbic acid (C).

Minerals are inorganic substances; they do not contain carbon atoms. They function to support the nervous system, water balance, and structure (skeletal system). Electrolytes are minerals and consist of sodium, potassium, magnesium, calcium, phosphorus and chloride. Trace minerals are also known as micronutrients or trace elements. Micronutrients are present in the body in small amounts (micrograms). Examples of trace minerals include; zinc, copper, chromium, selenium, manganese, iodide, and iron.

Water is another essential nutrient that serves the body as a solvent, lubricant, and vehicle for transporting nutrients and waste.

Other nutrients that have taken on more importance as knowledge of nutrition has evolved are phytochemicals. These are chemicals that are found in plants that if taken regularly may contribute to a reduced risk of diseases, such as cancer or cardiovascular disease.

Body Composition

Nutrients assimilated into the body contribute to its composition. Body composition refers to the distribution and size of the components of total body weight. When assessing nutritional status, the components of body weight important to consider are 'total', fat mass (FM) and fat-free mass (FFM). A body composition model described in Fig. **6**.

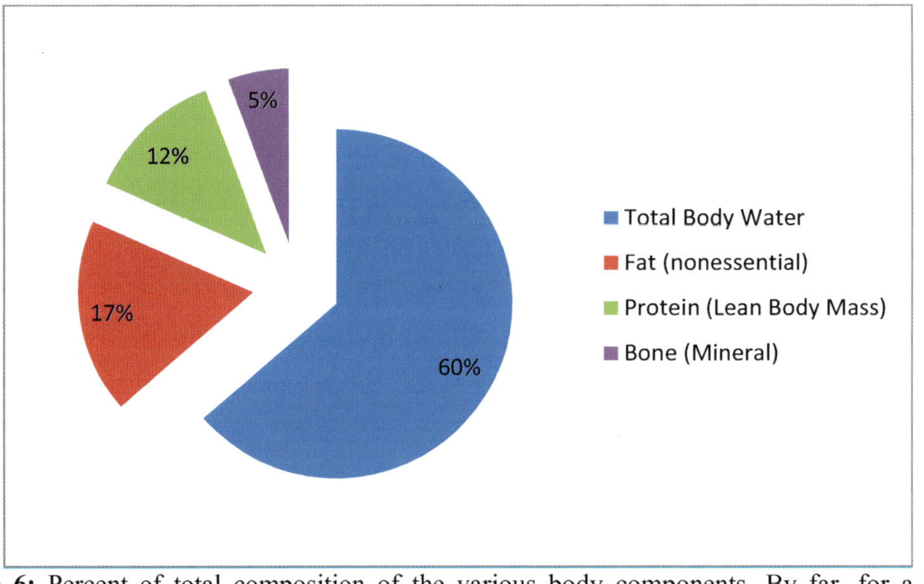

Figure 6: Percent of total composition of the various body components. By far, for a 70 kg individual water (42 kg) is the most abundant compartment of the body. Protein (10.6 kg) and bone (3.7 kg) make up the structural and organ components of the body. The other major compartment is Fat (12 kg).

Many methods have been used to assess the composition of the body and the effects nutrition has on the individual compartments. The overall goal of nutrition is adequate maintenance and replenishment of the lean body mass (protein, FFM) even though adequate water and structure (bone, minerals) is important as well. Anthropometrics include measurements of height and weight. The measured weight may also be termed, actual body weight. Height and weight are used to determine 'Ideal' weights by using the formulas noted below for males and females:

Ideal Body Weight Formulas

- Males: 106 lbs (48 kg) for the first 5 ft (152 cm) and add 6 lb (2.7 kg) for each inch (2.54 cm) over 5 ft.
- Females: 100 lbs (45 kg) for the first 5 ft and add 5 lbs (2.3 kg) for each inch over 5 ft.

The percent ideal body weight (% IBW) is then used to describe the measured weight in relation to the ideal (Table **2**).

- % IBW = Weight/IBW x 100.

Table 2. Body Compositions and Percent Ideal Body Weight of Various Healthy Individuals.

Source	Height (in)	Weight (lbs)	IBW (lbs)*	%IBW*
Football player (Lineman)	77	300	208	144
Football Player (Receiver)	68	180	154	117
Professor	68	182	154	118
Women Soccer Player	65	108	125	86
Malnourished				
• Mild				90
• Moderate				80-90
• Severe				<70
Obese				>130

*IBW = ideal body weight.

This chart compares the anthropometric measures for athletes (football players and a female soccer player), a university professor and criteria for malnourished individuals using % IBW as the parameter of assessment. When evaluating %IBW for the professor as compared with the football receiver there is likely to be significant differences in their body composition, especially as it relates to the fat mass and fat-free mass. When assessing the athletes' % IBW for the presence of malnutrition, the football lineman would be considered 'obese' and the women soccer player would be 'moderately malnourished'. However, it is likely that each is performing at an above average athletic workload. The lean body mass (LBM) (protein, FFM) is important to both athletic performance and health. However, the LBM is difficult to determine from just height and weight measures. Some techniques are being used in research that are more specific for LBM, but are not routinely available; hydro densitometry (underwater weighing), bioelectric impedance (resistance of tissues to flow of an electric current), isotopic dilution techniques, total body potassium and dual energy x-ray absorptiometry (DEXA).

Besides %IBW, the body mass index (BMI) is a weight-stature index used both as a measure of malnutrition and obesity (see formula below):

BMI Formula:

$$\text{BMI} = \text{Weight (kg)} \div \text{Height } (\text{m}^2)$$

The World Health Organization (WHO) has established a classification based on BMI for underweight, overweight and obese individuals (Table **4**).

The BMI classification began with broader categories noted in bold in Table **3** As nutrition knowledge expanded additional cutoff-points were added. These cutoff-points are used to delineate specific interventions related to nutrition, physical activity and lifestyle changes necessary to improve an individual's weight-stature to a healthier level.

In summary, pharmaconutrition (nutrition in health and disease) is concerned with nutrition concepts used to maintain or improve health and/or disease. In this context, health relates to growth and maintenance. Disease is considered either acute or chronic. Malnutrition as a consequence of disease is an important consideration. Nutrition in disease is intended to resolve malnutrition if present, maintain normal function and assist with correcting the cellular and functional disorders associated with disease. Nutrition in health and disease is an essential component of the human condition and must be considered in all aspects of life. As a health professional, a proper understanding of nutrition is necessary in order to provide optimal health service to people.

Table 3. Provides a simple classification based on BMI for underweight, overweight and obese individuals.

Groups	BMI (kg/m²)
Underweight	**<18.50**
Severe Thinness	<16.00
Moderate Thinness	16.00-16.99
Mild Thinness	17,00-18.49

Normal range	**18.50-24.99**
Overweight	**>25.00**
Pre-obese	25.00-29.99
Obese	**≥30.00**
Obese class I	30.00-34.99
Obese class II	35.00-39.99
Obese class III	≥40.00

Table 4. Classification of adult underweight, overweight and obesity according to body mass index (BMI).

Groups	BMI (kg/m^2)	
	Primary Cut-off Points	**Extra Cut-Off Points**
Underweight	**<18.50**	**<18.50**
Severe Thinness	<16.00	
Moderate Thinness	16.00-16.99	
Mild Thinness	17,00-18.49	
Normal range	**18.50-24.99**	**18.50-22.99**
		23.00-24.99
Overweight	**>25.00**	**>25.00**
Pre-obese	25.00-29.99	25.00-27.49
		27.50-29.99
Obese	**≥30.00**	**≥30.00**
Obese class I	30.00-34.99	30.00-32.49
		32.50-34.99
Obese class II	35.00-39.99	35.00-37.49
		37.50-39.99
Obese class III	≥40.00	≥40.00

Source: Adapted from WHO, 1995, WHO, 2000 and WHO 2004 @ http://apps.who.int/bmi/index.jsp?introPage=intro_3.html accessed August 24, 2012.

CONCLUDING REMARKS

The human body is a complex system that requires multiple nutrients in order to function properly. This chapter presented different types of nutrients that humans need to consume to be healthy. A balanced diet provides good nutrition and required nutrients in appropriate amounts. Nutrition is a key element in accomplishing good health. Hence, this chapter also presented an approach that can be pursued for disease prevention and management such as pharmaconutrition.

CONFLICT OF INTEREST

The authors confirm that this ebook contents have no conflict of interest.

ACKNOWLEDGEMENTS

The authors would like to thank you Mr. Preston Manwill for preparing the graphics of Fig. **2**.

REFERENCES

Center for Disease Control and Prevention. (1997). Lactic acidosis traced to thiamin deficiency related to nationwide shortage of multivitamins for total parenteral nutrition - United States. *The Journal of American Medical Association*, 278, 109-111.

Clayton, P. (2014). *Pharmaco-Nutrition, the new medicine*. Available at: http://www.immitec.com/care-pharma.net/home/dr.-pharm.-paul-clayton?stat=1 (accessed: 08.12.2014).

Davis, C. and Saltos, E., 1999, Dietary recommendations and how they have changed over time, *in* E. Frazao, ed., America's Eating Habits: Changes and Consequences: Wahinton, DC, Agriculture Information Bulletin No. 750, U.S. Department of Agriculture, Economic Research Service, p. 33-50.

Federal Security Agency, 1941, Characteristics of an effective nutrition education program, *in* Proceedings of the National Nutrition Conference for Defense, Washington, D.C.

Heyland, D. K. (2007, February 19). Pharmaco-Nutrition: An Emerging Paradigm. *Proceedings of the Society of Critical Care Medicine 36th Critcal Care Congress,* Orlando, FL.

Heyland, D., Jones, N., Cvijanovich, N. & Wong, H. (2008). Zinc supplementation in critically ill patients: a key pharmaconutrient? *Journal of Parenteral Enteral Nutrition*, 32, 509-519.

Howell, W. H., 1998, Anthropometry and body composition analysis, *in* L. E. Matarese and M. M. Gottschlich, eds., Contemporary Nutrition Support Practice: A Clinical Guide: Philadelphia, PA, W B Saunders Co, p. 33-46.

Jones, N., & Heyland, D. (2008). Pharmaconutrition: a new emerging paradigm. *Current Opinion in Gastroenterology*, 24, 215-222.

Kenney, W. L., Wilmore, J., and Costill, D., 1999, Obesity, Diabetes, and Physical Acitivity, *in* A. N. Tocco, K. Maurer, S. Calderwood, J. Sexton, eds., Physiology of Sport and Exercise: Champaign, IL, Human Kinetics, p. 545-572.

Mirtallo, J. (2013). Parenteral Nutrition: Can outcomes be improved? *Journal of Parenteral and Enteral Nutrition*, 37, 181-189.

Ryan, A. S. (2010). Exercise in aging: its important role in mortality, obesity and insulin resistance. *Aging Health*, 6, 551–563.

U.S. Department of Agriculture and U.S. Department of Health and Human Services (2005). Dietary Guidelines for Americans 2005. Available at: http://www.health.gov/dietaryguidelines/dga2005/document/pdf/DGA2005.pdf (accessed 05.12.2014).

U.S. Department of Agriculture and U.S. Department of Health and Human Services (2010). Dietary Guidelines for Americans 2010. Available at: http://www.health.gov/dietaryguidelines/dga2010/DietaryGuidelines2010.pdf (accessed 05.12.2014).

USDA (2011). A Brief History of USDA Food Guides. Available at: http://choosemyplate.gov/food-groups/downloads/MyPlate/ABriefHistoryOfUSDAFoodGuides.pdf (accessed 09.12.2014).

Wardlaw, G. M. and Smith, A. M., 2011, What You Eat and Why, *in* Contemporary Nutrition, 8th ed.: New York, NY, McGraw Hill, p. 3-34.

Welsh, S., Davis, C., and Shaw, A., (1992)., A brief history of food guides in the United States., Nutrition Today., p. 6-11.

Wischmeyer, P. E. (2008). Glutamine: role in critical illness and ongoing clinical trials. *Current Opinion in Gastroenterology*, 24: 190-197.

CHAPTER 2

Food Regulations in the United States

Melvin A. Pascall* **and Ken Lee**

The Ohio State University, Columbus, Ohio, USA

Abstract: Food laws and regulations within the United States are essential to food safety, commerce and improved national health. Understanding the differences between foods, drugs and dietary supplements is important for both regulatory and national health reasons. If these commodities are not defined properly and label claims about them are not in keeping with both good science and prevailing legislation, the packaged products could be in violation of the related laws or regulations. There are thirteen federal agencies that are associated with food regulation and safety in some manner. Of great interest across several agencies are specific regulations relating to food labeling. There is mandatory information that must be on all Food and Drug Administration (FDA) and United States Department of Agriculture (USDA) regulated labels, and there are new allowable label claims to help consumers understand the connection between food and health. This work focuses on special food ingredients and additives that have high public or scientific interest, with reference to selected categories of ingredients. These include direct, secondary direct and indirect ingredients, generally recognized as safe (GRAS) substances and color additives. The chapter discusses the rationalc behind the Infant Formula Act and provides an overview of FDA and USDA inspection strategies and enforcement actions.

Keywords: Dietary supplements, food, food laws/regulations, GRAS, health claims, US Federal Agencies.

INTRODUCTION

Food laws and regulations within the United States (US) are mainly focused on the manufacture, distribution and sale of foods. Federal regulations are usually associated with interstate food commerce. Within recent times, food laws and regulations were enacted to warrant the safety of foods imported into the US. In addition to these, all states, some cities, and municipalities have their own laws and regulations. Irrespective of the legal boundaries, all food laws and regulations within the US aim to prevent the commercialization of adulterated and misbranded foods.

***Corresponding author Melvin A. Pascall:** Food Science & Technology, The Ohio State University, Columbus, OH 43210, USA; E-mail: pascall.1@osu.edu

Esperanza J. Carcache de Blanco and Jay Mirtallo (Eds)

Adulteration is the contamination of food with filth and or other extraneous matter. In the case of infant formula, it also involves minimum quantities of nutrients and the proper quality control of the food. Recent laws and regulations have given regulatory agencies the authority to deem a food adulterated if it is manufactured, processed, transported or sold in environments that are unsanitary, even though proof of contamination in the food is not presented. If foods are not handled under conditions referred to as "good manufacture practices" (GMPs), the said foods could be declared adulterated. Foods containing ingredients, color additives and or animal drug residue that are not approved or used in accordance with stipulations of the relevant agencies could be deemed adulterated. The same applies to foods that are irradiated or meat and poultry products that were not subjected to anti and post-mortem inspection.

Misbranded is a false or misleading display or characterization of a food as it relates to its type, grade, composition, functionality or quality. Misbranding also extends to the marketing of a food as the product of one manufacturer when in fact the food is that of another manufacturer. If pertinent information about a food is misrepresented or omitted from the label, that omission or misrepresentation could cause the food to be deemed misbranded.

The main federal laws relating to food adulteration and misbranding are the Federal Food, Drug, and Cosmetic Act (FFDCA), the Federal Meat Inspection Act (FMIA), and the Poultry Products Inspection Act (PPIA) (FDA, 2011; Poultry and Poultry Products Inspection, 2014; Meat Inspection, 1999). Other laws of importance to adulteration and misbranding include the Infant Formulation Act (IFA) and the Nutrition Labeling and Education Act (NLEA) (FDA, 2014a; FDA, 2013). At the National level, The Food and Drug Administration (FDA), The United State Department of Agriculture (USDA) and The Environmental Protection Agency (EPA) are agencies with the main responsibilities for regulating the manufacture, processing, packaging, and distribution of safe and wholesome food within the US. State and Municipal agencies also participate in this exercise but at the local level. US Federal law prohibits the delivery of adulterated and misbranded foods into interstate commerce. The FDA and USDA are the main federal agencies responsible for the enforcement of these laws. Inspection is the main activity of these agencies in keeping adulterated and misbranded food products out of interstate commerce.

Section 502 of the FFDCA contains significant provisions about what is described as misbranding. In summary, this law states that foods can be designated as misbranded if one of the following criteria is met (FDA, 2011):

- Labeling is false or misleading,
- The name and address of the food manufacturer, packer, or distributor is not on the label,
- The net weight of the package is inaccurate,
- Required information about the product is not prominently displayed,
- There is not enough information about the direction of use when required,
- Mandatory warning statements are omitted,
- The food does not comply with the color additives provisions listed under Section 706 of the FFDCA, and
- The name of the packaged food is uncommon or unusual or that the name fails to meets the standard of identity provided for in section 401 of the FFDCA.

Current food good manufacturing practices (GMPs) are final rules developed by the FDA and can be found in Title 21 of the Code of Federal Regulations, Part 110 (21 CFR 110, 2014). These final rules are mandates projected to ensure that foods processed for consumption are wholesome and safe. It could be concluded that if foods are manufactured, processed, packaged, stored, transported and delivered according to GMP regulations, the likelihood of it becoming adulterated is significantly reduced. GMP regulations thus describe the equipment, facilities, methods, and controls for producing safe and wholesome processed foods. This also includes the decorum and practices of the human factor in food processing and handling. In its food inspection programs, GMP is one of the main areas of FDA's concerns.

DEFINITIONS

It is essential to distinguish between foods, drugs and dietary supplements since the inability to do so could give rise to violations of product misbranding. This would become evident during the discussion on label claims. For example, if a label claim is made that an item of food has the ability to cure a disease, that food product would be claiming the prerogatives of a drug and would be required to undergo all the legal requirements for drug approval.

Foods

A food is defined as an item that is consumed primarily for taste, aroma, or nutritive value, including chewing gum, and articles used as components of any other food or drink.

Drugs

A drug is defined as an item that is used in the diagnosis, cure, mitigation, prevention, or treatment of disease. It is also an item other than food that is used to affect the structure or function of the human body or beast.

Dietary Supplements

A dietary supplement is a product (other than tobacco) intended to supplement the regular diet. It must also contain at least one of the following: vitamins, minerals, amino acids, and concentrates, metabolites, extracts, *etc.* from herbs or other botanicals. A dietary supplement must not be displayed to be represented as a conventional food. Also, it cannot be the sole item of diet and it must be labeled as "dietary supplement".

MAIN FEDERAL AGENCIES ASSOCIATED WITH FOOD REGULATIONS

The Food and Drug Administration

The FDA is a regulatory agency that is under the Department of Health and Human Services (DHHS). It is headed by a Commissioner who reports to the Secretary of Health and Human Services. The Commissioner is appointed by the President of the United States, and must be approved by the United States Senate before the appointment is confirmed. The main office of the FDA is located in Silver Springs, Maryland and includes the Commissioner's office. All components of the FDA are supervised by the Office of the Commissioner and four directorates [Office of Foods and Veterinary Medicine (OFVM); Office of Global Regulatory Operations and Policy (OGROP); Office of Medicinal Products and Tobacco (OMPT); and Office of Operations (OO)]. These directorates are further subdivided into various centers and offices. The agency also comprises 223 field offices and 13 equipped laboratories located throughout the 50 states, the United States Virgin Islands, and Puerto Rico (FDA, 2014b).

The various offices and centers of the FDA are headed by Deputy Commissioners, Assistant Commissioners, Chief Counsel, Chief Scientist and Directors. Apart from the Office of the Commissioner, the main centers and offices involved with food regulations include:

- Center for Drug Evaluation and Research (CDER)
- Center for Food Safety and Applied Nutrition (CFSAN)
- Center for Veterinary Medicine (CVM)
- National Center for Toxicological Research (NCTR)
- Office of Regulatory Affairs (ORA)
- Centers of Excellence in Regulatory Science and Innovation (CERSI)

Many of these centers and offices are divided into sub-offices, divisions, and branches.

The main role of the FDA is to safeguard and promote the health of the citizens of the United States. This is done through the formulation of regulations, the issuance of advisory documents, educational exercises, and the enforcement of regulations intended to ensure the safety of the following products:

- Foods
- Tobacco products
- Dietary supplements
- Prescription and over-the-counter pharmaceutical products
- Drugs
- Biologics, including vaccines and blood products
- Medical devices
- Electromagnetic radiation emitting devices such as cellphones, lasers, microwaves, *etc.*
- Cosmetics

- Animal feed, drugs and other and veterinary products
- Non-specified red meat from bison, rabbit, game animals, zoo animals, deer, elk and moose
- Shell eggs
- Non-specified birds such as wild turkeys, wild ducks, wild geese and emus
- Products with less than 2% poultry on a wet basis
- Close-face sandwiches (Fig. **1**) with less than 35% cooked meat and poultry products not inspected by USDA and having bread that is less than 50% of the weight of the product
- Other products with less than 3% red meat, frozen fish dinners, alligator meat, shrimp, seafood (except catfish), *etc.*

The Center for Food Safety and Applied Nutrition (CFSAN) is a subdivision within the FDA that is mainly responsible for nutritional labeling and the safety of food. In conjunction with ORA, another subdivision within the FDA, CFSAN works to accomplish the following regulatory functions:

- Inspection and monitoring of food handling, transport and processing operations
- Analysis of food samples collected by ORA
- The pre-market approval food and color additives
- Studies consumers' responses to food safety issues relating to packaging, processing and bio-technology
- Works with ORA and other subdivisions (offices and centers) within FDA to take relevant corrective actions when warranted
- Provides educational outreach activities on various issues of public health concerns.

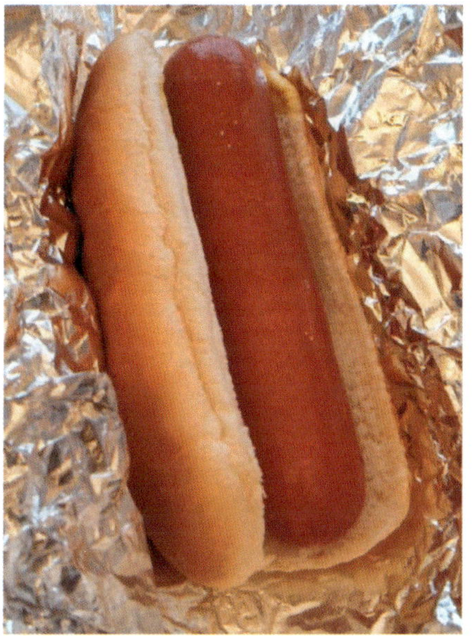

Figure 1: A close-face sandwich.

The Center for Food Safety and Applied Nutrition is divided into several offices. These in turn are subdivided into various divisions and branches that perform specific duties relating to food safety. These offices are:

- Office of Management
- Office of Analytics and Outreach
- Office of Food Safety
- Office of Cosmetics and Colors
- Office of Regulatory Science
- Office of Food Additive Safety
- Office of Compliance
- Office of Applied Research and Safety Assessment
- Office of Regulations, Policy and Social Sciences
- Office of Nutrition, Labeling and Dietary Supplements

The Office of Regulatory Affairs is a subdivision within the FDA and it is on the same level as that of CFSAN on FDA's organizational structure. However, unlike CFSAN that is headed by a director, ORA is headed by the Associate Commissioner for Regulatory Affairs. The Office of Regulatory Affairs is the lead office for FDA's field activities. Its main food safety function is to survey and inspect regulated companies in order to evaluate their compliance with public health laws and regulations. To help make this mandate possible, ORA helps to educate regulated companies on GMPs, highlights areas of significant violations during and after inspection visits, targets high-risk manufacturers and food handlers for subsequent scrutiny, works with state and local public health agencies to address issues of public health concerns, performs inspections of imported products into the US at the borders and on products in foreign countries that are destined for import to the US. To accomplish its mission, ORA has teams of employees called Consumer Safety Officers. These are referred to as inspectors or investigators. These officers are sometimes referred to as the "eyes and ears" of the agency. ORA is also responsible for providing advice and assistance on regulations and compliance policy issues, the evaluation of proposed legal actions against companies, individuals, *etc.*, and conducting criminal investigative activities in collaboration with other FDA centers and offices, including other federal (such as USDA, Customs and Border Protection, Consumer Product Safety Commission, *etc.*), state, and local enforcement agencies.

To provide these services to the entire US population, employees attached to ORA are spread throughout the continental US, Hawaii and its territories. The Office of Regulatory Affairs itself is divided into five regions. These are further divided into 13 districts and spread throughout the US. Each district has a main office and a number of Residence Posts. To support its work, ORA also has a number of laboratories that are capable of analyzing food samples under investigation. In cases of criminal activities involving food and other products regulated by the FDA, ORA collaborate with the Office of Criminal Investigations. If criminal charges must be filed for issues such as willful tampering of products, fraud, terrorism, *etc.*, it is done by the Justice Department since FDA does not have the authority to file these types of charges.

In the execution of its regulatory mandate to the US population, FDA approves new additives before they can be used in food. The agency also monitors the safety of dietary supplements and the nutritional content of infant formulas and medical foods. The agency is charged with ensuring that all ingredients used in foods are safe and free from contaminants or that levels are kept within approved limits. FDA is also responsible for the approval of all drugs used in animal and livestock feeds and that drug residues in these products are within safe limits. FDA also regulates labels on products and it seeks to ensure that they are truthful and are designed to assist consumers in decision making about the nutritional contents and nature of the product. FDA also monitors reports of adverse reactions to consumers after previously approved marketed products are purchased and used. In such cases, FDA may collaborate with the Centers for Disease Control (CDC) on epidemiological studies. Warranted by these investigations, FDA could ask manufacturers to recall a product, or the approval of the product could be withdrawn. Other actions that FDA could take include the requirements for label changes, seizure of products, quarantine, or they could seek an injunction, or prosecution from the court, especially in cases where federal laws and regulations were violated.

The US Department of Agriculture

The USDA is a subdivision of the federal government and is responsible for development and execution of policies on agriculture, farming, and food production. "Its main goals are to assist farmers and ranchers in meeting their needs, to promote food production and trade in agricultural goods, to uphold food safety principles, to promote sustainable agriculture and protect natural resources, to nurture rural communities, and end hunger in the US and abroad" (USDA, 2014).

In an attempt to meet its mission the USDA runs several programs. Examples of these programs include but are not limited to the following (USDA, 2014):

- The distribution of safe and wholesome food to citizens of the US
- Dissemination of nutrition educational materials in printed, media and electronic format to US citizens under the USDA Food and Nutrition Service
- Provide assistance to farmers and food producers with sales of crops and processed food on the domestic and foreign markets
- The USDA is also responsible for the management of overseas aid programs to developing countries, foreign governments, non-governmental agencies (NGO's) and international agencies such as World Food Program, for example. The USDA also manages the USAID program in the dissemination of funds for international aid programs.

Based on its programming activities, the USDA is divided into several internal agencies. These are:

- Cooperative State Research, Education, and Extension Service (CSREES)
- Agricultural Research Service (ARS)
- Animal and Plant Health Inspection Service (APHIS)
- Center for Nutrition Policy and Promotion (CNPP)
- National Institute of Food and Agriculture (NIFA)
- Economic Research Service (ERS)
- Farm Service Agency (FSA)
- Food and Nutrition Service (FNS)
- Food Safety and Inspection Service (FSIS)
- Foreign Agricultural Service (FAS)
- Forest Service (FS)
- Grain Inspection, Packers and Stockyards Administration (GIPSA)
- National Agricultural Statistics Service (NASS)
- National Finance Center (NFC)
- Natural Resources Conservation Service (NRCS)
- Risk Management Agency (RMA)
- Rural Development (RD).

The Food Safety and Inspection Services (FSIS) is the main agency within USDA that is responsible for food plant inspection. In general, this agency is responsible for ensuring that commercially produced meat, poultry, catfish and egg products are safe from poisonous and deleterious substances, that the food is wholesome, and correctly labeled and packaged. Currently, there are in excess of 8,000 USDA inspectors who are assigned the responsibility to inspect approximately 7,000 slaughter houses, food processing facilities, and ports of entry into the US. These officers are charged with the responsibility to verify that meat, poultry, catfish and egg products are safely processed, labeled properly and packaged in a wholesome manner. To meet this mandate, inspectors perform ante-mortem inspections (including humane stunning) on animals to verify that they are disease free, perform post-mortem examinations on carcasses to ensure the absence of diseases, and ensure that carcasses are handled and dressed in a way that minimizes microbial contamination (especially from organisms such as generic *E. coli* and *Salmonella*), they collect samples to test for specific animal diseases such as bovine spongiform encephalopathy (Mad Cow), Foot and Mouth Disease, Swine Fever and Encephalitis, for example. Samples are also collected for residual drug and chemical testing, to include items such as antibiotics, pesticides, industrial contaminants, *etc.* USDA inspectors also ensure that "hazard analysis for critical control point" (HACCP) requirements and standards of identity are met and that GMPs are followed by all regulated processors. Products regulated by USDA include red meat from animals such as cattle, sheep, swine, goat, horse, mules; poultry and poultry products from domesticated chicken, turkey, duck, geese, guineas; egg products from these birds; (Fig. **2**) open-face sandwiches (bread is unhinged) with greater than 3% meat and 2% poultry on a wet basis.

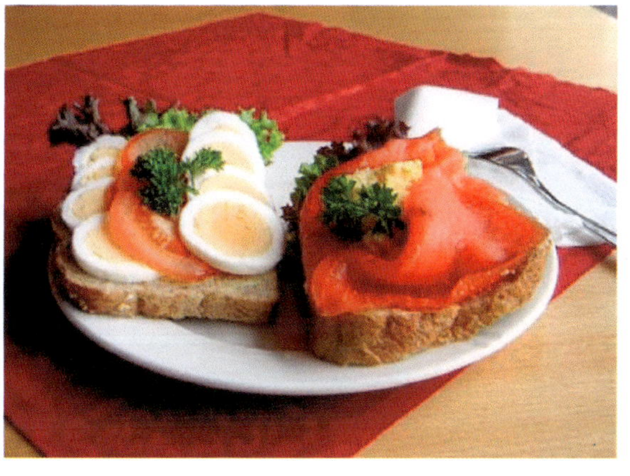

Figure 2: An open-face sandwich (Wikipedia, 2015).

The Environmental Protection Agency

The US Environmental Protection Agency (EPA) is a federal agency charged with the responsibility of protecting human health and the environment. The agency has an Administrator as its head. This person is appointed by the President of the

United States, but requires Congressional approval before the position is official. The EPA's headquarters is located in Washington, D.C. The agency is divided into ten regions scattered throughout the US. Each region has a regional office. The agency also has twenty seven testing laboratories where it conducts a variety of environmental assessments on samples relating to the use of pesticides, industrial contaminants, air pollution, chemical spills, surface cleaners, sanitizers, gasoline, *etc.* The agency conducts research and participates in programs designed to educate the public. The agency is also responsible for the maintenance and enforcement of national standards under a variety of environmental laws at the federal level, which includes consultation with state and local governments. The EPA works with industries to enforce environmental pollution prevention programs and the promotion of efforts to conserve energy. The EPA administers the Federal Insecticide, Fungicide, and Rodenticide Act (FIFRA) and is responsible for the registry of all pesticides, detergents, sterilants, and sanitizers for example, that are legally sold in the US. The EPA is also responsible for enforcing the Safe Drinking Water Act. It performs this function by setting standards and by ensuring that safe drinking water is made available to the public. This is done by inspecting injection wells (in order to ensure that underground sources of drinking water are safe) and surface water sources (EPA, 2014).

The Federal Trade Commission

The Federal Trade Commission (FTC) is a US governmental agency whose mission is to prevent business practices that are anticompetitive, deceptive or discriminating to consumers; to enhance informed consumer choices and public understanding of the competitive process; and to accomplish this without unjustifiably burdening legitimate business activity (http://www.ftc.gov/about-ftc). The FTC gets its authority from the Federal Trade Commission Act and it has the power to make rules and prosecute offenders in federal court. The work performed by the FTC is distributed by three bureaus within the agency. These are the Bureaus of Consumer Protection, Competition and Economics. These bureaus work in conjunction with the Office of General Counsel and seven regional offices distributed through the US (FTC, 2014).

The work of the Bureau of Consumer Protection focuses on the protection of consumers against unfair and deceptive acts or practices in business. The bureau accomplishes this through investigations, enforcement actions, and the dissemination of education material to the public. Specifically, this bureau focuses on issues such as false advertising, unfair or fraudulent marketing practices, improper financial products and practices, telemarketing fraud, privacy, and identity protection, including the US National Do Not Call Registry. The work of the Bureau of Consumer Protection is supported by that of the Bureau of Economics. The Bureau of Economics performs studies and provides information on the economic impact of the FTC's actions.

The Bureau of Competition is a subdivision within the agency mandated with the responsibility for eliminating or preventing anticompetitive business practices. This is accomplished by enforcing antitrust laws and prosecuting companies involved in illegal practices relating to business mergers. This bureau's activities also include the monitoring of illegal non-merger activities in business practices. These include practices that affect supply and demand, for example, including horizontal and vertical restraints involving agreements between competing businesses in the same industry.

FDA LABELING REQUIREMENTS

The Nutrition Labeling and Education Act of 1990 (NLEA) is largely responsible for the system of food labels in the US as we know it today. This legislation makes nutrition labeling mandatory on virtually all packaged foods and dietary supplements regulated by FDA. Currently, FDA is in the process of upgrading this legislation and it is expected that new labeling regulations will soon be put in place for all packaged foods and dietary supplements. In the absence of these new regulations, this chapter will focus on the requirements of the NLEA. These regulations place the responsibility of accurate food labeling on the manufacturer. The regulations state that all labels must have certain mandatory features and that nutrient values printed on labels must be based on the product composition. The regulations also state that analytical methods used to establish the nutrient values must meet standards adapted by the Official Methods of the Association of Official Analytical Chemists International (AOAC). Non-AOAC Official Methods are only allowed if valid AOAC methods are not available. The regulations also state exemptions that are allowed for certain foods and under certain conditions. For example, the labeling of infant formula has certain limitations not required for other types of foods. In the case of label claims and health messages, they must conform to strict guidelines stipulated by FDA. Food products not labeled in accordance with these requirements could be deemed as misbranded. The Food Drug and Cosmetic Act strictly prohibits the sale of foods that are deemed as adulterated and or misbranded. Such foods are subject to seizure and the manufacturer, packer or distributor could be prosecuted. This chapter will not go into the details of all label requirements but will provide a generalized overview to give the reader a working knowledge of FDA and USDA regulations regarding food labeling.

Mandatory Features Required on all FDA Regulated Labels

All FDA regulated labels must include a principal display panel (PDP) and an information panel.

The Principal Display Panel

Information about the product that must be on the PDP includes the name or identity of the product and the net weight. The information must be written in English although in some cases both English and a second language are allowed. Numeric characters that are identical in both languages do not have to be repeated. The PDP is the part of the label that must be displayed to consumers when they visit the grocery shelves of a store (Fig. **3**). Depending on the size and shape of the package, variations to the PDP are allowed within the limits of the FDA guidelines.

Only standardized, common or usual names must be used as prescribed in the regulations. If there is none, a descriptive name could be used but it must not be one designed to mislead consumers about the identity of the product. In certain circumstances, imitation or substitute foods could be named but it must be within the regulatory guidelines. Irrespective of the name selected to describe the packaged product, the type sizes and contrast with the background color of the label must make the label clearly legible to consumers. Artwork is allowed on the PDP of the label, however if used, it must not hide or detract from the relevant label statements about the product. The artwork also must not misrepresent the packaged food. For more details on the correct wording on the PDP, the reader is referred to FDA's website at www.FDA.gov.

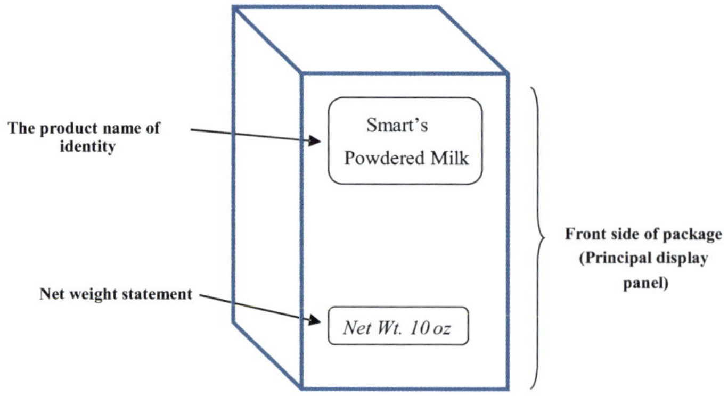

Figure 3: The principal display panel of an FDA regulated label.

The Information Panel

The information panel (Fig. **4**) is usually located to the right of the PDP and it must contain the name and address of the manufacturer, packer or distributor, the nutrition panel and the ingredient list. Depending on the size and shape of the package, the information panel could be on the same face of the package as the PDP. For some types of products, a handling statement is included. As is the case with the PDP, the regulations allow for variability due to the shape and size of the package. An ingredient statement is required when a product is fabricated from two or more ingredients. The ingredient list must be located on the same part of the label as the name and address of the manufacturer, packer or distributor of the product. Depending on the size and shape of the package, the ingredient statement could be located on the PDP. The type size of the lettering must be at least 1/16 of an inch in height and must contrast with the background color in a manner that makes it easily readable. The statement must list the ingredients in descending order of predominance. The regulations allow for variations in the ingredient list if the "2% or less rule" is used or for spices, colors and flavors. For ingredients identified as allergenic in the Food Allergen Act of 2006, the "2% or less rule" does not apply. Under the "2% or less rule" a manufacturer may not list an ingredient if it comprises 2% or less of the content of the product. Multi-ingredient components in a food product can be sub-listed in the ingredient statement. Some products require the display of warning statements. These must be prominently shown on the package as stipulated in the appropriate regulations.

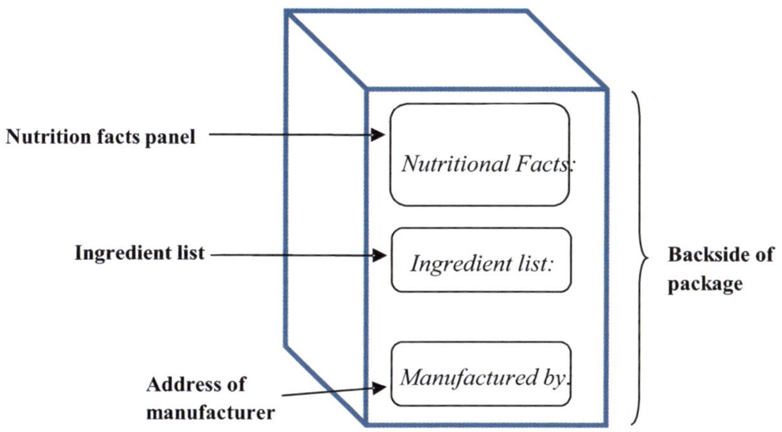

Figure 4: The information panel of an FDA regulated label.

The nutritional panel is shaped and structured as shown in Fig. **5** Depending on the size and shape of the package, variations of the shape are allowed, such as linear versions, for example. Fig. **6** shows the shape of a label that is allowed on rounded packages such as bottles. As shown in Fig. **5**, the panel is rectangular in shape and has the serving size and the number of servings in the package in the uppermost section. The serving size is explained by measuring terms such as cup, teaspoon, tablespoon, pieces, ounces, slices, *etc.* and its equivalent in metric units such as gram, milliliter, *etc.* Serving sizes are based on the reference amounts customarily consumed (RACC). The RACC was established by FDA for over 100 commonly consumed foods such as beverages (240 ml), cookies (30 g), snack foods (30 g), breads (50 g), breakfast cereal (1 cup prepared). This section is separated from the next lower section by a 7 point bar. This second section contains information on the amount of calories in a serving of the product

Nutrition Facts

Serving Size 2/3 cup (55g) cup
Servings Per Container 8

Amount Per Serving	
Calories 230	Calories from Fat 72
	% Daily Values*
Total Fat 8g	**12%**
Saturated Fat 1g	**5%**
Trans Fat 0g	
Polyunsaturated Fat 4g	
Monounsaturated Fat 3g	
Cholesterol 0mg	**0%**
Sodium 160mg	**7%**
Total Carbohydrate 37g	**12%**
Dietary Fiber 4g	**16%**
Sugars 1g	
Protein 3g	**6%**

Vitamin A 10%	•	Vitamin C 8%
Calcium 20%	•	Iron 45%

*Percent Daily Values are based on a 2,000 calorie diet. Your Daily Values may be higher or lower depending on your calorie needs.

	Calories	2,000	2,500
Total Fat	Less than	65g	80g
Sat Fat	Less than	20g	25g
Cholesterol	Less than	300mg	300mg
Sodium	Less than	2400mg	2400mg
Total Carbohydrate		300g	375g
Dietary Fiber		25g	30g

Figure 5: A typical nutritional panel.

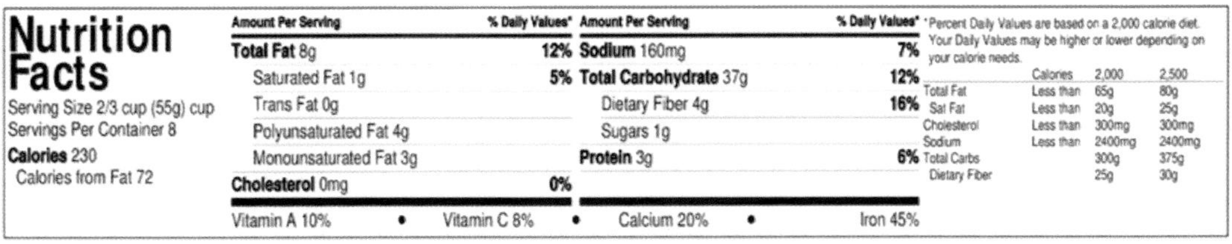

Figure 6: A nutritional panel allowed on rounded packages such as bottles.

and how much of that serving comes from fats. The third section contains information on the macro-molecular composition of the products and must contain data on the total fats, cholesterol, sodium, total carbohydrates and proteins of the product. The percent saturated and *trans* fat must be listed under the total fat heading and the dietary fiber and sugars under total carbohydrate. These must be indented with respect to their respective headings. The percentages of these compounds must be expressed as a percent of the daily reference value (DRV) of a postmenopausal woman. The DRV for the macromolecules was established by FDA as sources of energy that do not contribute calories. The DRV is based on a daily intake of 2000 calories. The DRVs for these energy-producing nutrients are based on daily calories intake. A six point bar separates the second from the third sections of the label. The fourth section is separated from the third by a 7 point bar and contains the percentages of vitamin A and C and that of calcium and iron in the product based on the Recommended Daily Intakes (RDI) established by FDA. The DRV and RDI are displayed on labels as the percent of the daily value (% DV). This was developed by FDA so that consumers could estimate the level of various nutrients in a normal serving of the packaged food and how it relates to the DV and the specific needs of the individual consumer. In the lower two sections of the nutrition facts panel manufacturers are allowed to put information (footnotes) on the DV (that it is based on a 2000 calorie diet) and calories. A full footnote may not be necessary depending on the size of the package or if a simplified label format is used. The NLEA also states that if the % DV for potassium or protein is provided under the % Daily Value heading, they must be included in the footnote. A footnote is not allowed on food labels for infants and children less than 4 years of age. FDA is currently in the process of updating its labeling regulations. Fig. **7** is a proposed nutritional panel that appears on FDA's website.

Disclosure Statements

A disclosure statement informs consumers that one or more of the nutrients in a product could influence a disease or health condition that is related to the diet.

Nutrition Facts

8 servings per container

Serving size	2/3 cup (55g)

Amount per 2/3 cup

Calories **230**

% Daily Value*

QUICK FACTS:

12%	**Total Fat** 8g
12%	**Total Carbs** 37g
	Sugars 1g
	Protein 3g

AVOID TOO MUCH:

5%	Saturated Fat 1g
	Trans Fat 0g
0%	**Cholesterol** 0mg
7%	**Sodium** 160mg
	Added Sugars 0g

GET ENOUGH:

14%	Fiber 4g
10%	Vitamin D 2mcg
20%	Calcium 260mg
45%	Iron 8mg
5%	Potassium 235mg

* Footnote on Daily Values (DV) and calorie reference to be inserted here.

Figure 7: FDA's proposed nutritional panel. (FDA, 2014c).

The statement is also required if the product has one or more nutrients in excess of a level referred to as the "reference amount customarily consumed per label serving". These are listed as follows: fat (13 g); saturated fat (4 g); cholesterol (60 mg) and sodium (480 mg). The regulations also allow for variations in the statement for products with small serving sizes. Disclosure statements are required on labels when certain claims about a product are made by the manufacturer. These claims include nutrient content, structure/function and health claims. Details on FDA approved label claims would be provided later on in this chapter. Disclosure statements must be prominently displayed on boldface type on the label and must be located adjacent to the label claim associated with it. FDA regulations also provide for variations in disclosure statements depending on the number of claims, and the size and shape of the package. The Food Allergen

Labeling and Consumer Act of 2004 requires a packaged product to be clearly labeled if it contains milk, eggs, fish, shellfish, tree nuts, wheat, peanuts and soybeans. In some foreign jurisdictions, sesame seeds are required to be listed as an allergy. All irradiated foods must carry the radura symbol on the label (Fig. **8**). The Food Drug and Cosmetic Act mandates that irradiation is considered as an ingredient when used to treat a food product.

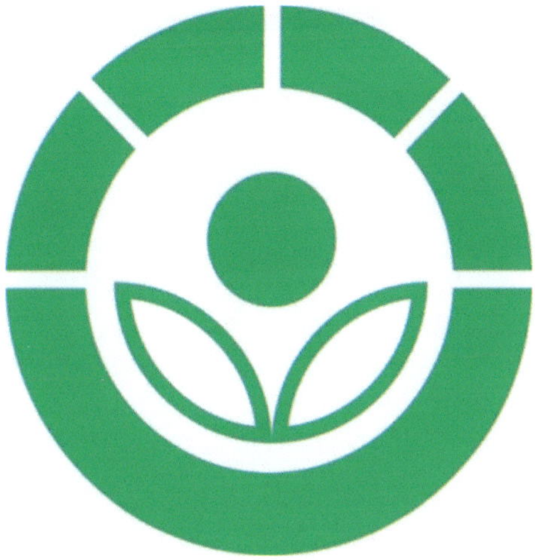

Figure 8: The Radura Symbol (FDA, 2013).

Mandatory Features Required on all USDA Regulated Labels

Labels required on USDA regulated products are similar to those on FDA regulated products. However, additional features are required on USDA labels. In this section of the chapter, the focus will not be on repeating the features already explained for FDA labels that are also on USDA ones, but the focus will be on the additional features. Thus, USDA labels must also have "Safe Handling Instructions" for meat or poultry products or for food with such portions when they are not ready-to-eat. In general, a handling statement is required for perishable foods. For USDA labels there is no requirement for 1/16" minimum type size. Metric units are not required in the net weight statement. All USDA labels must have an Inspection Legend & Establishment Number (Fig. **9**). For poultry processing plants, the establishment number begins with the letter "P". For packages having between 1 to less than 4 pounds of product, the net weight statement must be stated in ounces and pounds {example, NET WT. 16 OZ. (1 LB.)} and it must be located at the lower 30% of the PDP. For USDA labels, the signature line is the equivalent to the "Name and Place of Business" on FDA regulated labels.

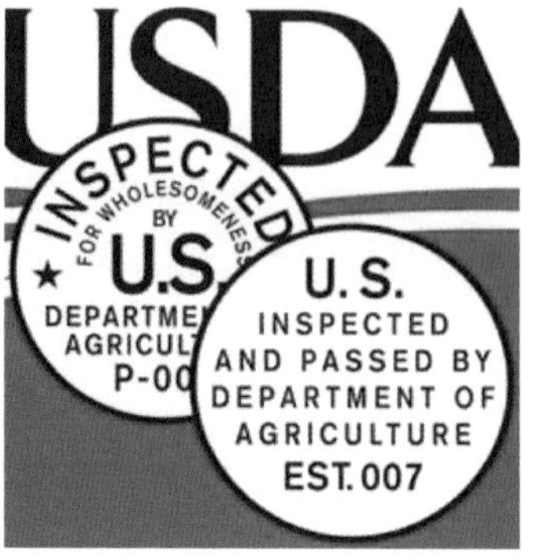
USDA
INSPECTED
FOR WHOLESOMENESS
BY
U.S.
DEPARTME
AGRICUL
P-00
U.S.
INSPECTED
AND PASSED BY
DEPARTMENT OF
AGRICULTURE
EST. 007

Figure 9: USDA Inspection Legend and Establishment Number (USDA, 2014).

FOOD CLAIMS

Food Label Claims

Before 1984, the food label told consumers about ingredients, convenience, taste, or how to store and prepare it, but not about its role in disease management. Health claims on food labels were forbidden by the FDA well into the 1980's. Prior to the internet, advertising was the major source of food information, and anyone making a health claim for food ran the risk of the product getting reclassified as a drug by FDA. This could mean a regulatory seizure of the advertised food as an unapproved new drug. Although it was known that some foods had specific health effects, it was left to the consumer to make these associations, a direct link was simply not allowed on the food package or in most forms of food advertising.

In October 1984 all of this changed. The Kellogg Corporation devoted the entire back of its All-Bran cereal box (Fig. **10**) and conducted a major ad campaign featuring the advice of the National Cancer Institute (NCI), stating dietary fiber "may reduce your risk of some kinds of cancer".

Kellogg worked closely with the NCI and with top officials at the Federal Trade Commission to get the words and message right, and most important, obtained *de facto* approval of two respected federal agencies. The FDA was blindsided, forcing a relatively quick liberalization of its health claim policies. Health claims soon appeared on many foods, not only replicating the NCI link of fiber to cancer, but also linking calcium to osteoporosis, and oat bran, fish oils, vitamin A or saturated fats to heart disease. Thirty years later, the FDA has reinvented itself with the well-earned tag line *"Protecting and Promoting Your Health"* that ironically is a health claim on this primary US federal food agency.

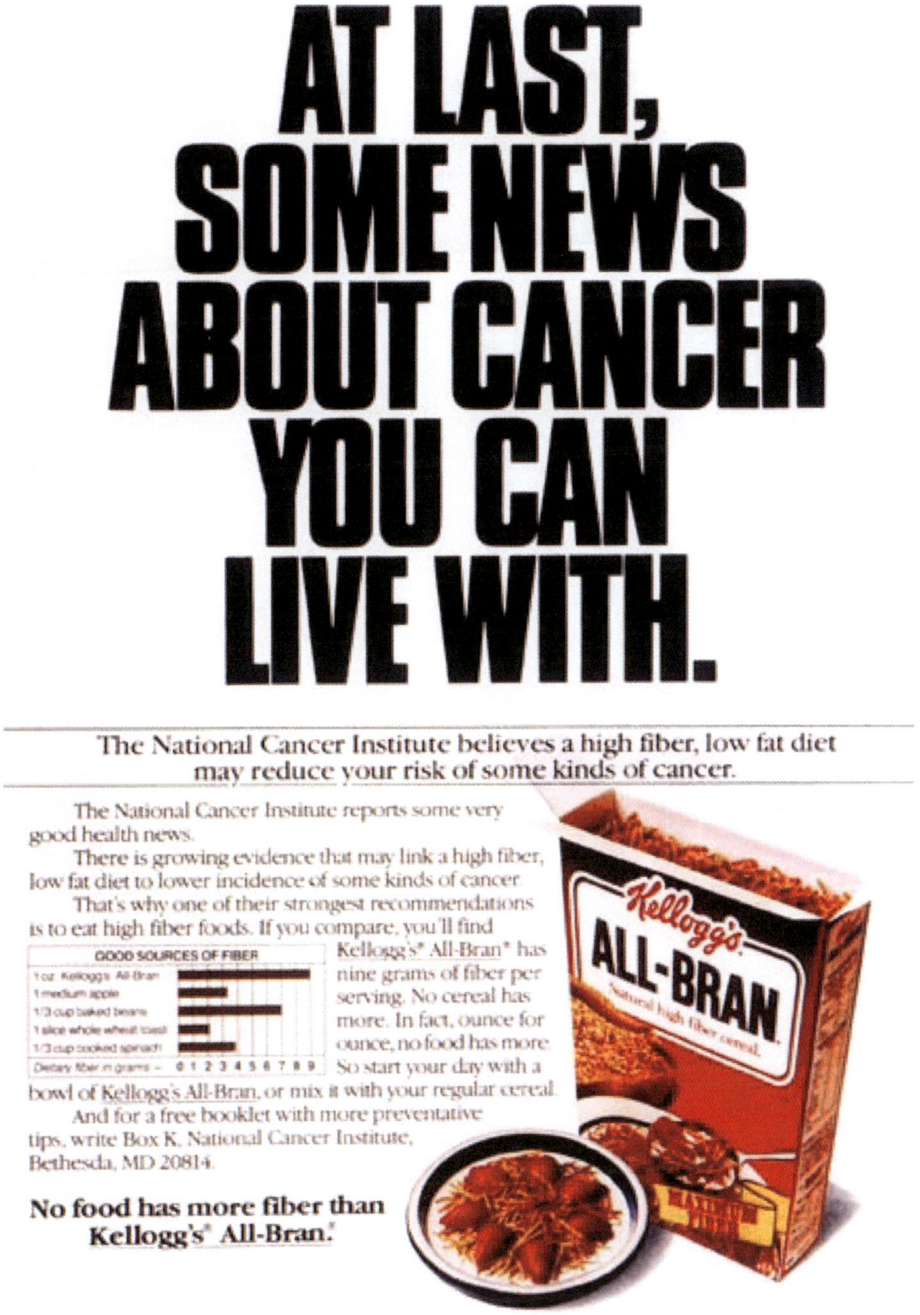
AT LAST, SOME NEWS ABOUT CANCER YOU CAN LIVE WITH.
The National Cancer Institute believes a high fiber, low fat diet may reduce your risk of some kinds of cancer.
The National Cancer Institute reports some very good health news.
There is growing evidence that may link a high fiber, low fat diet to lower incidence of some kinds of cancer.
That's why one of their strongest recommendations is to eat high fiber foods. If you compare, you'll find Kellogg's® All-Bran® has nine grams of fiber per serving. No cereal has more. In fact, ounce for ounce, no food has more. So start your day with a bowl of Kellogg's All-Bran, or mix it with your regular cereal.
And for a free booklet with more preventative tips, write Box K, National Cancer Institute, Bethesda, MD 20814.
GOOD SOURCES OF FIBER
1 oz. Kellogg's All-Bran
1 medium apple
1/3 cup baked beans
1 slice whole wheat toast
1/3 cup cooked spinach
Dietary fiber in grams – 0 1 2 3 4 5 6 7 8 9
No food has more fiber than Kellogg's® All-Bran.®
Kellogg's
ALL-BRAN
Natural high fiber cereal

Figure 10: An ad of Kellogg's All-Bran cereal. The ad states that National Cancer Institute research has shown "that a high fiber, low fat diet may reduce the risk of some kinds of cancer". (National Cancer Institute, 1984).

Four major categories of statements about beneficial food content are defined by FDA in today's food market;

1. Health claims,

2. Structure/function claims,

3. Nutrient content claims, and

4. Dietary guidance.

A health claim says a specific food or ingredient is related to a disease, such as "low sodium may reduce the risk of high blood pressure". Statements about a category of food, such as "vegetables maintain good health" are considered to be dietary guidance (FDA, 2013). Statements that say a specific food ingredient is related to a normal function or structure, such as "calcium builds strong bones" are known as structure/function claims (FDA, 2014). Statements that say a food contains more or less of a specific nutrient, such as "low in fat" are nutrient content claims (FDA, 2013). We take a brief look at each for their role in good health and disease management.

HEALTH CLAIMS

Today, most health claims on food labels and dietary supplements are regulated by the FDA, with some meat and poultry labels regulated by the USDA Food Safety Inspection Service or FSIS. Nutritional labelling is required on most foods and dietary supplements. Sometimes you might buy a food without a nutritional label; this was likely made by an exempt small business with less than 100 employees selling less than 100,000 units per year. But this exemption goes away if that small business makes a nutrition claim. Fresh produce, very small labels, or a small business selling dietary supplements with less than $0.5 million in gross annual sales is similarly exempt.

There are three ways that federal regulations ensure a health claim is truthful, beneficial, and not misleading. The first set of regulations comes from the 1990 Nutrition Labeling and Education Act (FDA, 1995). The NLEA required nutrition labeling on most foods, what is commonly known as the "Nutrition Facts panel," set standards for claims, and outlined how FDA approves health claims. It eliminated conflicting claims, like a "low cholesterol" claim on a food high in saturated fat. By defining low fat, high fiber, low sodium, light, or healthy, this both helped the consumer pick foods based on desired health outcomes, and motivated the industry to promote foods that meet these standards. In this way, the act reshaped the American diet. The NLEA required FDA review of substance-disease relationships, and only the eight below met the high standard of significant scientific agreement under the 1990 NLEA:

1. Dietary saturated fat and cholesterol -- risk of coronary heart disease (CHD)
2. Fruits, vegetables and grain products that contain fiber, particularly soluble fiber -- risk of CHD
3. Sodium -- hypertension
4. Dietary lipids -- cancer
5. Fiber-containing grain products, fruits, and vegetables -- cancer
6. Fruits and vegetables -- cancer
7. Calcium -- osteoporosis
8. Folate -- neural tube defects

NLEA enabled the industry to propose new health claims, and seven new claims leading to a total of 15 claims that meet the standard of significant scientific agreement were approved over several years:

1. Whole oat soluble fiber -- coronary heart disease (CHD)
2. Sugar alcohol -- dental caries
3. Psyllium seed husk -- CHD
4. Soy protein -- CHD
5. Sterol and stanol esters -- CHD
6. Oatrim -- CHD
7. Barley soluble fiber -- CHD

The second regulatory path comes from the 1997 FDA Modernization Act. The FDAMA allows a food health claim when a federal scientific body, such as the National Academy of Sciences (NAS) or the US Surgeon General authorizes it. This essentially put into law what the Kellogg Company did to circumvent FDA in 1984, as the NCI who endorsed the Kellogg cereal claim is a part of the National Institutes of Health. The required wording of the five claims enabled under FDAMA is explicit, such as:

1. "Diets rich in whole grain foods and other plant foods and low in total fat, saturated fat, and cholesterol may reduce the risk of heart disease and some cancers" (authorized by NAS).

2. "Diets containing foods that are a good source of potassium and that are low in sodium may reduce the risk of high blood pressure and stroke" (authorized by NAS).

3. "Drinking fluoridated water may reduce the risk of tooth decay" (authorized by the U.S. Surgeon General).

4. "Diets low in saturated fat and cholesterol, and as low as possible in *trans* fat, may reduce the risk of heart disease" (authorized by The Dietary Guidelines for Americans, a joint USDA and HHS policy document).

5. "Diets containing foods that are a good source of potassium and that are low in sodium may reduce the risk of high blood pressure and stroke" (authorized by the NAS).

The third and still evolving area of food regulations are **qualified health claims.** Health claims under NLEA or FDAMA require significant scientific agreement that made new claims very difficult. This is an issue of interesting societal and political debate, contrasting consumer protection with the consumer's right to choose based on incomplete evidence. A famous court decision, *Pearson v. Shalala (1999),* ruled FDA's strict enforcement was unconstitutional in a case involving four dietary supplements. Thus, the concept of qualified health claims was born, and moved from supplements to foods in 2003. A ranking system was created where the integrity of the claim was letter-graded A, B, C or D for significant, inconclusive, limited and very limited scientific evidence, respectively. The health claim text can vary, but the current standardized qualifying language is:

A. Significant scientific agreement: No qualifying language.

B. "… although there is scientific evidence supporting the claim, the evidence is not conclusive".

C. "Some scientific evidence suggests. However, FDA has determined that this evidence is limited and not conclusive".

D. "Very limited and preliminary scientific research suggests. FDA concludes that there is little scientific evidence supporting this claim".

As of this writing there are 28 authorized qualified health claims corresponding to the 28 rows in Table **1** below. These are based on the 17 food and disease relationships allowed by an FDA enforcement discretion letter on the indicated date, including a diabetes claim decision this year. Not shown are the 15 claim denials and one withdrawal. The letter grade assigned by these authors in the integrity column is based on the FDA allowed language. FDA does not publish a letter grade level less than "D" but they do provide language that makes it clear the food and disease relationship is quite poor, and these we note by (*) in this table. For highly questionable relations the FDA uses phrases such as "highly uncertain," "highly unlikely," or "FDA does not endorse" indicating the lowest level of integrity for a qualified health claim. How these statements affect consumer behavior and human health remains a matter of conjecture.

Table 1: Qualified health claims allowed on food or food supplements and the associated level of scientific integrity as of October 2014 (FDA, n.d.)*

Date	Food or Ingredient	Disease	Integrity	Eligible Foods
4/03/2001	0.8 mg Folic Acid	Neural Tube Birth Defects	*FDA does not endorse	Dietary supplements containing folic acid
5/15/2002	B Vitamins	Vascular Disease	**B**	Dietary supplements containing vitamin B6, B12, and/or folic acid
2/21/2003	Selenium	Cancer	**C**	Dietary supplements containing selenium
2/24/2003	Phosphatidylserine	Cognitive Dysfunction and Dementia	**D**	Dietary supplements containing soy-derived phosphatidylserine
7/14/2003	Nuts	Heart Disease	**B**	Almonds, hazelnuts, peanuts, pecans, some pine nuts, pistachio nuts, and walnuts

Table 1: contd…

3/09/2004	Walnuts	Heart Disease	**B**	Whole or chopped walnuts
9/04/2004	Omega-3 Fatty Acids	Coronary Heart Disease	**B**	Conventional foods and dietary supplements that contain EPA and DHA omega-3 fatty acids
11/01/2004	Monounsaturated Fatty Acids From Olive Oil	Coronary Heart Disease	**B**	Contain 6g or more olive oil and no more than 4g saturated fat
8/25/2005	Chromium Picolinate	Diabetes	*Highly uncertain	Dietary supplements
10/12/2005	Calcium	Colon/Rectal Cancer	**C**	Dietary supplements containing calcium
		Recurrent Colon/Rectal Polyps	**D**	
		Hypertension	**D**	
		Pregnancy-Induced Hypertension, and Preeclampsia	*Highly unlikely	
11/08/2005	Tomatoes and/or Tomato Sauce	Prostate Cancers	**D**	Cooked, Raw, Dried, or Canned Tomatoes; Tomato Sauces that contain at least 8.37 percent salt-free tomato solids
	Tomato Sauce	Ovarian Cancers	*Highly uncertain	
	Tomatoes	Gastric Cancers	*Unlikely	
		Pancreatic Cancers	*Highly unlikely	
10/06/2006	Unsaturated Fatty Acids from Canola Oil	Coronary Heart Disease	**C**	Contain 4.75g or more canola, low in saturated fat, low in cholesterol
3/26/2007	Corn Oil	Heart Disease	**D**	Contain 4g or more corn oil and no more than 4g saturated fat
6/19/2009	Antioxidant Vitamins	Cancer	**C**	Dietary supplements containing vitamin E and/or vitamin C
	Vitamin C	Gastric Cancer	*Highly uncertain	
	Vitamin E	Bladder Cancer	*Highly unlikely	
		Colorectal Cancer	*Highly unlikely	
		Renal Cancer	*Highly uncertain	

Table 1: contd...

2/24/2011	Green Tea	Cancer	**D**	Green tea and conventional foods and dietary supplements that contain green tea
5/24/2011	100% Whey-Protein Partially Hydrolyzed Infant Formula	Reduced Risk of Atopic Dermatitis	**D**	100% Whey-Protein Partially Hydrolyzed Infant Formula
6/24/2014	*Psyllium* Husk	Diabetes	**D**	Conventional foods Dietary supplements

*Information in this table was adapted from:
http://www.fda.gov/Food/IngredientsPackagingLabeling/LabelingNutrition/ucm073992.htm

NUTRIENT CONTENT CLAIMS

The content of a nutrient that has an FDA-established Daily Value can be explicitly stated. So content claims can be made for these 36 nutrients: total calories, total fat, saturated fat, cholesterol, sodium, potassium, dietary fiber, sugars, protein, vitamin A, vitamin C, calcium, iron, vitamin D, vitamin E, vitamin K, thiamin, riboflavin, niacin, vitamin B6, folate, vitamin B12, biotin, pantothenic acid, iodine, magnesium, zinc, selenium, copper, manganese, chromium, molybdenum, and chloride. There is no Daily Value for choline, ALA & DHA omega-3 fatty acids, but these three are allowed exceptions.

It seems fairly straightforward to just state the level of one or more of the above nutrients. But many words are used on labels to imply competitive benefit. FDA provides detailed rules when defining relative benefits from absence, such as free, low, less, little, fewer, only, reduced, light, no added, lean, extra lean, and zero. Similarly, FDA defines relative benefits from presence, such as a good source of, high, high potency, packed with, contains as much as, more, healthy, fortified, enriched, added, plus. For example, sodium-free means less than 5mg of sodium per serving and contains no added sodium ingredients; very low sodium means 35mg or less per serving; and low sodium means 140mg or less sodium per serving.

FDA has no claim definitions for sugars or carbohydrates, and for this reason "low carb" or "low sugar" are not allowed. Both "sugar free" and "no added sugar" is allowed as long as the calorie profile is disclosed and there is no ingredient that is a sugar. The claim "cholesterol-free" is valid if the cholesterol is normally present and a process removed it, but if the food is naturally so, the label must state that plainly, such as "peanut butter, a cholesterol-free food". There is much current interest in claiming "zero *trans* fat" but because *trans* fat is not a nutrient this is not allowed, whereas a simple statement of fact of 0g *trans* fat per service is okay.

Of specific interest for this text is the term "healthy" as it is considered an implied nutrient content claim. The food must be low in fat, low in saturated fat, contain 480mg or less of sodium, 60mg or less of cholesterol per serving, and contain at least 10% of the Daily Value of vitamin A, vitamin C, calcium, iron, protein or fiber. All the allowable nutrient content claims are detailed online (FDA, 2013b).

An excellent summary of nutrient content claims with examples of what is and what is not allowed by current US and Canadian regulations is published by Silliker Inc. and Food Consulting Company (Silliker, 2013). Although they provide this as a service to the food industry, the *"Silliker Nutrient and Health Claims US and Canadian Regulatory Guide"* is written at the consumer level and may be of value to anyone wishing to understand these complex set of regulations.

Structure/Function Claims (SFCs)

The 1994 Dietary Supplement Health and Education Act (DSHEA) enabled SFCs for dietary supplements, and since then these claims were extended to foods. These claims state the role a nutrient plays in normal body functions, body structures, or general health. They should not mention a disease state. So "calcium builds strong bones" is allowed, but "calcium prevents osteoporosis" is a health claim. SFCs are not recognized by the USDA so most meat and poultry products, some eggs, some pizzas and other USDA regulated foods cannot have them. Unlike the nutrient content claims, SFCs are not limited to just 36 nutrients, and include other food components such as prebiotics, probiotics, phytoestrogens, flavonoids and fatty acids.

SFCs do not require prior review by FDA as they are statements of fact about the effect of a food or dietary supplement on the function of the body. Disease claims require prior approval by FDA and may be made only for approved drugs or foods as noted above for health claims. Because the distinction between health claims and SFCs is sometimes difficult, the FDA published criteria to distinguish one from the other. Here in abbreviated form are the FDA's ten characteristics where if any one of the following tests is true it is not a SFC. Thus, it is a health claim requiring regulatory review when the statement claims:

1. An effect on a disease or class of diseases.

2. An effect on signs or symptoms of a disease.

3. An effect on a condition associated with a natural state, such as aging or menopause.

4. Uses a name, formula or picture to imply a disease (*e.g.*, CarpalHealth, CircuCure).

5. To diagnose, mitigate, treat, cure or prevent a disease.

6. To be a substitute for a therapy for a disease.

7. To augment a therapy or drug.

8. A role in the body's response to a disease.

9. To treat, prevent, or mitigate adverse events of a therapy for a disease.

10. Otherwise suggests an effect on a disease or diseases. This is a catch-all for any nuance not covered by the other nine criteria. (FDA, 2002).

So an allowable SFC for carotenoids, flavonoids and minerals like selenium would be "neutralizes free radicals". This would become a health claim requiring a petition for prior approval if it stated "neutralizes carcinogenic free radicals".

DIETARY GUIDANCE

Perhaps the least confounding statement is one of dietary guidance on a food label. Dietary guidance has neither of the two elements of a health claim; thus, it is not a specific food or food component and not a disease or health condition. It is a general statement of a pattern, practice or recommendation that is healthy. "Carrots are good for your health" qualifies, whereas "Carotenoids may prevent eye disease" does not. Dietary guidance can be given on food labels without FDA review and must meet the common requirement that the guidance is truthful and not misleading.

Social media and internet sources of food claims present a challenging mix of good and bad information, often unverified. The FDA requires information disseminated over the internet by or on behalf of a regulated company to meet the definition of labeling, so regulation of food claims apply to these online sites. An FDA letter to the Washington Legal Foundation provides more information on this issue (FDA, 2001). Misleading, false or harmful online food claims can be blocked by FDA if they are connected to a product or company, but other groups or individuals can intentionally mislead the public as a right of free speech. Most universities, particularly the land-grant institutions that have established food and agriculture disciplines, provide factual science-based food information online with the exclusive domain of EDU.

FOOD INGREDIENTS

The role of food ingredients in health and disease management is often misunderstood. Food ingredients include the wide category of food additives and preservatives that are often criticized for negative health impact rather than their role in ensuring food quality, safety and acceptance. This is perhaps due to the colorful evolution of additive regulation, including the trials of Harvey Washington Wiley's poison squad, where male volunteers documented reactions to eating questionable food ingredients. This led to the 1906 Food and Drugs Act and creation of the FDA. Due to stringent regulations, today's food additives are the most thoroughly tested substances that humans consume. Some have obvious health benefits like the vitamins and minerals, and some have functions that are under active investigation, like the role of antioxidants or pigments in the prevention of cancer.

A food ingredient is literally anything that becomes part of a food. This includes anything used in producing, processing, treating, packaging, transport or storage. So, if a food is wrapped in paper, the cellulose is an ingredient when present in the food. Interestingly, food irradiation is classified as an ingredient, probably from later disproven concerns about unique radiolytic products when the technology was approved in 1958. There is no residual radioactivity in the food and since unique products are negligible, there is no current way to test a food to see if it was irradiated.

Food ingredients can be categorized as direct additives that are intentionally added, as secondary direct additives that may become part of a food such as color additives, generally recognized as safe ingredients (GRAS), or prior-sanctioned substances. The FDA approves most additives except some GRAS determinations that are independent of FDA. It may make sense to just compile one approved list of everything intentionally added to food in the USA as that is what most people want to know. There are more than 3000 total substances now in an inventory maintained by FDA, appropriately named EAFUS (Everything Added to Food in the United States) (FDA, 2011).

Contaminants are not ingredients, as the intent is to eliminate these unwanted materials from food. These undesirables range from elements like mercury that are environmental hazards, to complex chemicals like acrylamide that may result from frying, to bio-products like aflatoxin from mold growth, to microorganisms like salmonella from infected food. In some cases contaminants may be present in food despite all efforts to prevent or eliminate them. These are referred to as unavoidable contaminants. These could be natural contaminants, others associated with various industries, run-off from animal farms, chemicals used in crop production or from other environmental sources. Irrespective of the source, when added contaminants cannot be avoided by Good Manufacturing Practice (GMP) an action level is set by FDA in the interest of consumer safety. In the case of USDA regulated plants, the reliance is on FDA regulations for action levels in meat and poultry processing. A list of FDAs action level for minimum levels of unavoidable contaminants could be found in the "Defect Levels Handbook" (FDA, 2014d). This should not be an excuse for food companies to have unnecessary contaminants in their products because it could cause the food to be adulterated. However, all necessary efforts must be made to remove or prevent contamination. This is one of the benefits of a workable hazard analysis for critical control point (HACCP) plan. A HACCP plan is required for all juice and seafood processing regulated by FDA and for all facilities inspected by USDA.

Indirect Additives

In contrast with contaminants, indirect additives are not intended to be food but will become an ingredient in a food due to direct or incidental contact. Thus the total amount of indirect additive in food is quite small. Food packaging is an obvious indirect source, so manufacturers must prove to the FDA that all materials coming in contact with food are safe before approval. Indirect additives are not included in the EAFUS list (FDA, 2011).

Coatings and films keep food fresh by keeping unwanted stuff out and keeping desirable stuff in the food, most often moisture. If you ever tried to make pickles from grocery store cucumbers, you know they are coated with an anti-wilting wax that makes this impossible. Many foods are packaged in plastic, and rarely is the plastic container eaten. However, in 2010 attention was focused on an ingredient in the plastic, bisphenol A (BPA) that could migrate into the food. BPA is found in polycarbonate plastics that are often used for water bottles. The plastic also provides an important coating between a metal container and our food. There may be adverse health effects from high level BPA exposure, particularly of concern to infants and children. The FDA notes that BPA is safe at the very low levels in food but continues its review and research. Alternative consumer products have emerged that are labeled as BPA-free, so some consumers avoid coated metal canned foods, and food containers marked with recycle codes 3 or 7.

Food Additives with Health Benefits and Health Risks

Direct additives are needed in four broad categories;

1. to maintain food quality,
2. to assist in food processing,
3. to make food more appealing, or
4. to improve nutritional value.

Food additives add flavor, color, texture, consistency, health value, or shelf-life, among other benefits. If something is not beneficial it should not be in food. This point leads to ongoing debates about the health benefits of artificial color additives and artificial sweeteners, as examples.

There are more than 3000 direct additives now approved and listed in EAFUS, with the average person consuming about 160 pounds of additives each year. That same person consumes about a ton (1,996 pounds to be exact) of total food each year. So the average consumer eats 8% in additives, a figure that sounds high until we understand that this includes 150 pounds of added sweeteners (like sucrose) and two pounds of salt (sodium chloride). This leaves 8 pounds or less than a half percent for all the rest, minimizing potential health impacts. However, consuming those quantities of sugars and salt remain significant health concerns that are covered elsewhere in this text.

The amount of a direct additive allowed in food varies by substance. Its quantity must not exceed the amount reasonably required to accomplish its intended effect. A deviation from this could mean that the food was not manufactured under GMP. For example, sodium nitrite is added to cured meats to prevent botulism at 156 ppm (this odd figure is actually an easy to use ¼ ounce per pound). Any more than this will not further prevent botulism, so this processed meat product would be deemed adulterated. All additives must be food-grade, which means it is sanitary and meets the safety and wholesomeness requirements for food.

It would require more than eight single spaced pages to list the names in the EAFUS (FDA, 2011). The majority of these names are flavors. The FDA also provides the name and function of all food additives permitted for direct addition to human food in Title 21 of the Code of Federal Regulations, 2014.

It would be unnecessary to examine the human health consequences of each direct additive because in most cases there is none and the ingested levels are quite small. We highlight here those additives that either science or popular belief has implied an impact on human health and disease management.

Food preservatives include antioxidants like butylated hydroxyanisole (BHA) or ethylene diamine tetraacetic acid (EDTA) and sodium nitrite used for curing meats. Nitrites and nitrates provide safety against pathogens, particularly against deadly *Clostridium botulinum* that produces a very potent neurotoxin that kills several people yearly. Nitrites gained much publicity in the 1980's as it could react chemically to form nitrosamines, a cancer causing chemical. As a result, a special committee was appointed by the National Academy of Sciences (NAS) to examine this issues. The NAS recommended continued use of nitrite as it is so effective against botulism, and noted that salt-curing and smoking of meats be minimized. Although people assumed all nitrite in food was added by the industry, only about 40% of the nitrite is a direct additive and the majority is naturally occurring. Work by Lee *et al.* (1986) showed the human body produces its own nitrate, so what we make can exceed the amount of nitrate and nitrite in the diet. Added *versus* natural presence of a chemical is a recurrent theme with many food additives. What is added to food is often a natural component of food or of the human body, greatly complicating attempts to regulate or assign a particular health outcome. Although the risk of cancer from added nitrite is quite small, it is balanced by the risk of botulism when it is not added, a concept popularly discussed as the risk-benefit equation.

Caffeine is on the GRAS list, permitted as an additive to cola beverages at a limit of 0.02 percent. It is a natural component of coffee and tea and at much smaller amounts in cocoa. At one time pregnant women were warned to avoid it, but it has since been proved that there are no adverse effects on the developing fetus. Even though the caffeine additive is approved only for cola drinks, creative marketers added it to alcoholic beverages, energy drinks, chewing gum, and a host of unregulated foods. The manufacturers of energy drinks have used a loophole around this 0.02 percent safety limit by claiming the drinks to be dietary supplements, and not be subject to food safety regulations. Thus, the safety of high dose caffeinated drinks is now an uncontrolled experiment. From 2004 to

2012, five people died after consuming Monster energy drinks according to FDA, and in Canada, three deaths were attributed to consumption of Red Bull in the same period (DeNoon, 2012). With so many more added caffeine foods and drinks emerging, FDA is expected to be busy tracking this additive and investigating the health consequences associated with its consumption.

The primary benefit of color additives is in the appearance of the food. For this reason many have questioned the approval of food coloring since some are associated with adverse health side effects. This has led to a confusing regulatory landscape, where the most common global food color, FD&C Red 2, is banned in the US based on questionable studies, but it is accepted as an ingredient in imported products. The nine FD&C certified colors approved in the US are man-made, and have widespread use due their high tinctorial value. This means that much less is needed to get the right color. This helps to reduce the cost of production and improve marketability since these have no taste, and produce a more uniformly colored product when compared with natural colors. Both the very small amounts of certified colors used and the extensive testing done over several decades have shown that FD&C colors are mostly safe. In 2007 a British study linked FD&C yellow 5 (tartrazine) to an increase risk of hyperactivity in kids, resulting in clear labeling of yellow 5 and calls for further studies. In 2014, the safety of caramel (that is used to color cola beverages), was questioned for high levels of 4-MEI (4-methylimidazole) and many companies reduced its concentration in their products. The FDA found that "eliminating 4-MEI in food is virtually impossible" as it is formed during the normal cooking process. Nonetheless, fear of artificial colors has been a boon to natural colorants, exempt from certification. Vegetable extracts, minerals and animal products are all used to add natural coloration to today's food supply. They are more expensive, add unintended flavors, have low tinctorial value (so more must be used), vary in color, and are less tested for health effects than certified colors. Perhaps a serendipitous benefit is a growing body of research that shows some natural colorants may have long term health benefits. The resveratrol in red wine is associated with improved heart health, although most of this benefit is attributed to the alcohol content. There is good evidence that some natural pigments such as lycopene, the color of tomatoes, watermelon, and grapefruit may help reduce cancer risk.

All additives are tested for safety and the most thoroughly tested class of additives are the high-intensity sweeteners. Of these, aspartame, or Nutrasweet, may hold the record with thousands of research publications, reviews and editorials. All of this attention resulted in a clean bill of health showing aspartame is a safe food ingredient. It is basically a dipeptide of two naturally occurring amino acids, and the human body treats it as it would any protein. However, public preoccupation with the safety of any high-intensity (aka, non-nutritive, artificial) sweetener is likely to continue particularly with the explosion of misleading opinions on social media. Six high-intensity sweeteners are FDA-approved today. These include saccharin, aspartame, acesulfame K, sucralose, neotame and advantame. Stevia may be next. Each has its own social controversy based on questionable theories. Prior to the internet, an attempted ban on saccharin in 1972 was deferred by a special act of the US Congress, aware of voters' desire for this sugar substitute. This unending ambivalence about natural *versus* synthetic sweetness is perhaps driven by a nation that wants to curtail sugar consumption while still craving sweets.

Consumption of natural caloric sweeteners exceeds synthetic non-caloric sweeteners more than 100-fold, so health effects are much more likely, just based on total dose. The USDA reports that the total caloric sweetener consumption in the US increased 39% from 110 pounds in the 1950's to 152 pounds per person per year in 2000. Sucrose (table sugar) dropped 32% during that same period, leaving a remarkable increase in high fructose corn syrup from zero to 64 pounds per person per year. Studies associate high simple sugar intakes with higher triglycerides, lower HDL cholesterol, and with select chronic diseases such as obesity and diabetes. The proposed changes to the required FDA nutrition facts label for year 2015 will require information about added sugars, based on a need for more nutrient-rich foods, although it is argued that added simple sugars are identical to that which is naturally present. Nonetheless, the specific health consequences of a large increase in simple sugar consumption over the past half century remain an active investigation.

Salt (sodium chloride) is simultaneously an essential nutrient, food preservative, key flavor ingredient, and health risk. The average consumption of two pounds of salt per year, corresponding to about 2500 milligrams per day, is considered high by medical professionals, as it can cause hypertension in one out of five people. As the oldest known food additive, salting enables preservation of perishable foods for year round consumption, and was so highly valued that it was used as currency, spawning words like "salary" and compliments like "salt of the earth". The mineral sodium is needed for water balance, blood, and nerve function, and its absence could be fatal. Nonetheless, most Americans consume more sodium than needed for essential functions, and The Dietary Guidelines for Americans likely to be published in 2015 will recommend a lower daily value than the current 2300 mg/day. About 75% of the sodium consumed in the US today is from processed or prepared foods, so meaningful salt reduction depends upon industry response to competitive or regulatory incentives.

Monosodium glutamate (MSG) is simultaneously an essential amino acid, key flavor ingredient and alleged health risk. MSG is GRAS and sometimes referred to as the fifth taste. It was accused of an allergy-like reaction called the Chinese restaurant syndrome (Tu, 2014). A questionable bit of research in the 1960's showed damage to lab rats when they were injected with this additive (a very poor experimental design for any food). Although the overwhelming scientific verdict was "not guilty" the public remembers the accusation and proposals by New York City regulatory agencies to ban MSG. With MSG a key ingredient in most Asian cuisine, we can just imagine a regulatory raid in New York Chinatown restaurants. Fifty years later New York City sought to ban large sugar sweetened soft drinks, illustrating again how food health perception can drive public food policy.

Infant Formula Act

The FDA gets its authority to regulate the manufacture, labeling, and inspection of food for infants from the Infant Formula Act of 1980. This act also establishes quality control rules for the manufacturing process, defines adulteration, recall procedures, recording keeping mandates and inspection guidelines. All manufacturers of infant formula must register with FDA and all new or modified formula must get FDA approval prior to marketing. In addition to these requirements, the results of all tests done on a new formula must be submitted to FDA before the said formula is marketed into interstate commerce. In 1985, the Infant Formula Act of 1980 was revised and it now includes the minimum concentrations of 9 nutrients and maximum concentrations of 9 nutrients that must be in the formula. When establishing or modifying its rules and regulations on infant formula, FDA considers recommendations from the Committee on Nutrition. Recommendations and policy statements from this committee are usually published in the Pediatric Nutrition Handbook, (2014). Examples of such statements include iron fortification of infant formula (1979, 1989, 1999), the use of hypoallergenic infant formulas (2000), breastfeeding and the use of human milk (1997), soy-protein-based formulas (1998, 2001), and the use and misuse of fruit juice (2001). The main difference between the regulation of infant formula and food for the rest of the population is the issue of what could cause an infant formula to become adulterated. The Infant Formula Act states that a formula could be deemed adulterated for the following reasons, including those outlined for other types of food:

- If the formula fails to provide the nutrients required under the Act,
- The formula will be deemed adulterated if each batch is not tested for its required nutrient content,
- The formula must be manufactured in batches and not by a continuous process,
- If regularly scheduled testing is not done on the formula,
- If the formula is not manufactured under GMP,
- If the formula fails to meet expected quality requirements,
- If continuous monitoring devices are not used for in-process controls during its manufacturer,
- If regular scheduled audits are not implemented to ensure that the formula is manufactured according to specification.

The Infant Formula Act also requires manufacturers to retain records for a specified period of time. This is to ensure the need for traceability if required by FDA personnel or the manufacturer itself. During an FDA inspection the need to inspect records may arise to ensure that the company demonstrated compliance with the regulations. FDA inspectors will also want to review the results of all testing (including those for microbial and packaging safety), and that all ingredients used are accompanied by certification of guarantees from their suppliers. Labeling requirements for infant formula are similar to those mentioned earlier in this chapter. However, all labels on infant formulas must receive FDA approval before the product could be marketed. Manufacturers are not allowed to make nutrient content label claims, especially for food for infants less than 2 year of age, except those for claims that state the nutrient content and an indication of no salt and no sugar in the formula. All other claims are disallowed by the regulations.

If an infant formula is deemed to be adulterated or misbranded, the manufacturer is required to recall the product. The Food Safety Modernization Act of 2012 (FSMA) gives FDA more power to order a recall even if the manufacturer is hesitant to do so. Irrespective of the circumstances, the manufacturer is required to notify FDA of the recall. The actual recall will be supervised by FDA including the decision to end it.

These new regulations require that the manufacturer keep all records for an extended period of time so that they could be examined by the FDA.

FDA and USDA Enforcement

The main goal of federal enforcement agencies is to prevent food borne illnesses and diseases and to keep adulterated and misbranded products out of interstate commerce. To assist this process, both FDA and USDA use inspection as a major tool. This effort is also augmented by state and municipal agencies that operate within their individual jurisdictions. During an inspection, the main areas of focus include personnel, equipment and facilities, sanitation, sewer and waste disposal, water supply, and the food handling and processing methods in detail. FDA regulated plants are inspected randomly while USDA plants cannot operate without inspection or exemption to do so from USDA. In cases of violations, the agencies have the authority to issue warning letters, perform seizures, quarantine, administration detention, emergency permit, obtain injunctions from the court, or take other actions as allowed under the law. The USDA has the added leverage of withdrawing inspection as a method of demanding compliance. In the case of criminal activities, FDA can collaborate with the Justice Department in order to have individuals arrested and if convicted be subjected to fines and imprisonment. As was mentioned earlier, the agencies now have the authority to order a mandatory recall of a product if the situation warrants it. In the case of imported food, the agencies have the authority to refuse entry of the product if it is even suspected of being adulterated or misbranded. The FSMA now gives FDA the authority to inspect foreign manufacturers who export products to the US. Since the agency'-s' actions are public knowledge (except that of FTC), it is usually in the best interest of food manufacturers to cooperate with the inspecting agency and seek to resolve the situation instead of adopting an adversarial posture.

CONCLUDING REMARKS

United States laws relating to food safety, health and nutrition are mainly found in the Food Drug and Cosmetic Act, the Infant Formula Act, the Nutrition Labeling and Education Act of 1990, FDA Modernization Act of 1997, and the Dietary Supplements Health and Education Act of 1994. These federally enforced laws help ensure the United States diet is wholesome, healthy and safe. Two agencies mainly responsible for food, drugs and dietary supplement regulations are the FDA and USDA. Other agencies with some oversight include the Federal Trade Commission, Environmental Protection Agency, Bureau of Alcohol Tobacco and Firearms, and the Customs Department.

CONFLICT OF INTEREST

The authors confirm that this chapter contents have no conflict of interest.

ACKNOWLEDGMENTS

Declare None.

REFERENCES

Code of Federal Regulations (2014). *Food additives permitted for direct addition to food for human consumption.* Title 21, chapter 1(B) part 172. Available at: http://www.accessdata.fda.gov/scripts/cdrh/cfdocs/cfcfr/cfrsearch.cfm (accessed: 15.1.2015).

Denoon, D.J. (2012). *FDA: 5 Death Reports for Monster Energy Drink.* WebMD Heath News, [Online] Available at: http://www.webmd.com/food-recipes/news/20121023/death-reports-monster-energy-drink (Accessed: 9.1.2015).

Food and Drug Administration (1995). *Nutritional Labeling and Education Act (NLEA) Requirements (8/94 - 2/95)* [Online]. Available at: http://www.fda.gov/ICECI/Inspections/InspectionGuides/ucm074948.htm (Accessed: 9.1.2015).

Food and Drug Administration (2002). *Guidance for Industry: Structure/Function Claims, Small Entity Compliance Guide)* [Online] Available at: http://www.fda.gov/Food/GuidanceRegulation/GuidanceDocumentsRegulatoryInformation/ucm103340.htm (Accessed: 9.1.2015).

Food and Drug Administration (2011a). *Everything Added to Food in the United States (EAFUS)* [Online] Available at: http://www.fda.gov/Food/IngredientsPackagingLabeling/ucm115326.htm (Accessed: 9.1.2015).

Food and Drug Administration (2011b). *Federal Food, Drug and Cosmetic Act* [Online] Available at: http://www.fda.gov/regulatoryinformation/legislation/FederalFoodDrugandCosmeticActFDCAct/default.htm (Accessed: 21.8.2014).

Food and Drug Administration (2013). *Food Labeling Guide* [Online] Available at: http://www.fda.gov/Food/GuidanceRegulation/GuidanceDocumentsRegulatoryInformation/LabelingNutrition/ucm2006828.htm (Accessed: 23.8.2014).

Food and Drug Administration (2013a) *Guidance for Industry: A Food Labeling Guide (11. Appendix C: Health Claims)* [Online] Available at: http://www.fda.gov/Food/GuidanceRegulation/GuidanceDocumentsRegulatoryInformation/LabelingNutrition/ucm064919.htm (Accessed: 9.1.2015).

Food and Drug Administration (2013b). *Guidance for Industry: A Food Labeling Guide (9. Appendix A: Definitions of Nutrient Content Claims)* [Online] Available at: http://www.fda.gov/Food/GuidanceRegulation/GuidanceDocumentsRegulatoryInformation/LabelingNutrition/ucm064911.htm (Accessed: 9.1.2015).

Food and Drug Administration (2014). *Qualified Health Claims* [Online] Available at: http://www.fda.gov/Food/IngredientsPackagingLabeling/LabelingNutrition/ucm2006877.htm (Accessed: 9.1.2015).

Food and Drug Administration (2014a). *Infant Formula Guidance Documents & Regulatory Information* [Online] Available at: http://www.fda.gov/Food/GuidanceRegulation/GuidanceDocumentsRegulatoryInformation/InfantFormula/default.htm (Accessed: 23.8.2014).

Food and Drug Administration (2014b) *FDA Organization* [Online] Available at: http://www.fda.gov/aboutFDA/Centersoffices/default.htm (Accessed: 31.7.2014)

Food and Drug Administration (2014c) *Proposed Changes to the Nutrition Facts Label* [Online] Available from: http://www.fda.gov/Food/GuidanceRegulation/GuidanceDocumentsRegulatoryInformation/LabelingNutrition/ucm385663.htm#images [Accessed: 8th January 2015].

Food and Drug Administration (2014d) *Defect Levels Handbook.* [Online] Available from: http://www.fda.gov/food/guidanceregulation/guidancedocumentsregulatoryinformation/sanitationtransportation/ucm056174.htm. US Government Printing Office. Washington, DC (Accessed: 10.8.2014).

Food and Drug Administration 2015. Food Advisory Committee Meeting On Infant Formula: Briefing Materials. [Online] Available from: http://www.fda.gov/ohrms/dockets/ac/02/briefing/3852b1_01.htm (Accessed: 1.4.2015).

Food and Drug Administration (n.d.) *Summary of Qualified Health Claims Subject to Enforcement Discretion* [Online] Available from: http://www.fda.gov/Food/IngredientsPackagingLabeling/LabelingNutrition/ucm073992.htm [Accessed: 9th January 2015].

Kleinman, R.E., Greer, F.R (2013). In: Pediatric Nutrition Handbook, 7th Edition. American Academy of Pediatrics. Elk Grove, IL. [Online] Available at: https://www.aap.org/en-us/about-the-aap/Committees-Councils-Sections/pages/Committee-On-Nutrition.aspx (accessed: 5.9.2014).

Lee, K., Greger, J.L., Consaul, J.R., Graham, K.L., Chinn, B.L. (1986). Nitrate, Nitrite balance and *de novo* synthesis of nitrate in humans consuming cured meats. *Am. J. Clin. Nutr.* 44:188-194.

Meat Inspection (1999). *Title 9 CFR, part 416, sections 1-17* [Online] Available at: http://www.gpo.gov/fdsys/pkg/CFR-2011-title9-vol2/pdf/CFR-2011-title9-vol2-sec416-2.pdf. US Government Printing Office: p. 605-607 (Accessed: 31.7.2014).

National Cancer Institute (1984). *All-Bran Cereal Ad.* [Online] Available at: https://visualsonline.cancer.gov/details.cfm?imageid=2157 (Accessed: 9.1.2015).

Pearson v Shalala (1999). 164 F.3d 650, US Court of Appeals, District of Columbia.

Poultry and Poultry Products Inspection (2014). *USCODE 2011 Chapter 10* [Online] Available at: http://www.gpo.gov/fdsys/pkg/USCODE-2011-title21/pdf/USCODE-2011-title21-chap10.pdf. US Government Printing Office: p. 449-469 (Accessed: 18.8.2014).

Sanchez, M. C. 2015. Introduction to Statutory Framework and Case Law. *In* Food Law and Regulations for Non-Lawyers – A US Perspective. P. 12-24. Springer Cham Heidelberg. New York, NY.

Silliker (2013). *Silliker Nutrient and Health Claims U.S. and Canadian Regulatory Guide.* [Online] Available at: http://www.foodlabels.com/pdf/RegulatoryGuide.pdf (Accessed: 9.1.2015).

Termini, 2013a. Chapter 5 Human Drugs: Approval Process, Prescription, Generic, Over the Counter Products. Promotion and Adverse Events. In Food and Drug Law: *Federal Regulation of Drugs, Biologics, Medical Devices, Foods, Dietary Supplements, Cosmetics, Veterinary and Tobacco Products.* p. 178. Forti Publications. Wynnewood, PA.

Termini, 2013b. Chapter 10 Dietary Supplements: Herbs, Botanicals and Neutraceuticals. In Food and Drug Law: *Federal Regulation of Drugs, Biologics, Medical Devices, Foods, Dietary Supplements, Cosmetics, Veterinary and Tobacco Products*. p. 499-501. Forti Publications. Wynnewood, PA.

The Environmental Protection Agency (2014). *Environmental Protection Agency Organization* [Online] Available at: http://www2.epa.gov/aboutepa (Accessed: 10.8.2014).

The Federal Trade Commission (2014). *The Federal Trade Commission Organization* [Online] Available at: http://www.ftc.gov/about-ftc (Accessed: 10.8.2014).

Title 21 of The Code Of Federal Regulations, Part 110 (2014). *Current Good Manufacturing Practice in Manufacturing, Packing, or Holding Human Food* [Online] Available at: http://www.accessdata.fda.gov/scripts/cdrh/cfdocs/cfcfr/CFRSearch.cfm?CFRPart=110&showFR=1. US Government Printing Office. (Accessed: 23.8.2014).

Tu, C. (2014). *Is MSG Bad for Your Health?* October 20, 2014 Science Friday, [Online] Available at: http://www.sciencefriday.com/blogs/10/02/2014/is-msg-bad-for-your-health.html?series=28 (Accessed: 9.1.2015).

United States Department of Agriculture (2014). *United States Department of Agriculture Organization* [Online] Available at: http://www.usda.gov/wps/portal/usda/usdahome?navtype=MA&navid=ABOUT_USDA (Accessed: 31.7.2014).

Wikipedia (2015). *Open Sandwich* [Online] Available at: http://en.wikipedia.org/wiki/Open_sandwich (Accessed: 13.8.2015).

CHAPTER 3

Macronutrients

Esperanza J. Carcache de Blanco*

College of Pharmacy, The Ohio State University, Columbus, Ohio, USA

Abstract: The human body is a complex system that requires energy to function properly. The most common sources of energy for the human body and that are called nutrients come from plant and animal origin. The nutrients include carbohydrates, proteins, and lipids. This chapter focuses on the three major groups of nutrients that the human body uses to obtain energy in order to perform its functions.

Keywords: Amino acid, carbohydrates, disaccharide, fats, glicerophospholipids, glucose, glycerides, histidine, isoleucine, lactose, leucine, lipids, lysine, maltose, methionine, oils, phenylalanine, polysaccharide, proteins, sucrose, threonine, tryptophan, valine.

INTRODUCTION

Nutrition and health directly affect the overall performance of the human body. In order to perform well, the human body needs not only sources of energy, but also other nutrients (Wardlaw and Smith, 2011). Sources of energy are directly correlated to body activity. The major sources of energy used by the human body include carbohydrates, proteins and lipids. Carbohydrates are divided into simple and complex categoriesdepending on the number of sugar units (Graham Solomons *et al.*, 2013). Lipids are organized depending on the number and types of glycerides units as well as on the presence of phosphorus or nitrogen, *etc.* (Graham Solomons *et al.*, 2013). Proteins are classified depending on the type of amino acids present as part of the molecules (Graham Solomons *et al.*, 2013). The main content of this chapter will focus on the description of the three major sources of energy that the body uses to obtain the energy.

3. SOURCES OF ENERGY

The human body uses three major groups of nutrients for fuel: 1) carbohydrates, 2) fats and oils, and 3) proteins (Wardlaw and Smith, 2011). The energy produced

***Corresponding author Esperanza J. Carcache de Blanco:** College of Pharmacy, The Ohio State University, Columbus, OH 43210, USA; E-mail: carcache-de-blan.1@osu.edu

by these food sources are often expressed as calories. Calorie values given on food labels are technically kilocalories.

3.1. Carbohydrates

Carbohydrates (CHOs) are chemical organic compounds containing carbon, hydrogen, and oxygen. Carbohydrates are the most frequently macronutrients consumed by humans as part of the diet. All CHOs are primarily molecules of sugars (*e.g.*, glucose) that are used as source of energy by the body (Wardlaw and Smith, 2011). They are synthesized through the process of photosynthesis that occurs in green plants, making green plants the main source of CHOs in our food. Photosynthesis is the process by which plants use energy from the sun to synthesize compounds that generate energy, such as glucose (Dictionary/Thesaurus, 2014). In this process, six molecules of carbon dioxide (CO_2) combine with six molecules of water H_2O) to form one molecule of glucose ($C_6H_{12}O_6$) and six molecules of oxygen (O_2) (Fig. **1**).

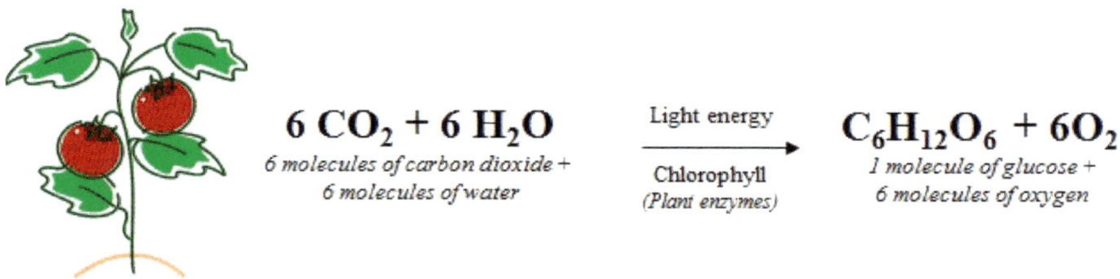

Fig. (1). Photosynthesis scheme.

3.1.1. Classification

Carbohydrates are classified as simple and complex (Fig. **2**) (Graham Solomons *et al.*, 2013; Wardlaw and Smith, 2011). Simple CHOs are called sugars and are either monosaccharides or disaccharides. Complex CHOs are either called starches or fibers depending on their digestibility by the enzymes found in the gastrointestinal tract.

3.1.1.1. Simple Carbohydrates

Simple CHOs are also classified as simple sugars (Wardlaw and Smith, 2011). They are formed by a single sugar molecule (monosaccharides) or two sugar molecules (disaccharides) that have bond together and occur naturally in food, such as in fruits. Simple CHOs have simple structures (Fig. **3**) with small number of sugar units that can be separated into glucose (monosaccharide) quickly and

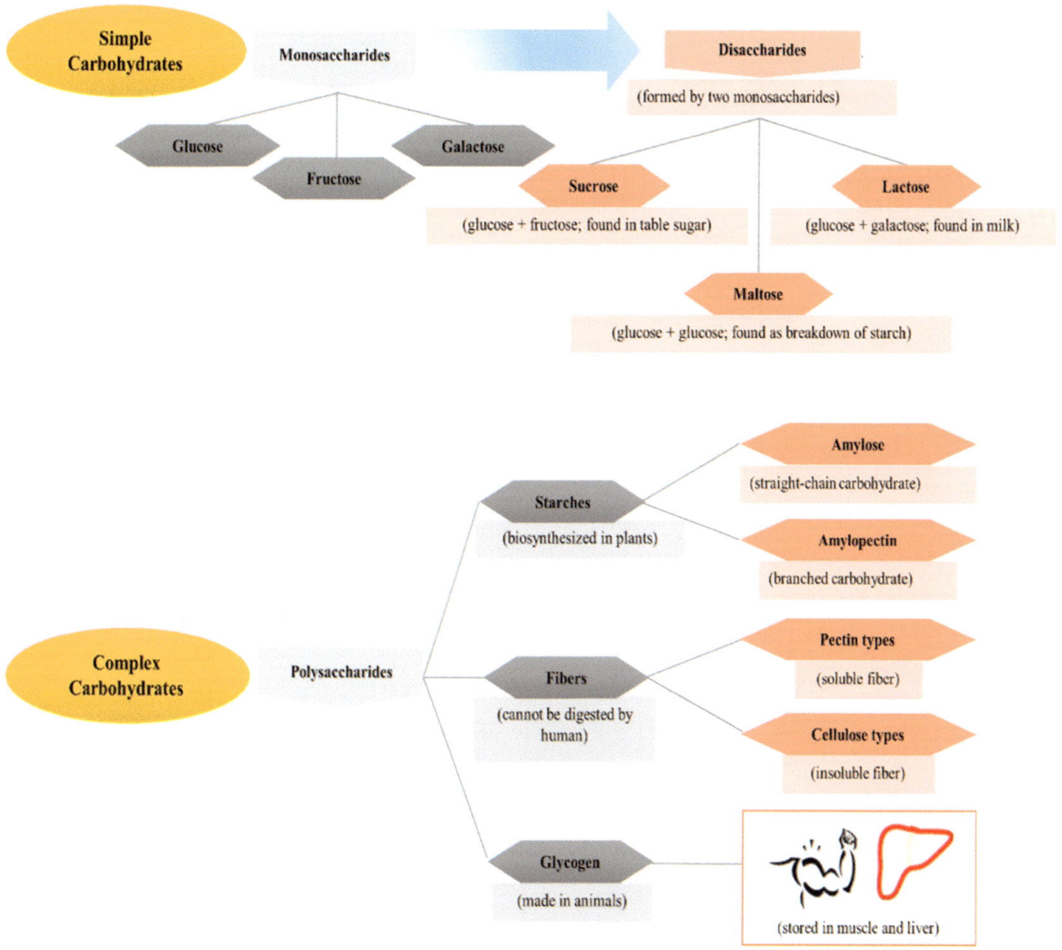

Fig. (2). Classification of carbohydrates. (Morrison and Boyd, 1987; Solomons *et al.*, 2013).

easily. They can be converted in energy readily after intake. However, this chemical process gives an increase of energy by rising rapidly blood glucose levels (glucose), which is rapidly followed by a severe drop of blood glucose levels, and; therefore, a descent in energy levels. The overall process can ultimately leave us feeling more tired than before sugar intake took place. Sucrose (disaccharide) is a classic example of this type of simple CHOs (Wardlaw and Smith, 2011). Sucrose is formed when one molecule of glucose is bonded together with fructose (Fig. **3**) (Graham Solomons *et al.*, 2013). Other examples of disaccharides are lactose (formed by one molecule of glucose and one molecule of galactose) and maltose (formed by one molecule of glucose and one molecule of glucose) (Graham Solomons *et al.*, 2013).

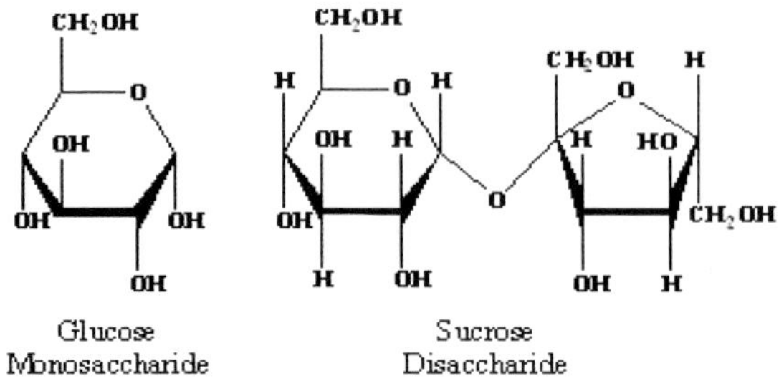

Fig. (3). Examples of simple carbohydrates (Graham Solomons *et al.*, 2013).

Sucrose is a sugar used to sweeten beverages. It is found naturally in sugarcane, beets, honey, and maple sugar. Sucrose is also used to prepare cakes, pastries, soft drinks, and sweets. It is also found in other processed foods. Simple sugars are often associated with diabetes, hunger, lack of concentration, mood swings, tooth decay, weight gain, and hyperactivity, especially in children. The major food source of lactose is milk. In the beer and liquor industry, maltose plays a key role where starches found in various cereals grains are converted into simpler CHOs by enzymes present in these grains (Wardlaw and Smith, 2008).

Sugars found in fruits (fructose) and milk (lactose) may not have the same rapid rise of serum glucose as fruits contain other substances (more complex sugars and oily substances) that prevent the quick release of glucose into the bloodstream (Carbohydrates, 2014). Sucrose alone is metabolized and absorbed too quickly, causing unbalanced levels of blood glucose, which is not beneficial to the body. The human body does not need such a large amount of sugars or energy at once as the body only converts certain amount of sugars into glycogen to be stored for later use; hence, the excess is converted into lipids/fat and stored as such. This stored fat is then more difficult to be converted back into sugar for use. Most natural sugars found in fruits in combination with other substances release energy slowly, contain low levels of simple sugars than sucrose/the refined table sugar alone and do not contribute equally to weight gain (Slavin *et al.*, 2008). These natural sugars found in fruits are also high in fiber (complex carbohydrates) and vitamins (Wardlaw and Smith, 2011).

3.1.1.2. Complex Carbohydrates

Single units of sugars are bonded together to form a chain, known as polysaccharide (poly means many). Complex CHOs are also known as starchy CHOs or polysaccharides (Graham Solomons *et al.*, 2013). Complex CHOs can be found in bread, brown rice, cereals, legumes, most grains, potatoes, pasta, and certain fruits and vegetables (Swann, 2006; Wardlaw and Smith, 2011). Due to the more complex chemical structure (may contain 1000 or more glucose units), complex CHOs are not fragmented down or digested as fast as simple CHOs (Fig. **4**) (Wardlaw and Smith, 2011).

The energy generated from these foods containing complex carbohydrates is released at a slow and constant rate, suggesting balance in energy and blood glucose levels all day. Thus, complex CHOs are healthier than simple CHO containing foods. Most foods containing complex CHOs are often considered lower in fat than simple CHOs as high consumption of the latter is associated with high triglycerides. Complex CHOs found in foods sources are often found together with other nutrients; hence, complex CHOs are said to also contain vitamins and fiber, which are indispensable body nutrients. Most foods rich in CHOs contain mixtures of soluble and insoluble fibers (Slavin *et al.*, 2008; Wardlaw and Smith, 2011). The major sources of fibers include whole grains, all plants, wheat products, rye, rice, vegetables, citrus fruits, apples, oat products, carrots, barley, and beans (Swann, 2006; Wardlaw and Smith, 2011).

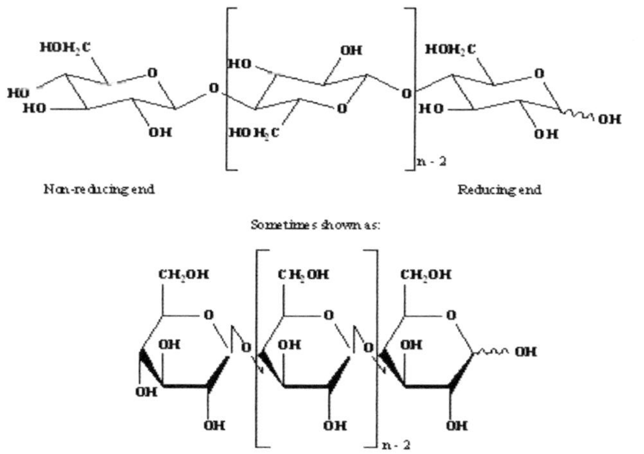

Fig. (4). Representation of cellulose (fiber), example of a complex carbohydrate (Graham Solomons *et al.*, 2013).

Plants store complex carbohydrates in the form of digestible starches such as amylose and amylopectin (Fig. **5**). Amylose is a straight chain of glucose units that comprises about 20% of digestible starch. Plant sources of amylose include vegetables, beans, breads, pasta and rice. Amylopectin, on the other hand, is a highly branched chain molecule and comprises about 80% of the digestible starches. Cellulose (Fig. **4**) is a fiber also found in plants that is classified as a complex carbohydrate (Graham Solomons *et al*., 2013). It cannot be digested by humans despite its similarity in structure to amylose.

Glucose plays a key role in the breakdown of carbohydrates since all enzymes involved in the breaking down of glucose and other related sugars act at the end of a glucose chain. Amylopectin is branched (Fig. **6**); it has more end terminal chains for enzyme action. Amylopectin, therefore, is digested more rapidly than amylose, raising blood sugar more readily than amylose (Graham Solomons *et al*., 2013; Wardlaw and Smith, 2011).

Glycogen consists of a chain of glucose units with many branches ready for enzyme action making it more readily available than amylopectin for digestion and energy production.

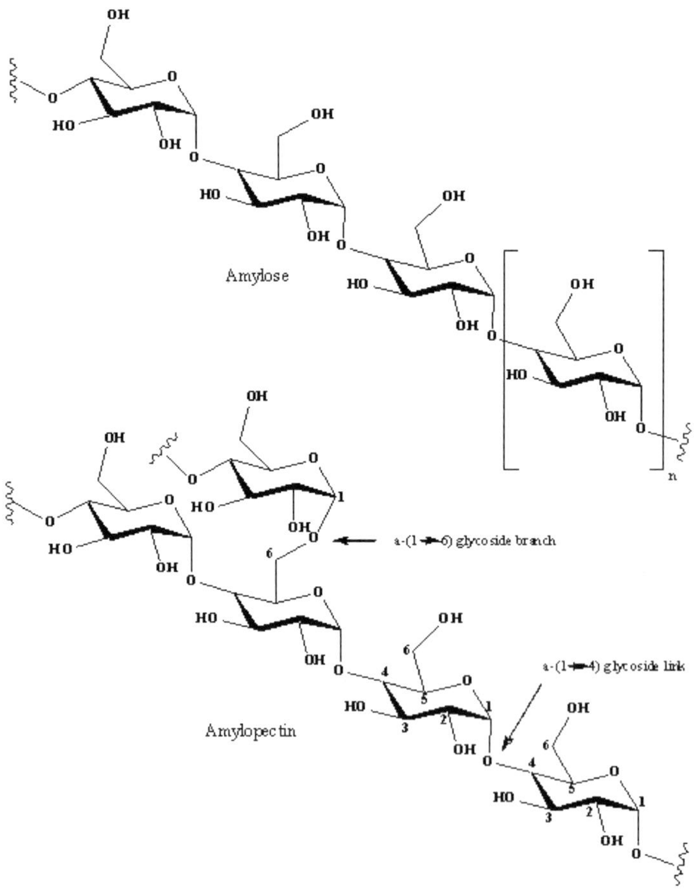

Fig. (5). Digestible complex carbohydrates (Graham Solomons *et al*., 2013).

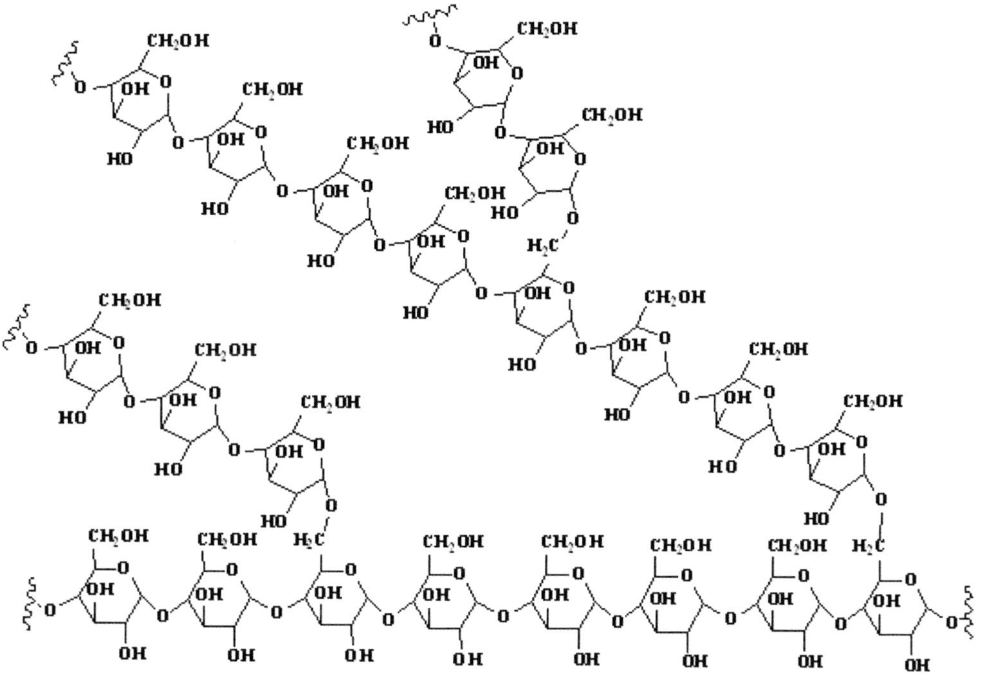

Fig. (6). Glycogen, an ideal form of glucose storage in human body (Graham Solomons *et al.*, 2013).

3.1.2. Role of Carbohydrates

Carbohydrates are a source of calories and energy for the body, which is needed to carry out daily activities and exercise. Any additional energy obtained from the carbohydrates consumed as part of our diet is stored in the body for later use. The human body needs a continuous supply of energy to function properly; hence, lack of adequate intake of CHOs can cause exhaustion or weariness, lack of endurance and stamina, and poor mental function. Foods considered high in CHOs provide not only calories, but also many important health benefits, especially fiber-rich foods such as fruits, vegetables, legumes, and whole-grain breads and cereals (Swann, 2006). Fiber is crucial for the elimination of waste materials and toxins, and helps to preserve the intestines with lower risk of chronic diseases and clean, as some polysaccharides exhibit anti-inflammatory properties (Slavin *et al.*, 2008). The Adequate Intake for fiber in adults is 25 g/day for women and 38 g/day for men (Food and Nutrition Board, 2005). Adequate Intake falls to 21 g/day for women and 30 g/day in men, after age 50 (Food and Nutrition Board, 2005). In North America, fiber intake average is below the recommended Adequate Intake (Wardlaw and Smith, 2011). Even though CHOs come from different sources and some are more beneficial than others, CHOs should be a major part of our diet. Carbohydrates are also important energy sources of the brain, heart, and nervous digestive and immune systems.

3.1.3. Carbohydrates as Source of Energy

Digestible CHOs are the main source of energy of our body. CHOs provide on average 4 kcal per gram. The RDA for CHOs is 130 grams per day for adults (Food and Nutrition Board, 2005). The recommendation for CHOs intake is based in the amount required to provide sufficient glucose for the brain and nervous system, without counting on ketone bodies resulting from fat breakdown as caloric source (Wardlaw and Smith, 2011). When CHOs are digested and metabolized, they are converted to glucose (in turn into blood sugar). Glucose is then utilized or stored to be used later as energy. If the converted glucose is not needed for immediate use, it will be kept in the liver and muscles in the form of glycogen. This can be used as an immediate source of energy when needed by the body.

3.1.3.1. Type of Carbohydrates in a Healthy Diet

Carbohydrates are an essential part of a balanced and healthy diet, and of the calorie intake needed daily. The main source should be complex CHOs, preferably the whole grain meal varieties, as well as fruit and vegetables (Swann, 2006; Wardlaw and Smith, 2011). Simple CHOs should be limited, particularly of the refined kind, including sucrose (refined sugar). Simple sugars have no nutritional value. Additionally, limiting the consumption of simple sugars has been correlated with reduced risk of developing certain chronic diseases such as diabetes, obesity, and dental caries. It has also been correlated to a higher quality diet (Consumer Report, 2005).

3.1.3.2. Examples of "Good" Carbohydrates Sources

When a source of CHOs contains a high amount of complex CHOs, it is considered a “Good” source. Examples of these sources include all types of pasta but especially whole meal pasta, barley, beans, bran, brown rice, chickpeas, corn, lentils, oats, peas, potatoes, sweet potatoes, wheat germ, whole meal bread, wholegrain cereals such as Weetabix, muesli, All bran, brown breads, root vegetables such as carrots, leeks, radishes, and turnips. Sources of different types of CHOs from six different categories (Table **1** for main sources) include cooked carrots (8 g covers 6% RDA), cooked corn (21 g covers 16% RDA), plain M&M (30 g covers 23% RDA), orange (16 g covers 12% RDA), pineapple chunks (1 g covers 8% RDA), Spaghetti noodles (19 g covers 15% RDA), seven grain bread (12 g covers 9% RDA), fat-free milk (12 g covers 9% RDA), and peanuts (6 g covers 5% RDA) (Wardlaw and Smith, 2011).

Table 1. Dietary sources of carbohydrates. (USDA, 2016).

Product	Carbohydrate (grams)	% RDA	Category
Baked Potato, 1 each	63	48%	Vegetables
Cola Drink, 12 fluid oz	25	19%	Empty calories
Banana, 1 each	27	21%	Fruits
Cooked Rice, 1 cup	45	34%	Grains
Light Yogurt, 1 container	6	5%	Dairy
Kidney Beans, 1 cup	110	86%	Protein
RDA	**130**	**100%**	

3.1.3.3. Examples of "Bad" or Less Recommended Carbohydrates Sources

Sources of CHOs containing large amount of simple sugars are considered a "Bad" source of energy. Examples of these sources include uncontrolled intake of biscuits, cakes, candies, cereals, chocolate, fizzy drinks, sugary breakfast pastries, syrup, and table sugar (sucrose).

3.1.4. Digestion and Absorption

Digestion of CHOs can take two routes (Fig. 7). Physical and chemical digestion occurs during food preparation while enzymatic digestion occurs in the body. Cooking softens the connective plant tissues. Heating starch granules while soaking them in water makes them much easier to digest. Enzymatic digestion of CHOs begins in the mouth. **Amylase** is an enzyme found in the saliva secreted by serous cells of the salivary glands. Amylase breaks down the more complex CHOs into simpler types such as disaccharides (maltose) and monosaccharide. The food after broken down moves to the esophagus and enters the stomach where the acidic environment inactivates the enzyme amylase. Thus, no CHOs digestion occurs in the stomach. Then, the food mixture (chyme) enters the duodenum (upper part of small intestine), where a form of amylase secreted by the pancreas converts starch into maltose in the small intestine. Amylase is released from the pancreas in response to the presence of CHOs in the chyme. Enzymes (**maltase**, **lactase** and **sucrase**) found on the wall of the small intestine break down the corresponding disaccharides (maltose, lactose and sucrose) into monosaccharides (glucose, fructose and galactose). Simple CHOs are more easily absorbed and are finally converted to glucose. They are absorbed through the intestinal walls into the bloodstream and taken to the liver *via* portal vein.

Absorption of some CHOs needs specific carrier and energy input to be taken by the absorptive cells in the small intestine. Glucose and galactose are pumped into the cells along with sodium, undergoing active absorption. Fructose is taken up by the cells through facilitated diffusion, using a carrier but no requiring energy input. The liver transforms monosaccharides into glucose and a) releases it into the bloodstream for transport to organs (adipose tissues, brain, kidneys, and muscles), b) produces glycogen for storage, c) produces fat (when CHOs are consumed in large amounts and the overall calorie needs are exceeded).

Any undigested CHO, including viscous fiber, travels to the large intestine to be fermented there to various acids and gases by bacteria. Acids and gases produced are then absorbed into the blood stream. The glucose released into the bloodstream and taken to the liver is stored or dispersed to cells for its use as energy. Non-fermentable fiber escapes enzymatic digestion and is excreted in the feces.

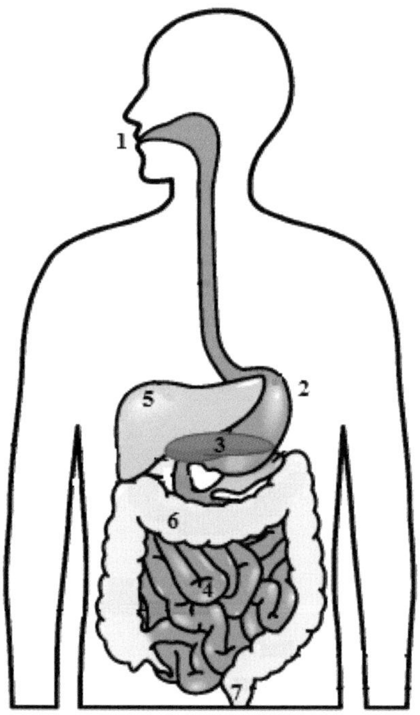

1. Mouth: amylase breaks down some starch to maltose
2. Stomach: no digestion occurs in the stomach because amylase is inactivated by strong acid and chyme moves to small intestine
3. Pancreas: amylase from pancreas breaks down starch in small intestine
4. Small intestine: disaccharides are broken down into monosacharides by enzymes in the wall of the intestine
5. Monosaccharides are absorbed into blood to be taken to the liver via portal vein
6. Large intestine: bacteria ferments viscuos fiber into acids and gases
7. Rectum and anus: non-fermentable fiber is excreted in feces

Fig. (7). Digestion of carbohydrates scheme.

Hence, the liver controls blood glucose levels by providing enough energy for all body functions. For example, surplus glucose is converted to glycogen in the liver (glycogenolysis) in response to the hormone insulin, and stored; otherwise, it could be a cause of hyperglycemia. Using a similar mechanism, if blood sugar levels fall below normal levels (*e.g.* between meals), the glycogen is re-converted to glucose (glycogenolysis) in response to messages sent by the hormone glucagon, to avert hypoglycemia (Wardlaw and Smith, 2011).

In summary, the chemical nature of the CHO itself affects the speed of carbohydrate digestion, and resistance to enzymes. A simple sugar, therefore, is digested or metabolized much faster than a starch since it is much less resistant to enzymatic digestion and absorption. Conditions that can affect the speed of digestion include: the presence of acid (from gastric juices or the food itself), and the presence of soluble fiber.

3.1.5. Sweeteners

Sweeteners are classified into two main categories: nutritive sweeteners and alternative sweeteners (FDA, 2006; Wardlaw and Smith, 2011). Nutritive sweeteners provide calories for the body and are classified as sugars (*e.g.*, fructose, glucose, invert sugar, lactose, maltose, and sucrose). Fructose not only provides calories, but it also serves as the standard against which all other sweeteners are measured (Wardlaw and Smith, 2011). Sugars most commonly used in foods are listed below.

Brown sugar	Fructose	Invert sugar	Molasses	Sugar
Caramel	Fruit sugar	Lactose	Polydextrose	Turbinado sugar
Corn syrup	Glucose	Levulose	Powdered sugar	
Date sugar	High-fructose corn syrup	Maltodextrins	Sorbitol	
Dextrose	Honey	Maple syrup	Sucrose	

Sugar alcohols are also used as nutritive sweeteners, but contribute fewer calories than sugars per gram (2.6 kcal/gram). Examples include sorbitol and xylitol. These are used in candies, breath mints, and sugarless gums. Sugar alcohols are not easily metabolized by bacteria in the mouth; hence do not promote tooth decay. Because of their chemical composition, they are also absorbed and metabolized to glucose more slowly than simple sugar. Therefore, they remain in the intestinal tract for longer time, and can cause diarrhea if found in large quantities (Wardlaw and Smith, 2011; Warshaw, 2004).

Alternative sweeteners, also called artificial sweeteners, include acesulfame-K, aspartame, cyclamate, neotame, saccharin, sucralose, and tagatose (ADA, 2004; FDA, 2006). Sacharin is the oldest alternative sweetener, once was thought to increase the risk of bladder cancer, but is not listed as potential cause of cancer (FDA, 2006; Wardlaw and Smith, 2011). Aspartame is used in over 90 countries and has filed complaints on headaches, dizziness, seizures, and nauseas. Individuals with phenylketonuria should avoid aspartame due to its high content of phenylalanine, an amino acid. Aspartame (methyl L-α-aspartyl-L-phenylalaninate), therefore, is considered more a protein than a carbohydrate. Acceptable Daily Intake (ADI) for aspartame is 50 mg/kg body weight, which is equivalent to 14 cans of soda or 80 packages of Equol (4',7-isoflavandiol) (Wardlaw and Smith, 2011). Neotame ((3*S*)-3-(3,3-dimethylbutylamino)-4-[[(2*S*)-1-methoxy-1-oxo-3-phenylpropan-2-yl]amino]-4-oxobutanoic acid) is structurally similar to aspartame, but it does not break down in the body to amino acids; hence it is not harmful for individuals suffering from phenylketonuria (FDA, 2006) (Wardlaw and Smith, 2011). Tagatose ((*3S,4S,5R*)-1,3,4,5,6-pentahydroxy-hexan-2-one) is poorly absorbed and yield only 1.5 kcal/g (FDA, 2006; Wardlaw and Smith, 2011). Sucralose (1,6-Dichloro-1,6-dideoxy-β-D-fructofuranosyl-4-chloro-4-deoxy-α-D-galactopyranoside) is very stable and does not break down under high heat conditions, it is excreted as such in the feces (FDA, 2006; Wardlaw and Smith, 2011). These sweeteners provide little or no calories when consumed as part of food products. Cyclamate (sodium N-cyclohexylsulfamate) is used in Canada in medicines and as table sweetener, but it was banned in the United States in 1970. FDA indicate the safety of sweeteners by an ADI guideline that is based on animal studies and it is set in a similar way a therapeutic index of a regular drug is determined at a level 100 times less than the level at which no harmful effects were observed in the animal model. The ADI is calculated to be the amount of alternative sweetener considered safe for daily use over one's lifetime (FDA, 2006).

3.2. Proteins

Proteins form the major part of lean body tissue, about 17% of body weight. Proteins are the structural material for the body, muscle, blood, cells enzymes and immunity. The body requires protein to repair tissues and maintain function. Proteins are the building blocks of life (Fig. **8**). The basic structure of protein is a chain of amino acids (a.a. or AA). AA contain N bonded to C. AA link *via* peptide bonds to form proteins. The sequence of covalently linked a.a. is known as the primary structure of a protein. Hence, a protein is a polypeptide, a linear polymer of many a.a., linked by peptide bonds (Graham Solomons *et al.*, 2013; Wardlaw and Smith, 2011).

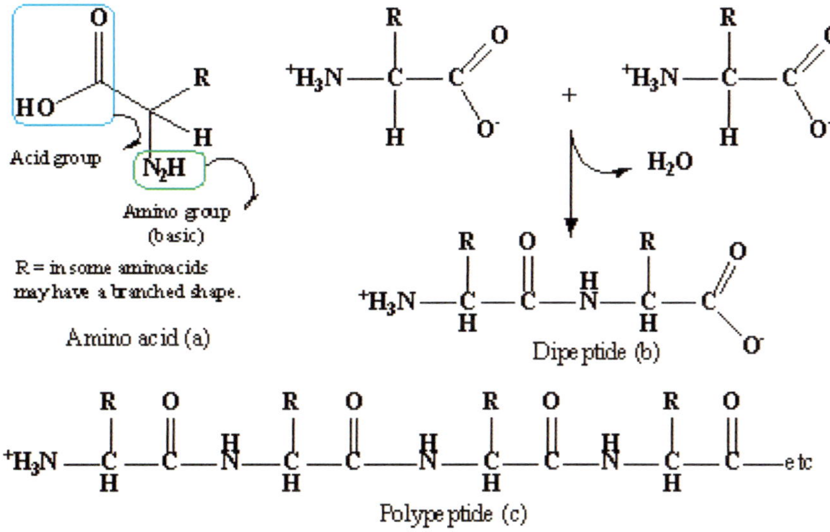

Fig. (8). Generic amino acid (a), dipeptide (b), and protein structures (c) (Graham Solomons *et al.*, 2013).

The body needs 20 different amino acids to function properly. Peptide bonds occur between the carboxylic group of one a.a. and the basic amino group of the next a.a. Peptide bonds are broken by acids or enzymes during digestion. Thc production of proteins is affected by the limiting factor called limiting amino acid. The **limiting amino acid** is the a.a. or essential a.a. in smallest amount in a food or diet in relation to the body needs. It limits the amount of protein the body can synthesize (Graham Solomons *et al.*, 2013; Wardlaw and Smith, 2011).

3.2.1. Classification

In the body, the synthesis of proteins begins with a.a. from both protein-containing foods and those synthesized from other compounds within the body. Amino acids do not need to be consumed all in one meal, but balance over the entire day accounts more accurate for the protein synthesis (Wardlaw and Smith, 2011).

Amino acids are classified into three groups:

- Essential, also called indispensable
- Nonessential, also known as dispensable
- Conditional

Both essential and nonessential a.a. can be found in foods that contain proteins. Lack of enough essential amino acids slows production of new proteins. Health can deteriorate if your body breaks down protein faster than you can make them (Lemke and Williams, 2008; Wardlaw and Smith, 2011).

3.2.1.2. Essential Amino Acids

Essential amino acids cannot be made by the human body, and must be provided by food. The chemical structures of some amino acids are branched and are called branched-chain amino acids (see ones with asterisks). These branched-chain amino acids are used by muscles for energy needs. A main source of these types of amino acids is milk (*e.g.*, whey proteins). Proteins from milk are popular with strength-training athletes (Lemke and Williams, 2008; Wardlaw and Smith, 2011). The nine essential amino acids are:

- Histidine
- Isoleucine
- Leucine
- Lysine
- Methionine
- Phenylalanine
- Threonine
- Tryptophan
- Valine

3.2.1.3. Nonessential Amino Acids

Nonessential amino acids are made by the body from essential amino acids or in the normal breakdown of proteins (Lemke and Williams, 2008; Wardlaw and Smith, 2011). Nonessential amino acids include:

- Alanine
- Asparagine

- Aspartic acid
- Glutamic acid

3.2.1.4. Conditional Amino Acids

Conditional amino acids are typically not essential, except in times of sickness and stress (Lemke and Williams, 2008; Wardlaw and Smith, 2011). These a.a. are as follow:

- Arginine
- Cysteine
- Glutamine
- Glycine
- Ornithine
- Proline
- Serine
- Tyrosine

3.2.2. Protein Synthesis

Protein synthesis (Fig. **9**) is a complicated process where a section of DNA in the nucleus is copied and sent to ribosomes in the cytoplasm. The ribosome uses the information to combine amino acids in the proper sequence to form protein molecules. First, a process called transcription takes place. Protein synthesis begins in the nucleus, where a section of DNA is copied. The copy, usually about 8000 bases, is known as messenger RNA (mRNA) that contains the DNA code to be used for the synthesis of a specific protein and is transported to the cytoplasm where the protein synthesis occurs. RNA, unlike DNA, is composed of a single strand of nucleotides and can pass through the pores of the nuclear membrane into the cytoplasm. Once in the cytoplasm, the mRNA is transported for translation (the next step in the process) of the mRNA code into a specific protein molecule to a ribosome, and binds to the ribosome. Translation is the process where a specific sequence of amino acids is formed along the mRNA in accordance with

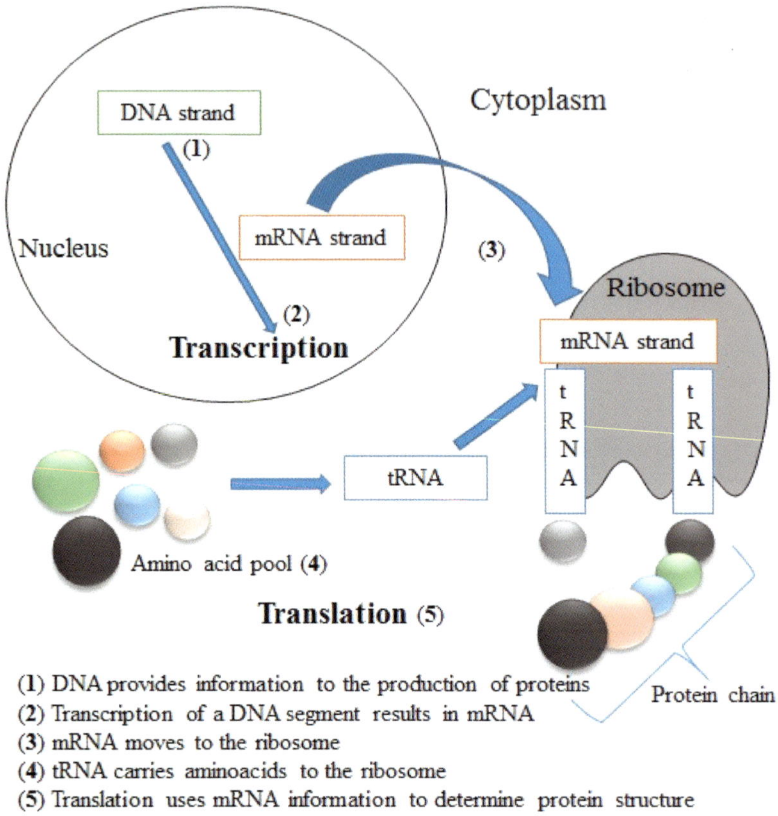

Fig. (9). Protein synthesis scheme.

the codons transcribed on it. The mRNA provides a sequence of triplet codes – set of three bases transcribed from the DNA – for the synthesis of a particular protein. Each three-base set, or triplet, is called a codon. Each codon codes for one of twenty amino acids. Amino acids are carried to the ribosome by transfer RNA (tRNA) and a polypeptide chain is built according to the sequence of codons on the mRNA. Each molecule of tRNA has three bases (anticodon) which bind to the mRNA triplet codes (codon) following the rules of complementary base pairing. The ribosome moves along the mRNA and uses the codons to select amino acids as they arrive. A polypeptide chain, linked by peptide bonds, is formed. Polypeptide chains, once formed, twisted and folded, are assembled into protein molecules (Lemke and Williams, 2008; Wardlaw and Smith, 2011).

3.2.3. Role of Proteins

Proteins play a crucial role in many body processes since some processes such as blood clotting, fluid balance, hormone and enzyme production, visual processes, transport of substances in the bloodstream, as well as cell repair and function, require specific proteins (Fig. **10**). Every cell in the human body contains proteins. Proteins are also major part of the glands, skin, muscles, and organs. Proteins are distributed in all body fluids, except bile and urine. Hence, proteins are needed as part of the diet to assist the body build and repair cells, and cellular function. Proteins are also essential for growth and development during childhood, adolescence, and pregnancy (Wardlaw and Smith, 2011).

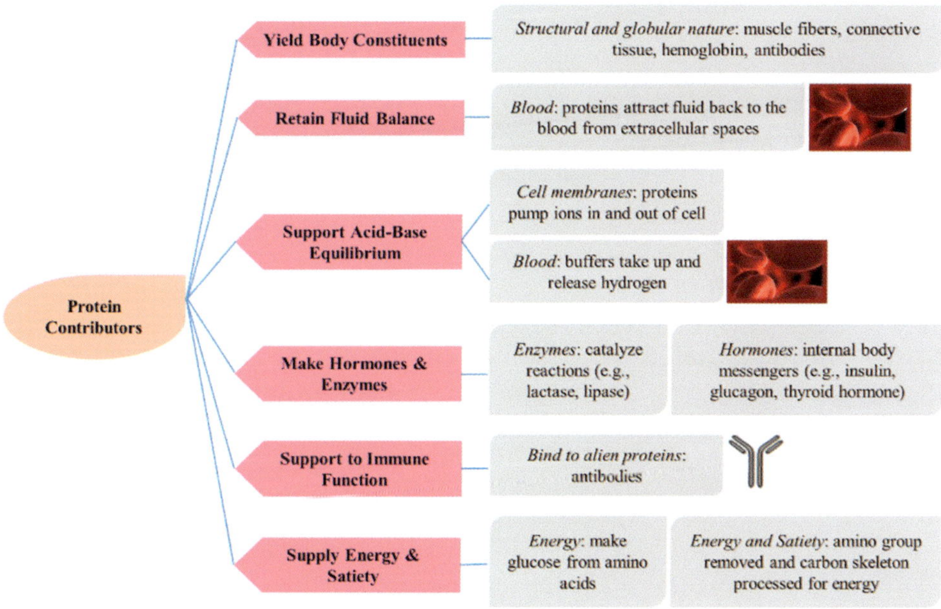

Fig. (10). Role of proteins in the body. (Wardlaw and Smith, 2011).

In healthy people, protein needs can be determined by achieving equilibrium between protein intake and protein losses from protein breakdown. Protein equilibrium or protein balance is key in good health. The amount of protein breakdown can be calculated by quantifying the amount of urea and other nitrogen compounds in the urine, feces, hair, nails, *etc.* If the body is growing or recovering from a disease, a positive protein balance is needed to supply the basic components required for building new tissues. Negative protein balance is the result of consuming less protein than needed, as occurs during acute illness which induces a reduction in the desire to eat or just the mere fact of losing more protein than consumed. The RDA for adults to maintain protein equilibrium is 0.8 grams of protein per kilogram of healthy body weight, which translates into about 10% of total calories (Food and Nutrition Board, 2005; Trumbo *et al.*, 2002). The body cannot store excess protein, converting excess a.a. into glucose or fat for energy needs. In adults, it is required that 11% of protein requirement be provided by essential amino acids. Infants and pre-school children require 40% of protein supplied by essential amino acids, which is reduced later childhood to only 20% (Wardlaw and Smith, 2011).

3.2.4. Proteins as Source of Energy

According to previous reports, 70% of proteins in North America diet come from animal sources. Worldwide only about 35% of proteins come from animal sources and Africa and East Asia only 20% of proteins come from animal sources. Amino acids, though, are left as a result of protein digestion (Wardlaw and Smith, 2011). The human body uses a number of amino acids to break down food. Amino acids need to be consumed in large enough and diverse quantities for optimal health. Amino acids are found in animal sources as well as in plant sources. People do not need to eat animal products to g*et al*l the protein needed for a balanced diet. Consuming too little protein calories can cause protein-calorie malnutrition (PCM), also known as protein-energy malnutrition (PEM). Hence, it is crucial to have an adequate intake of proteins. Proteins can also be broken down to provide energy for the body, yielding an average of 4 kcal/g (Food and Nutrition Board, 2005; Wardlaw and Smith, 2011). Lack of enough protein synthesis increases the risk of diseases and even death (Key *et al.*, 2006; Sabate, 2003).

3.2.5. Type of Proteins in a Healthy Diet

Proteins are grouped in three types including complete or high-quality proteins, incomplete or low-quality proteins, and complementary proteins. Complete or high-quality proteins include sources that contain the nine essential a.a. in sufficient quantities. Animal sources contain all nine essential a.a. and composition of human tissue resembles animal tissue (Chao *et al.*, 2005; Wardlaw and Smith, 2011). Incomplete or low-quality proteins include sources that lack adequate amounts of one or more essential a.a. A single plant source may have only some essential a.a. in adequate amounts (Sabate, 2003; The Vegetarian Resource Group, 2008). Complementary proteins result when one or more proteins combine to compensate for deficiencies in essential a.a. content in each protein. Mixed diets provide high-quality proteins due to the complementary protein pattern that result (Wardlaw and Smith, 2011).

3.2.5.1. Examples of "Good" Protein Sources

A “Good” source of protein contains a high amount of all nine essential a.a. Examples of these sources include animal sources such as eggs, fish, meats, milk, and quinoa (ADA, 2003; Wardlaw and Smith, 2011). Soy is considered a high-quality source of protein since it also contains all essential a.a. Quinoa is another plant source rich in proteins and in essential a.a. In addition to these single sources, some combinations of plant sources of proteins can provide high-quality proteins (WebWatch, 2008; Xiao, 2008). Sources of different types of proteins from five different categories (Table **2** for main sources) include apple (0.5 g covers 1% RDA), beans (8.1 g covers 14.5% RDA), beef chuck (15.3 g covers 27% RDA), broiled chicken (21.3 g covers 38% RDA), cheddar cheese (7 g covers 12.5% RDA), egg (5.5 g covers 10% RDA), kidney 1% low fat milk (8 g covers 14% RDA), pasta (1.2 g covers 2% RDA), peanuts (7.3 g covers 13% RDA), and white rice (2.1 g covers 4% RDA) (Wardlaw and Smith, 2011).

3.2.5.2. Examples of "Bad" or Less Recommended Protein Sources

Plant sources that contain little or no proteins such as fruits are considered "Bad" sources of proteins. These plant sources lack essential a.a. or contain inadequate amounts (ADA, 2003).

Table 2. Examples of sources of proteins. (USDA, 2016).

Product	Protein (grams)	% RDA	Category
Canned tuna, 1 ounce	8	15%	Meats &Beans
Yogurt, 1 container	17	30%	Dairy
Corn, 1 cup	16	30%	Vegetables
Whole wheat bread, 1 slice	4	7%	Grains
Banana, 1 unit	1.3	2%	Fruits
RDA	**56***	**100%**	

*RDA for a 70 kg man.

3.2.6. Digestion and Absorption

Hydrochloric acid and pepsin present in the stomach begin the enzymatic digestion of proteins (Fig. **11**). Pepsin is an enzyme that breaks polypeptides into shorter chains. The release of this enzyme is controlled by the hormone gastrin. Some seven or more factors influence how fast the enzymes act on proteins. These factors include a) the concentration of the enzyme; b) the amount of protein food needing to be digested or absorbed; c) the pH of the food and that of the stomach; d) the temperature of the food; e) time; and f) the presence of any digestion inhibitors or pH adjusting agents, such as antacids. Cooking and chewing aid in unfolding and denaturing proteins, but protein digestion does not start in the mouth, as CHO metabolism does. The hydrochloric acid in the stomach is necessary to denature proteins in order for pepsin to break the protein bonds. The protein-containing foods are broken apart to smaller units such as proteins; then, proteins are broken into their constituent parts, the amino acids (Wardlaw and Smith, 2011).

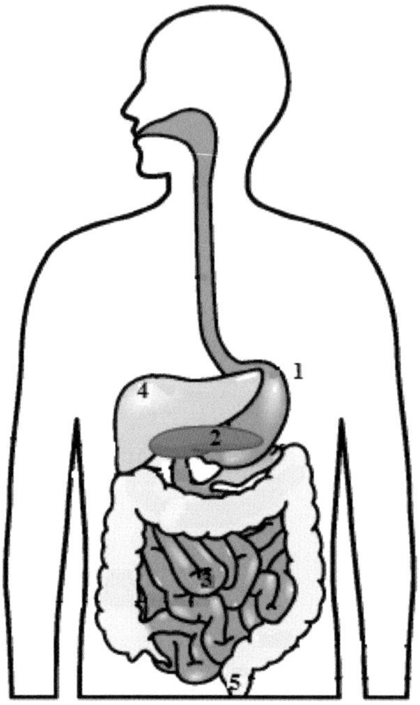

1. Stomach : pepsin and stomach acid participate in partial protein digestion
2. Pancreas : released enzymes further digest polypeptides
3. Small intestine: digestion of aminoacid chains to single aminoacid occur inside cells of small intestine
4. Liver: absorbed aminoacids through the portal vein are transported to the liver and then enter the general bloodstream
5. Rectum and anus: small amount of dietary proteins are present in feces

Fig. (11). Digestion of proteins scheme.

Chyme moves to the small intestine and activate the release of the hormone cholecystokinin (CKK) from the walls of the small intestine. CKK travels to the pancreas through the bloodstream to cause the release of protein splitting-enzymes, such as trypsin. Protein digestion continues in the upper section of the small intestine under the action of the pancreatic enzymes, trypsin and chymotrypsin. These enzymes further divide the chains of a.a. into smaller segments (2-3 units) of a.a. or even single a.a. The amino acids are absorbed in the small intestines by the blood capillaries, carried through the liver, and then go into the general blood circulation. Once in the blood, the a.a. are carried by both the red blood cells and by the plasma. The a.a. are thereby distributed in all body tissues, where the corresponding cells select the needed substrate to repair and reform the necessary protein structures (Wardlaw and Smith, 2011).

3.2.7. Protein Diets

A typical diet supplies an average of 50% of protein in the form of essential a.a (Wardlaw and Smith, 2011). However, several health problems may result if a high-protein diet is followed for an extended period of time, such as:

- Some high-protein diets control CHO intake to an extent that nutritional deficiencies of certain nutrients such as vitamins found in plants (folate), minerals (magnesium), and phytochemicals can develop.
- High-protein diets limit CHO intake to an extent that insufficient fiber intake results, which can cause health issues such as constipation and diverticulitis.
- Some high-protein diets encourage the consumption of foods such as red meat and full-fat dairy products, which may increase the risk of heart disease, calcium losses, and colon cancer due to excessive fat and low-fiber content.
- A high-protein diet might deteriorate kidney function in people with kidney disease because a) animal protein may contribute to kidney stone formation, b) kidneys are overburdened with excretion of extra nitrogen as urea and other nitrogen containing compounds, c) elimination of all the waste products of protein metabolism can be an issue for the body, and d) this type of diet can cause increase in urine output, posing a risk for dehydration.

Low-protein diets on the other hand slow the decline of kidney function, particularly important in diabetes (Aronson, 2005).

3.2.7.1. Warning

A diet with high meat intake can contribute to high cholesterol levels or other diseases such as gout. A diet high in protein may also put a strain on the kidneys. If we do not consume adequate amount of proteins, many metabolic processes slow down and due to the lack of key proteins there would be an increased risk of infections, disease, and death (Chao *et al*., 2005; Food and Nutrition Board, 2005; Trumbo *et al*., 2002; Wardlaw and Smith, 2011).

3.2.8. Food Label

Information found in nutrition labels can help to choose nutritious food by answering the following questions (Fig. **12**). Which product is better choice for a meal? What is the amount of protein in the product? How much of my daily requirement will be provided by the consumption of one serving size of this product?, *etc.*

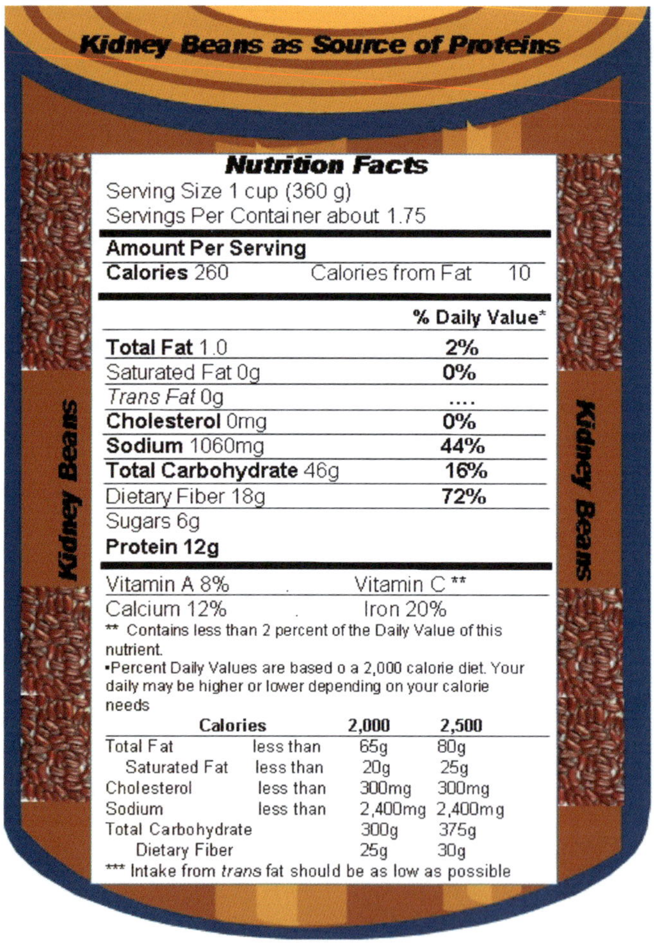
Kidney Beans as Source of Proteins
Kidney Beans
Kidney Beans
Nutrition Facts
Serving Size 1 cup (360 g)
Servings Per Container about 1.75
Amount Per Serving
Calories 260 Calories from Fat 10
% Daily Value*
Total Fat 1.0 2%
Saturated Fat 0g 0%
Trans Fat 0g ....
Cholesterol 0mg 0%
Sodium 1060mg 44%
Total Carbohydrate 46g 16%
Dietary Fiber 18g 72%
Sugars 6g
Protein 12g
Vitamin A 8% Vitamin C **
Calcium 12% Iron 20%
** Contains less than 2 percent of the Daily Value of this nutrient.
•Percent Daily Values are based o a 2,000 calorie diet. Your daily may be higher or lower depending on your calorie needs
Calories 2,000 2,500
Total Fat less than 65g 80g
Saturated Fat less than 20g 25g
Cholesterol less than 300mg 300mg
Sodium less than 2,400mg 2,400mg
Total Carbohydrate 300g 375g
Dietary Fiber 25g 30g
*** Intake from trans fat should be as low as possible

Fig. (12). Food label (Values used in this figure may not be accurate; they serve filling purposes only).

3.3. Lipids

Lipids are a broad group of naturally-occurring chemicals that include fats, fat-soluble vitamins (such as vitamins A, D, E and K), sterols, monoglycerides, diglycerides, phospholipids, waxes, and others. Hence, the chemical structure of lipids is diverse and is mostly formed of C, H, and O. The main biological functions of lipids involve energy storage, as structural components of cell membranes, and as important signaling molecules (Wardlaw and Smith, 2011).

3.3.1. Classification

The classification of lipids is chemically based on the distinct hydrophobic and hydrophilic elements that compose the lipid. Lipids, in general, do not readily dissolve in water (Graham Solomons *et al.*, 2013). Fatty acids are long chain of carbons that in the alpha end have an acid group and in the omega end have a methyl group (Graham Solomons *et al.*, 2013). In the body and in foods, fatty acids are found in the main form of lipids, triglycerides. In this book, only lipids most relevant to Pharmaconutrition will be discussed.

3.3.1.1. Fatty Acyls

Fatty acyls, their conjugates and derivatives, are a diverse group of compounds biosynthesized by chain-elongation of an acetyl-CoA group with malonyl-CoA or methylmalonyl-CoA groups (Dewick, 2009). The structural composition of fatty acids contains a polar, hydrophilic end, and a hydrophobic end that is non-polar and insoluble in water (Graham Solomons *et al.*, 2013). The fatty acid structure (see Fig. **13**) is one of the most essential components of biological lipids, and is commonly utilized as a building block in lipids with more complex structure. The carbon chain typically contains between four and 24 carbons. The chain can be saturated or unsaturated, and may have attached functional groups such as oxygen, halogens, nitrogen, and sulfur. Numbering of the chain starts from the omega end (Graham Solomons *et al.*, 2013). Fatty acids can be monounsaturated (only one double bond) and polyunsaturated (two or more double bonds). Double bonds in the carbon chain can be either "*cis*" or "*trans*", which significantly affects the molecule's arrangement. "*Cis*"-double bonds cause the fatty acid chain to bend, and the effect is more pronounced in longer chains containing more *cis* double bonds. This chemical arrangement plays a significant role in the structure and function of cell membranes. Most naturally occurring fatty acids are of the "*cis*" configuration, even though the "*trans*" configuration can also be found in some natural and partially hydrogenated fats and oils. The type of double bond in the fatty acids not only affects the configuration, but also their roles on cell membranes and when attaching to X, N, and S groups (Wardlaw and Smith, 2011).

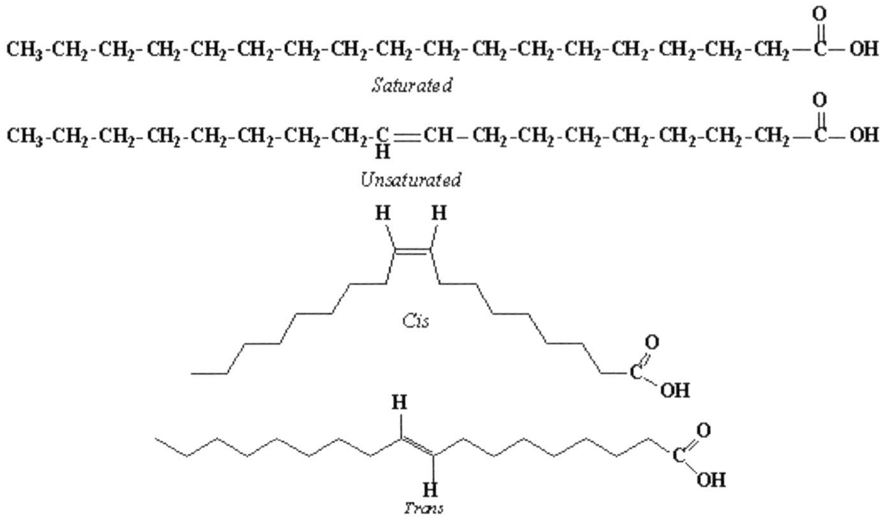

Fig. (13). Generic fatty acid structures (Graham Solomons *et al.*, 2013).

Examples of fatty acyls include the eicosanoids, derived primarily from arachidonic acid and eicosapentaenoic acid, which include prostaglandins, leukotrienes, and thromboxanes. This group plays important roles in inflammatory processes. Other important classes of lipids in the fatty acid category are the fatty esters and fatty amides. Fatty esters are key biochemical intermediates that include fatty acid carnitines, fatty acid thioester coenzyme A derivatives, fatty acid thioester ACP derivatives and wax esters. The fatty amides include neurotransmitters such as the cannabinoid anandamide that belong to the N-acyl ethanolamines (Wardlaw and Smith, 2011).

3.3.1.2. Glycerolipids (Triglycerides)

Glycerolipids include mono-, di- and tri-substituted glycerols. The triacylglycerols (fatty acid esters of glycerol) are the most well-known, also known as triglycerides (Fig. **14**) (Dewick, 2009; Wardlaw and Smith, 2011). These are the most common type of lipids found in the body and foods. In triacylglycerols, the three hydroxyl groups of glycerol are esterified, typically by different fatty acids. Glycerol serves as backbone for the three attached fatty acids. These types of lipids cover the majority of storage fat in animal tissues (Wardlaw and Smith, 2011). The presence of two fatty acid chains attached forms a diglyceride, while having only one attached to the backbone forms a monoglyceride (Graham Solomons *et al.*, 2013). Fat mobilization occurs when ester bonds of the triacylglycerols are hydrolyzed, and glycerol and fatty acids are released from adipose tissue (Wardlaw and Smith, 2011). Additional subclasses of glycerolipids are represented by glycosylglycerols, which have attached *via* a glycosidic linkage one or more sugar residues to glycerol. Digalactosyldiacylglycerols found in plant membranes and seminolipid from mammalian sperm cells are good examples of this type of glycerolipids. During digestion, triglycerides are converted into monoglycerides. After absorption, fatty acids and monoglycerides are reformed into triglycerides (Wardlaw and Smith, 2011).

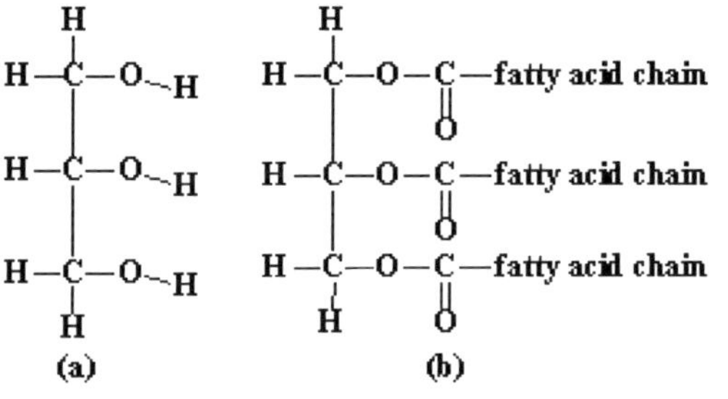

Fig. (14). Glycerol (a) and the generic structure of a triglyceride (b) (Graham Solomons *et al.*, 2013).

3.3.1.3. Glycerophospholipids

There are many different types of glycerophospholipids in the body, especially in the brain. They are also built on a backbone of glycerol and at least one of the fatty acids is replaced by a compound containing P and sometimes N (Dewick, 2009; Graham Solomons *et al.*, 2013). The body is able to produce all phospholipids it needs and they participate in fat digestion. Glycerophospholipids, also referred to as phospholipids (Fig. **15**), are abundant in nature and are important components of the lipid bilayer of cells. They are also highly involved in metabolism and cell signaling. Neural tissue (including the brain) is rich in glycerophospholipids, and variations in composition have been associated with various neurological disorders (Wardlaw and Smith, 2011). Glycerophospholipids classification is based on the nature of the polar headgroup at the “sn”-3 or the “sn”-1 position of the glycerol backbone in the case of eukaryotes/ eubacteria and archaebacterial, respectively. Three classical examples of glycerophospholipids found in biological membranes include phosphatidylcholine (also known as PC, GPCho or lecithin), phosphatidylethanolamine (PE or GPEtn) and phosphatidylserine (PS or GPSer). Some glycerophospholipids such as phosphatidylinositols and phosphatidic acids serve as precursors of second messengers that are membrane-derived in eukaryotic cells. Sometimes, they also serve as second messengers themselves. They even serve as a primary component of cellular membranes and binding sites for intra- and intercellular proteins. Typically in archaebacterial, one or both of these hydroxyl groups are acylated with long-chain fatty acids, including variations such as alkyl-linked, Z-alkenyl-linked (plasmalogen) glycerophospholipids, and dialkylether variants (Dewick, 2009; Wardlaw and Smith, 2011).

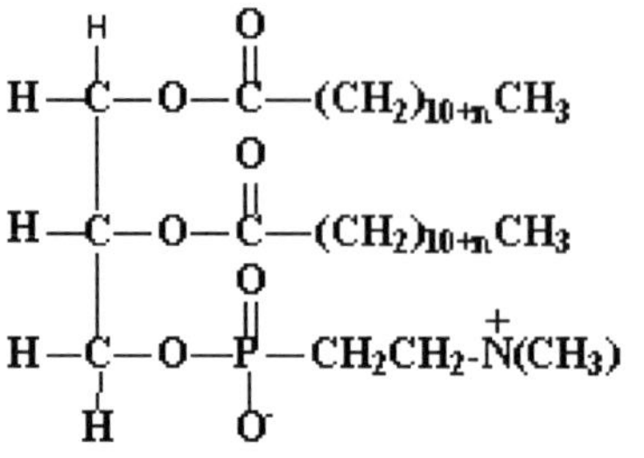

Fig. (15). Generic structure of a phospholipid (Graham Solomons *et al.*, 2013).

3.3.1.4. Sphingolipids

Sphingolipids, share a common structural feature, a sphingoid base backbone that is biosynthesized "*de novo*" from a long-chain fatty acyl CoA and the amino acid serine, then converted into ceramides, phosphosphingolipids, glycosphingolipids and other compounds (Dewick, 2009). Sphingosine is the major sphingoid base of mammals. A major subclass of sphingoid base derivatives with an amide-linked fatty acid includes ceramides (N-acyl-sphingoid bases). The fatty acid units usually contain chain lengths from 16 to 26 carbon atoms that can be saturated or mono-unsaturated. In mammals, the major phosphosphingolipids are sphingomyelins (ceramide phosphocholines). In insects, ceramide phosphoethanolamines are the predominant ones, while in fungi, phytoceramide phosphoinositols and mannose-containing headgroups are the main types (Dewick, 2009; Wardlaw and Smith, 2011). The glycosphingolipids belong to a family of diverse compounds in which one or more sugar residues are linked to the sphingoid base *via* a glycosidic bond. Cerebrosides and gangliosides are classified as simple and complex glycosphingolipids, respectively (Dewick, 2009; Graham Solomons *et al.*, 2013).

3.3.1.5. Sterol lipids

Sterol lipids (Fig. **16**) are built as multi-ring structures which makes them different from other lipids (2008; Graham Solomons *et al.*, 2013; Lemke and Williams, 2008). The most common example is cholesterol which is not soluble in water. Sterol lipids, glycerophospholipids and sphingomyelins are an important component of membrane lipids. The steroids, such as cholesterol and its derivatives, all derived from the same fused four-ring core structure, have

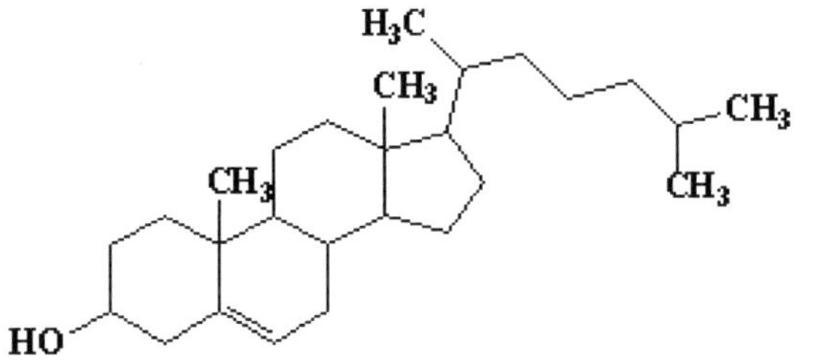

Fig. (16). Generic structure of a sterol (Graham Solomons *et al.*, 2013; Lemke and Williams, 2008).

different biological roles as hormones and signaling molecules. Cholesterol is used to form certain hormones and bile acids. Some of the hormonal related functions include those of the estrogen family, androgen, and vitamin D. The estrogen family includes the eighteen-carbon steroids (C-18) whereas the C-19 steroids comprise the androgens such as testosterone and androsterone. The glucocorticoids, mineralocorticoids, and progestogens are categorized as part of the subgroup with C-21. The secosteroids are characterized by the cleavage of the B ring on the core structure, including various forms of vitamin D. Oxidized derivatives of cholesterol in mammals that are synthesized in the liver include bile acids and their conjugates. The corresponding equivalent phytosterols in plant include β-sitosterol, stigmasterol, and brassicasterol; the latter compound is also utilized as a biomarker for algal growth. Ergosterol is the prime sterol in fungal cell membranes (Lemke and Williams, 2008; Micallef and Garg, 2008; Wardlaw and Smith, 2011).

3.3.1.6. Prenol Lipids

Carotenoids contain simple isoprene units connected head-to-tail that function as antioxidants and as precursors of vitamin A. The quinonoid core of non-isoprenoid origin in quinones and hydroquinones also have an isoprenoid chain attached. Vitamin E and vitamin K, as well as the ubiquinones, are also examples of this group of lipids. The terminal isoprenoid unit attached to the oxygen remains unsaturated in polyprenols (called bactoprenols) that are biosynthesized by prokaryotes, whereas the terminal isoprenoid is reduced in animal polyprenols (dolichols) (Dewick, 2009; Graham Solomons *et al.*, 2013; Wardlaw and Smith, 2011). Prenols are biosynthesized from the 5-carbon precursors isopentenyl diphosphate (IPP) and dimethylallyl diphosphate (DMAPP) (Dewick, 2009). The simple isoprenoids (linear alcohols, diphosphates, *etc.*) are formed by the successive addition of C5 and C10 units, and are classified according to number of these units. Structures containing 40 carbons or more are known as tetraterterpenes or polyterpenes, respectively (Dewick, 2009).

3.3.1.7. *Saccharolipids*

Saccharolipids are compounds with fatty acid units directly connected to a sugar backbone, making structures that are compatible with membrane bilayers. In the glycerolipids and glycerophospholipids, a monosaccharide replaces the glycerol backbone (Lemke and Williams, 2008).

3.3.1.8. Polyketides

Polyketides found in dietary products include a large number of secondary metabolites and nutrients that have great structural diversity. They are naturally biosynthesized. The classic, iterative, and multimodular enzymes that polymerize the acetyl and propionyl subunits share mechanistic features with the fatty acid synthases. Many polyketides are cyclic molecules usually modified by glycosylation, methylation, hydroxylation, oxidation, and/or other processes. Many anti-microbial, anti-parasitic, and anti-cancer agents are polyketides or polyketide derivatives (erythromycins, tetracyclines, avermectins, and antitumor epothilones) (Dewick, 2009; Lemke and Williams, 2008; Wardlaw and Smith, 2011).

3.3.2. Role of Lipids

According to Dietary Guidelines, it is recommended that 20-35% of total calories (44-78 g/day of total 2000 kcal/day including 5% of essential fatty acids such as omega-3 and-6) come from lipid sources (Fig. **17**) (Wardlaw and Smith, 2011) (Food and Nutrition Board, 2005). American Heart Association (AHA) recommends <7% total calories from saturated fat, <1% from *trans* fat, and a maximum of 300 mg/day of cholesterol (Lichtenstein *et al.*, 2006). The major dietary lipids for humans come from animal and plant sources such as triglycerides, sterols, and membrane phospholipids (Micallef and Garg, 2008; Wardlaw and Smith, 2011). Most of the lipid found in food is in the form of triacylglycerols, cholesterol, and phospholipids. A minimum amount of dietary fat is needed for transport to the small intestine and absorption of fat-soluble vitamins (A, D, E and K) and carotenoids (Wardlaw and Smith, 2011).

Even though recommendations are made for reduced consumption of fats, it is important to have an insulating layer of fat in cold climates. Fat tissue also surrounds and protects some organs from injury. Hence, extra fat provides energy storage for times when food is scarce (Lau *et al.*, 2005; Micallef and Garg, 2008).

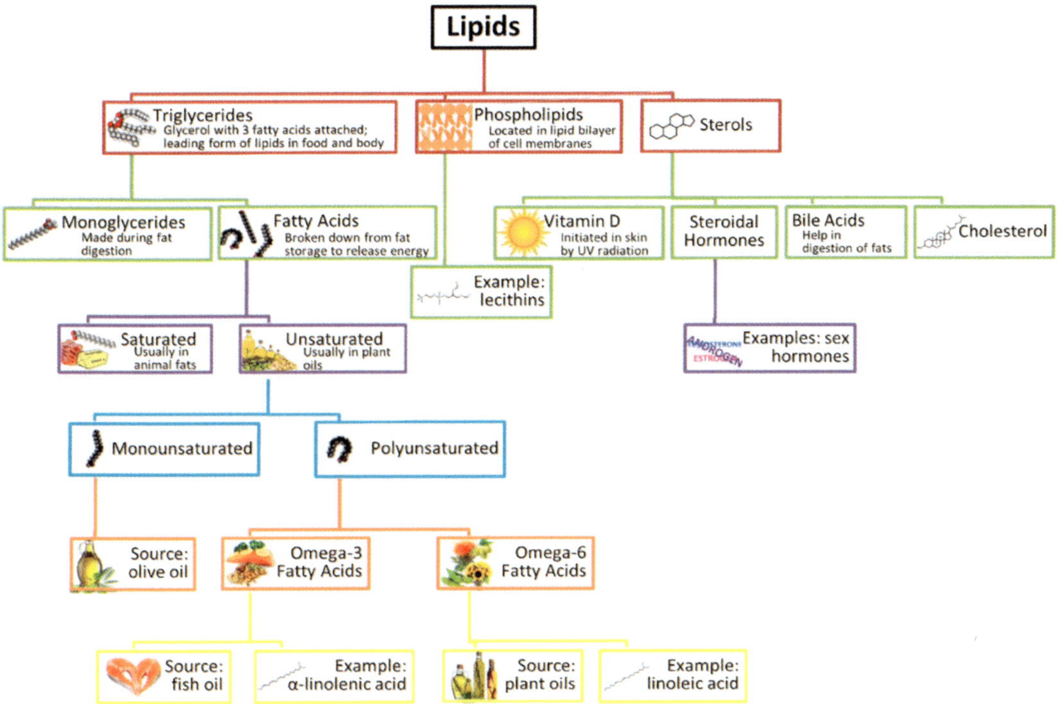

Fig. (17). Types and roles of lipids. (Wardlaw and Smith, 2011).

3.3.3. Lipids as Source of Energy

Lipids provide energy for body functions. Half of the energy used by the entire body at rest and during light activity comes from fatty acids. Lipids do not react with other cell constituents; hence, it is a safe form of energy storage which is in the form of triglycerides (Lau *et al.*, 2005; Wang *et al.*, 2006). Some fatty acids afford 8.6 kcal/g whereas some longer chain fatty acids deliver 9.6 kcal/g. Not all fats in our diet have the same energy content, but fat provides an average of 9 kcal/g (Food and Nutrition Board, 2005). The different classes of lipids have diverse functions in the body and the body needs little fat to maintain health, including essential fatty acids. All are necessary for health, but many can be made by the body and therefore are not needed in our diet (ADA, 2005). Only certain polyunsaturated fatty acids are essential parts of a diet, such as linoleic acid (omega-6 fatty acid type) and alpha-linolenic acid (omega-3 fatty acid type) (Kris-Etherton and Hill, 2008). Sources of different types of lipids from six different categories (Table **3** for main sources) include mixed nuts (16 g fat have 78% calories from fat and 23% AHA), hamburger with bun (12 g fat have 39% calories from fat and 17% AHA), margarine (12 g fat have 100% calories from fat and 17% AHA), whole milk (8 g fat have 49% calories from fat and 11% AHA), chicken breast with skin (7 g fat have 36% calories from fat and 10% AHA), whole-milk yogurt (7 g fat have 28% calories from fat and 10% AHA), baked beans (7 g fat have 31% calories from fat and 10% AHA), flax seeds (3 g fat have 62% calories from fat and 4% AHA), and fig Newton cookies (3 g fat have 23% calories from fat and 4% AHA) (Wardlaw and Smith, 2011).

Table 3. Natural sources of lipids. (USDA, 2016).

Product	Fat (grams)	% AHA	Category
T-bone steak, 1 ounce	5	7	Meats and beans
Canola oil, ½ tablespoon	7	10	Oils
Avocado, 1 cup	22	33	Vegetables
Cheddar cheese, 1 ounce	10	14	Dairy
Snack crackers, 1 cup	14	20	Grains
M&M milk chocolate candies, 1 ounce	20	30	Optional calories
AHA Recommendation	**70**	**100**	

Another way of grouping fat sources from highest to lowest content of calories from fat is as follow: salad oils and spreads (100%), avocados, bacon, bologna, and nuts (about 80%), cheddar cheese and peanut butter (about 75%), hamburgers and steak (about 60%), chocolate bars, doughnuts, ice cream, and whole milk (50%), eggs, pancakes, lean cuts of meat, and pumpkin pie (35%), and bread (15%). Even though salad oils have higher fat content than cheese, it is recommended to be careful with the consumption of cheese based on the amount consumed and the type of fat.

3.3.4. Essential Fatty Acids

Humans and other mammals have a nutritional requirement of certain essential fatty acids, because they cannot be synthesized from simple precursors in the diet (Fig. **18**) (Kris-Etherton and Hill, 2008; Wang *et al.*, 2006). The body must obtain linoleic acid and alpha-linolenic acid from foods to preserve health, so they are called *essential* fatty acids. The recommended intake per day of omega-3 fatty acids (alpha-linoleic acid) is 1.6 g for men and 1.1 g for women and of omega-6 fatty acids is 17 g for men and 12 g for women. These fatty acids are categorized as 18-carbon polyunsaturated fatty acids that differ in the number and position of the double bonds. The position of the double bonds determines the type of essential fatty acid (omega-3, -6, and -9) (Kris-Etherton and Hill, 2008; Wang *et al*., 2006; Wardlaw and Smith, 2011).

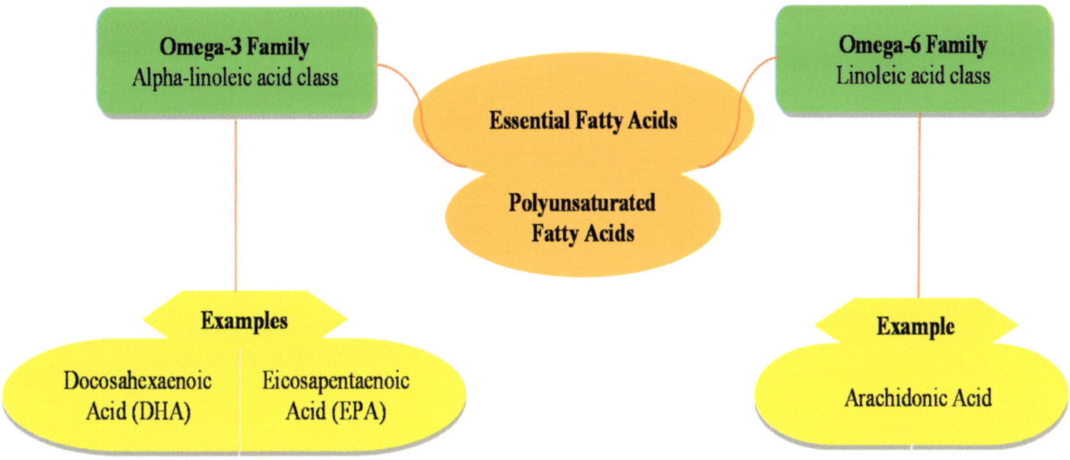

Fig. (18). Essential fatty acids.

These essential fatty acids participates in parts of vital body structures, carry out significant roles in immune system function and vision, aid to form cell membranes, and participates in the production of hormone-like compounds (Kris-Etherton and Hill, 2008). They are also involved in inflammation such as arachidonic acid. Omega-6 and omega-3 fatty acids must be obtained through the diet because human cells lack the enzymes needed to produce these fatty acids. The body can synthesize other fatty acids, such as omega-9 fatty acids, and therefore they are not essential components of the diet. Most vegetable oils contain high amount of linoleic acid (safflower, sunflower, and corn oils). Green leaves of plants, selected seeds, nuts and legumes (particularly flax, rapeseed, walnut and soy) contain alpha-linolenic acid. Fish oils (Table **4**) are predominantly rich in the longer-chain omega-3 fatty acids such as eicosapentaenoic acid (EPA) and docosahexaenoic acid (DHA) (He and Daviglus, 2005; Micallef and Garg, 2008).

Benefits of having adequate intake of essential fatty acids include: 1) products containing omega-3 decrease blood clotting, have a favorable effect on heart rhythm, and decrease inflammatory processes, 2) large amounts of omega-3 from fish (2-4 d/day) lower triglycerides, 3) ingestion of fish (240 g) twice a week lowers risk of heart attack, 3) consumption of baked fish is recommended since fried fish decreases the ratio of omega-3 and -6, may produce *trans* fatty acids, and oxidize lipid products (increase cardiovascular disease risk) (Kris-Etherton and Hill, 2008; Kuller, 2006).

Table 4. Essential fatty acids (Omega-3) in fish content. (USDA, 2016).

Omega-3	DHA (g) 20:6	EPA (g) 20:5
Atlantic Salmon	0.4	0.1
Anchovy	0.3	0.2
Bluefish	0.2	0.1
Catfish, channel	0.04	0.03
Coho salmon	0.3	0.1
Halibut	0.1	0.2
Rainbow trout	0.2	0.06
Sardines in sauce	0.3	0.2
Striped bass	0.2	0.05
Tuna, white, canned	0.2	0.07

*Grams per ounce of serving. **Recommended intake per day 1.6 g for men and 1.1 g for women of Omega-3.

3.3.5. Diets and Sources of Lipids

In North America, the typical diet contains about 33% of calories from total fat, 13% from saturated fat, and between 180 and 320 mg per day of cholesterol. The major source of the fat content in North American diet includes animal sources, whole milk, pastries, cheese, margarine, and mayonnaise. Other diets with lower rates of chronic diseases such as the Mediterranean diet includes large amounts of olive oil instead of small amount of animal fat (animal flesh and dairy products). To help follow dietary guidelines come lipids sources have been recommended for increased intake *versus* other lipids sources (Table **5**) (Micallef and Garg, 2008; Wardlaw and Smith, 2011).

Plant oils supply most of the essential oils in this diet. Other lipid sources such as phospholipids include wheat germ, peanuts, egg yolk, soy beans, and organ meats. Phospholipids as lecithin found in egg yolk are added to salad dressing as an emulsifier to keep vegetable oil suspended in water (Micallef and Garg, 2008).

3.3.5.1. Warning

Fats rich in saturated fatty acids are usually solid at room temperature (Table **6**). Unsaturated fatty acids are found as liquids at room temperature. A large number of studies on dietary intake of omega-3 fatty acids (unsaturated fatty acids) have shown positive health benefits associated with cancer, cardiovascular diseases, infant development, and various mental disorders, such as attention-deficit hyperactivity disorder, dementia, and depression. In contrast, the consumption of *trans* fats is considered a risk factor for cardiovascular disease. *Trans* fats can be formed during food processing and can be found in partially hydrogenated vegetable oils. Since it

Table 5. Lipids in diet. (Health.gov, 2016).

Recommend:	reduce intake*	increase intake
Dairy	• Butter • Ice cream • Fat-rich cheese • Whole milk	• Fat-free and low-fat milk • Low-fat frozen desserts (e.g., yogurt) • Low-fat/part-skim cheese
Fruits	• Fruit pies • Fruit marmalades	• Fresh or frozen fruits
Grains	• Bakery goods • Pasta dishes with cheese or cream sauces	• Brown rice • Dry beans, peas or lentils • Whole-grain breads • Whole grain crackers • Whole-grain pasta
Lipids	• Lard/solid fats • Hard margarine • Shortenings	• Vegetable oils • At the table - margarine (in small amounts)
Protein	• Bacon • Egg yolks • Organ meats (e.g., liver) • Sausage	• Egg whites/egg substitutes • Baked fish/shellfish • Lean meat/poultry (with fat trimmed away) • Soy products
Vegetables	• Fries • Potato chips • Fried or cooked in butter or oily dairy	• Fresh, frozen, steamed vegetables

*Products high in fat content

seems structurally similar to saturated fats (straight chain), it is also suggested to limit its intake. A few studies have suggested that high total dairy fat intake is also associated to an increased risk of obesity and diabetes. Additional issues with the consumption of lipids include: 1) high consumption of omega-6 and saturated fatty acids increases clotting and inflammation risks, 2) fish oil should be limited in individual with bleeding disorders and those taking anticoagulants, and 3) lack of enough consumption is correlated to flaky and itchy skin as well as restriction in growth and wound healing (Getz, 2009; Hansson, 2005).

Table 6. Health effects of lipids, sources, and state. (Wahrburg, 2004).

Fat Acid Type - Health Impact	Sources	Physical State*
Saturated – Negative Impact		
Significantly increase cholesterol Long chain C12-C16 Does not cause significant increase Medium and short chain (C4-C10)	 Animal fat (beef, pork, and lamb) Plant oils (coconut, palm, and palm kernel), and milk fat (butter)	 Solid Soft or liquid
Monounsaturated – Positive Impact		
Decrease blood levels of cholesterol	Plant oils (olive, canola, peanut)	Liquid
Polyunsaturated Fatty Acids		
Decrease blood cholesterol levels	Corn oil, fish oil, safflower oil, and sunflower oil	Liquid
Essential – Protective Effects		
Omega 3: alpha-linolenic acid class Reduces inflammation responses, blood clotting, and plasma triglycerides Omega 6: linoleic acid class Regulates blood pressure and increases blood clotting	Canola oil, fish (salmon, tuna, sardines, mackerel), flax seed, hemp oil, soybean oil, walnuts Beef, poultry, safflower oil, sunflower oil, corn oil	Liquid Solid to liquid
Trans		
Increase LDL and lower HDL	Hardened fats: Pastries, chips, fried and convenience foods	Soft to very solid

*Physical state at room temperature

It is also important to be careful with hidden fat in dietary products. Some examples of products containing hidden fat include: whole milk, pastries, cookies, cakes, hotdogs, crackers, French fries, and ice cream (Getz, 2009).

It is also important to understand the difference in meaning of terms used in Nutrition. For instance, the use of low-fat by North Americans refer to reduced fat versions of pastries, cookies, and cakes while the use of the same term by health professionals in low-fat diets refer to fruit, vegetables, whole grain, bread, and cereals (Wardlaw and Smith, 2011).

3.3.6. Lipid Metabolism

The process of lipid metabolism generates, modifies, and degrades the lipid storage to produce the structural and functional lipids characteristic of individual tissues. The excess CHO from over consumption of dietary CHO is converted to a type of lipid such as triacylglycerol type. This involves a process called lipogenesis; comprising the synthesis of fatty acids from acetyl-CoA and the esterification of fatty acids in the production of triacylglycerol. Fatty acid synthases polymerize and then reduce acetyl-CoA units during the catalysis in the production of fatty acids. Extension of the acyl chains in the fatty acids occurs by a cycle of enzyme reactions that add acetyl groups, reduce them to alcohol groups, dehydrate them to alkene groups and then reduce them again to an alkane groups. The fatty acids may be next converted to triacylglycerols that are bundled in lipoproteins and later secreted from the liver (Wardlaw and Smith, 2011)

In the synthesis of unsaturated fatty acids the introduction of a double bond in the fatty acyl chain includes a desaturation reaction. For instance, the unsaturation of stearic acid by stearoyl-CoA desaturase-1 produces oleic acid in humans. The doubly and triply unsaturated fatty acids, linoleic and linolenic acid, cannot be synthesized in mammalian tissues, and must, therefore, be obtained from the diet (Wardlaw and Smith, 2011)

The synthesis of triacylglycerol occurs in the endoplasmic reticulum. Acyl groups in fatty acyl-CoAs are transferred to the hydroxyl groups of glycerol-3-phosphate and diacylglycerol as part of the metabolic pathways used in the biosynthesis (Wardlaw and Smith, 2011).

Isoprenoids, such as terpenes including the carotenoids, are made from isoprene units donated from the reactive precursors IPP and DMAPP that can be utilized in different ways. The process involves the assembly and modification of the isoprene units. The precursors use pyruvate and glyceraldehyde 3-phosphate as substrates. One important biosynthetic pathway that uses these activated isoprene units as contributors is the steroid biosynthesis. Here, the isoprene contributors are arranged to form squalene and then folded up and cyclized to obtain lanosterol. Lanosterol can then be transformed to other steroidal analogs such as cholesterol and ergosterol (Lemke and Williams, 2008; Wardlaw and Smith, 2011).

Beta oxidation is the metabolic process by which fatty acids generate acetyl-CoA after they are broken down in the mitochondria and/or in peroxisomes. For the most part, the mechanism of oxidation of fatty acids is similar to, but not identical to the reversal route of fatty acid synthesis. Fragments of two-carbons are detached consecutively from the carboxyl end of the acid after steps of dehydrogenation, hydration, and oxidation to form a beta-keto acid, which is fragmented by thiolysis. The acetyl-CoA is eventually converted into ATP, CO_2, and H_2O through the citric acid cycle and the electron transport chain. For instance, the complete oxidation of the fatty acid palmitate yields 106 ATP.

Unsaturated and odd-chain fatty acids may involve supplementary enzymatic steps for degradation (Wardlaw and Smith, 2011).

3.3.7. Digestion and Absorption

Most dietary fats are not soluble in water; hence, they are not easily broken down by fat-digesting enzymes (lipase) found in the watery content of the gastrointestinal tract (Fig. **19**). Thus, fats have a tendency to take longer to be digested and absorbed than CHOs or proteins. As a result, the small amount of enzyme lipase secreted by Ebner's glands on the tongue and by the stomach have not significant digestive actions on these dietary fats. Therefore, the real breakdown of fat occurs when the fats reach the duodenum in the form of gastric chyme (Wardlaw and Smith, 2011).

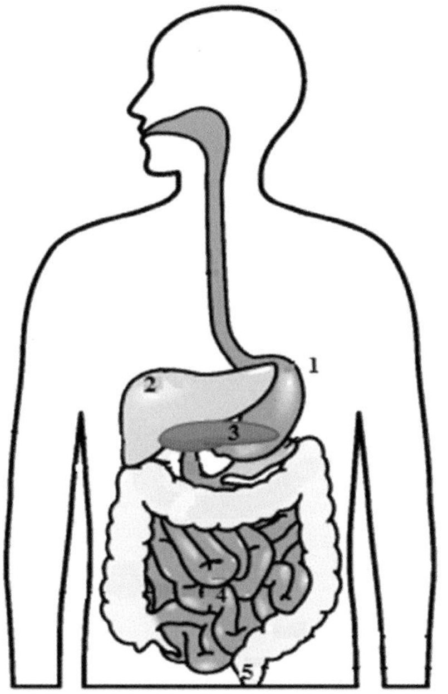

1. Stomach : minor digestion of fat occur in the stomach by the action of lipase enzymes
2. Liver: bile from liver emulsify lipids in digestive juices for fat digestion and absorption
3. Pancreas : secrets enzymes (e.g., lipase) into the small intestine
4. Small intestine: primary site for digestion and absorption of lipids (long-chain fatty acids are transported through the lymph and bloodstream while short-chain are absorbed directly into portal circulation)
5. Large intestine: small amount (<5%) of ingested fat is excreted in feces

Fig. (19). Absorption and digestion of lipids scheme.

Fat digestion and absorption convert complex fat molecules into smaller molecules. Pancreas is the main source of enzymes for fats and proteins digestion. The digestive enzyme lipase that enters the duodenum from the pancreas mixes with the fats and breaks down lipid molecules into both fatty acid molecules and glycerol molecules. Lipase is miscible in water and can only interact with the polar part of the fat molecules. Fat molecules are not soluble in water and enter the duodenum in a gelatinous mass, making it challenging for the pancreatic lipase enzymes to break down the fat molecules. The digestive system also utilizes in this process a substance called bile, produced in the liver but stored in the gallbladder that enters the duodenum *via* the bile duct. Bile emulsifies fats to allow lipase improve access to fat molecules, accelerating breakdown and digestion (Wardlaw and Smith, 2011).

In the human body, absorption of fat takes between 10 and 15 minutes. The process occurs on the finger-like projections that cover the small intestine walls, named the villi. Each villus comprises a series of lymph vessels (lacteals) and blood vessels (capillaries). The lacteals drive the fatty acids and glycerol into the lymphatic system from where they are transferred into the bloodstream. The fatty acids that are stored or oxidized for energy, are first transported *via* the bloodstream to the membranes of adipose or muscle cells. Even though glucose is the body ideal source of energy, only about 5 percent of absorbed fat can be transformed into glucose. An important portion of the digested fat is usually stored in the adipose cells as body fat. The glycerol portion of the fatty acid is either converted into glucose (gluconeogenesis) or used to help breakdown glucose into energy (glycolysis) after it is absorbed by the liver (Wardlaw and Smith, 2011).

3.3.8. Food Label

Nutrition labels are key in finding the presence of hidden fat in dietary products (Fig. **20**). On labels, high fat products are listed first. Low-fat products contain less than three grams of fat per serving. Fat free products contain less than 0.5 grams of fat per serving. Reduced fat products contain at least 25% less fat than usually found in the same type of product. Hence, information found in nutrition labels can help on daily food choices.

Nutrition Facts **Label A**

Serving Size	1 cup (55g/2.0 oz.)
Servings Per Container	10

Amount Per Serving	Cereal	Cereal with Vz Cup Vitamins A & D Skim Milk
Calories	170	210
Calories from Fat	10	10
	% Daily Value**	
Total Fat 1.0 g*	**2%**	**2%**
Sat. Fat 0g	**0%**	**0%**
Trans Fat 0g	*	
Cholesterol 0mg	**0%**	**0%**
Sodium 300mg	**13%**	**15%**
Potassium 340mg	**10%**	**16%**
Total		
Carbohydrate 43g	**14%**	**16%**
Dietary Fiber 7g	**28%**	**28%**
Sugars 16g		
Other Carbohydrate 20g		
Protein 4g		
Vitamin A	15%	20%
Vitamin C	20%	22%
Calcium	2%	15%
Iron	65%	65%

"Amount in cereal. One half cup skim milk contributes an additional 40 calories, 65mg sodium, 6g total carbohydrate (6g sugars), and 1g protein.
""Percent Daily Values are based on a 2,000 calorie diet. Your daily values may be higher or lower depending on your calorie needs:

		Calories:	2,000	2,500
Total Fat	Less than		65g	80g
Sat Fat	Less than		20g	25g
Cholesterol	Less than		300mg	300mg
Sodium	Less than		2,400mg	2,400mg
Potassium			3,500mg	3,500mg
Total Carbohydrate			300g	375g
Dietary Fiber			25g	30g

Calories per gram: Fat 9 • Carbohydrate 4 • Protein 4

"Intake of trans fat should be as low as possible.

Ingredients: Wheat bran with other parts of wheat, raisins, sugar, corn syrup, salt, malt flavoring, glycerin, iron, niacinamide, zinc oxide, pyridoxine hydrochloride (vitamin B_6), riboflavin (vitamin B_2), vitamin A palmitate, thiamin hydrochloride (vitamin B_1), folic acid, vitamin B_{12}, and vitamin D.

Nutrition Facts **Label B**

Serving Size	3/4cup (30g)
Servings Per Container	About 17

Amount Per Serving	Cereal	Cereal With72 cups skim milk
Calories	170	210
Calories from Fat	0	5
	%Daily Value**	
Total Fat 0g*	**0%**	**1%**
Saturated Fat 0g	**0%**	**1%**
Trans Fat 0g	*	
Cholesterol 0mg	**0%**	**1%**
Sodium 60mg	**2%**	**4%**
Potassium 80mg	**2%**	**8%**
Total Carbohydrate 35g	**9%**	**11%**
Dietary Fiber 1 g	**4%**	**4%**
Sugars 20g		
Other Carbohydrate 13g		
Protein 3g		
Vitamin A	25%	30%
Vitamin C	0%	2%
Calcium	0%	15%
Iron	10%	10%

"Amount in cereal. One half cup skim milk contributes an additional 40 calories, 65mg sodium, 6g total Carbohydrate (6g sugars), and 1g protein.

""Percent Daily Values are based on a 2,000 calorie diet. Your daily values may be higher or lower depending on your calorie needs:

		Calories:	2,000	2,500
Total Fat	Less than		65g	80g
Sat Fat	Less than		20g	25g
Cholesterol	Less than		300mg	300mg
Sodium	Less than		2,400mg	2,400mg
Potassium			3,500mg	3,500mg
Total Carbohydrate			300g	375g
Dietary Fiber			25g	30g

Calories per gram: Fat 9 • Carbohydrate 4 • Protein 4

"Intake of trans fat should be as low as possible.

Ingredients: Wheat, Sugar, Corn Syrup, Honey, Caramel Color, Partially Hydrogenated Soybean Oil, Salt, Ferric Phosphate, Niacinamide (Niacin), Zinc Oxide, Vitamin A (Palmitate), Pyridoxine Hydrochloride (Vitamin B_6), Riboflavin, Thiamin Mononitrate, Folic Acid (Folate),Vitamin B12 and Vitamin D.

Fig. (20). Improvised labels A and B.

CONCLUDING REMARKS

The human body requires a balanced nutrition to function properly. A balanced diet is composed by multiple components that include macronutrients and micronutrients. This chapter have discussed the three major classes of macronutrients that the body needs as part of a balanced diet, including carbohydrates, proteins, and lipids. The chapter also discussed the sources of these nutrients and how these nutrients can be absorbed and metabolized by the human body. In summary, this chapter presented elements that are essential in understanding the importance of macronutrients in a balanced diet to have an adequate nutrition for the proper function of a healthy human body.

CONFLICT OF INTEREST

The authors confirm that this chapter contents have no conflict of interest.

ACKNOWLEDGMENTS

The author would like to thank you Michelle OgavaIgual for preparing some figures and tables. The authors are also thankful to Roshamur C. Forestrania for formatting some references.

REFERENCES

American Dietetic Association. (2003). Position of the American Dietetic Association and Dietitians of Canada. Vegetarian diets. Journal of American Dietetic Association, 103: 748-65.

American Dietetic Association. (2004). Position of the American Dietetic Association: use of nutritive and nonnutritive sweeteners. Journal of American Dietetic Association, 104: 255-75.

American Dietetic Association. (2005). Position of the American Dietetic association: fat replacers. Journal of American Dietetic Association, 105: 266-75.

Aronson, D. (2005). Vegetarian Nutrition. *Today's Dietitian*, 7: 3.

Horn, R. S. (2014). What is so special about carbohydrates? Available at: http://www.medbio.info/ (Accessed: 2.26.2015).

Chao, A., Thun, M. J., Connell, C. J., McCullough, M. L., Jacobs, E. J., Flanders, W. D., Rodriguez, C., Sinha, R. & Calle, E. E. (2005). Meat consumption and risk of colorectal cancer. JAMA, 293: 172-82.

Consumer Report. (2005). Sweeteners can sour your health: *Consumer Reports on Health*, 17: 8.

Dewick, P. M. (2009). *Medicinal Natural Products: A Biosynthetic Approach*. 3rd ed. University of Nottingham, UK: John Wiley & Sons, Ltd..

Photosynthesis. (2014) *American Heritage® Dictionary of the English Language*. 5th ed. Huntington Valley, PA: Farlex, Inc.

FDA. (2006). Artificial sweeteners: no calories...sweet!. *FDA Consumer Magazine*. 40 (4): 27-28.

Food and Nutrition Board, I. O. M. (2005). *Dietary Reference intakes for energy, carbohydrate, fiber, fat, fatty acids, cholesterol, protein, and amino acids*. Washington, DC: National Academies Press.

Getz, L. (2009). A Burger and Fries (Hold the Trans Fats). Today's Dietitian, 11: 36.

Graham Solomons, T. W., C. B. Fryhle, & Snyder, S. A. (2013). *Organic Chemistry*. 11th ed. Hoboken, NJ: John Wiley and Sons, Inc.

Hansson, G. K. (2005). Inflammation, atherosclerosis, and coronary artery disease. The New England Journal of Medicine, 352: 1685-1695.

He, K. & Daviglus, M. L. (2005). A few more thoughts about fish and fish oil. Journal of American Dietetic Association, 105: 350-351.

Health.gov (2016). Choose sensibly. Available at: http://health.gov/dietaryguidelines/dga2000/document/choose.htm (accessed 02.19.2016).

Key, T. J., Appleby, P. N. & Rosell, M. S. (2006). Health effects of vegetarian and vegan diets. Proceedings of the Nutrition Society, 65: 35-41.

Kris-Etherton, P. M. & Hill, A. M. (2008). n-3 fatty acids: Food or supplements?. Journal of the American Dietetic Association, 108: 1125-1130.

Kuller, L. H. (2006). Nutrition, lipids, and cardiovascular disease. Nutrition Reviews, 64: S15-26.

Lau, V. W., Journoud, M. & Jones, P. J. (2005). Plant sterols are efficacious in lowering plasma LDL and non-HDL cholesterol in hypercholesterolemic type 2 diabetic and nondiabetic persons. American Journal of Clinical Nutrition, 81: 1351-8.

Lemke, T. L. & Williams, D. A. (2008). Foye's Principles of Medicinal Chemistry. 6th ed.: Baltimore, MD, Lippincott Williams & Wilkins, a Wolters Kluwer business.

Lichtenstein, A. H., Appel, L. J., Brands, M., Carnethon, M., Daniels, S., Franch, H. A., Franklin, B., Kris-Etherton, P., Harris, W. S., Howard, B., Karanja, N., Lefevre, M., Rudel, L., Sacks, F., Van Horn, L., Winston, M., Wylie-Rosett, J., & A. H. A. N. Committee. 2006, Diet and lifestyle recommendations revision 2006: a scientific statement from the American Heart Association Nutrition Committee. Circulation, 114: 82-96.

Micallef, M. A. & Garg, M. L. (2008) The lipid-lowering effects of phytosterols and (n-3) polyunsaturated fatty acids are synergistic and complementary in hyperlipidemic men and women. Journal of Nutrition, 138:. 1086-90.

Morrison, R. T., and R. N. Boyd. (1987). Química Orgánica. 5th ed. Boston, M. A., Addison-Wesley Iberoamericana.

Sabate, J. (2003). The contribution of vegetarian diets to human health. Forum of nutrition, 56: 218-20.

Slavin, J., Klosterbuer, A. & Willis, H. (2008) How fiber affects weight regulation. Food Technology, p. 34-41.

Swann, L. (2006) Educate your brain about whole grain. Today's Dietitian, 8: 36.

The Vegetarian Resource Group. (2008). Who's the Veggie-Friendliest of Them All?. Vegetarian Journal, 27: 14.

Trumbo, P., Schlicker, S., Yates, A. A. & Poos, M. (2002) Dietary reference intakes for energy, carbohydrate, fiber, fat, fatty acids, cholesterol, protein and amino acids. Journal of the American Dietetic Association, 102: 1621-1630.

USDA (2016). National Nutrient Database for Standard Reference. Available at: HYPERLINK "http://ndb.nal.usda.gov/ndb/search/list?qlookup=11674" http://HYPERLINK "http://ndb.nal.usda.gov/ndb/search/list?qlookup=11674" ndb.nal.usda.gov/ndb/search/list?qlookup=11674, 14400, 09040, 20445, 01256, 16027, HYPERLINK "http://ndb.nal.usda.gov/ndb/search/list?qlookup=15118" 15118, 01256, 20314, 18075, 09040, HYPERLINK "http://ndb.nal.usda.gov/ndb/search/list?qlookup=13473" 13473, 04582, 09037, 01009, 18229 , 19141 (accessed 02.02.2016).

USDA (2016). National Nutrient Database for Standard Reference. Available at: http://ndb.nal.usda.gov/ndb/nutrients/report/nutrientsfrm?max=25&offset=0&totCount=0&nutrient1=621&nutrient2=629&nutrient3=204&subset=0&fg=15&sort=c&measureby=m 15209, 15239, 15189, 15126, 15240, 15004, 15038, 15233, 15089, 15001 (accessed 02.02.2016).

Wang, C., Harris, W. S., Chung, M., Lichtenstein, A. H., Balk, E. M., Kupelnick, B., Jordan, H. S. & Lau, J. (2006). n-3 fatty acids from fish or fish-oil supplements, but not alpha-linolenic acid, benefit cardiovascular disease outcomes in primary- and secondary-prevention studies: a systematic review. American Journal of Clinical Nutrition, 84: 5-17.

Wahrburg, U. (2004). What are the health effects of fat? *European Journal of Nutrition*, 43(1S): 6-11.

Wardlaw, G. M., and A. M. Smith. (2008). Contemporary Nutrition. 5th ed. New York, N. Y., McGraw Hill. Higher Education.

Wardlaw, G. M., and A. M. Smith. (2011). Contemporary Nutrition. 8th ed. New York, N. Y., McGraw Hill, Inc. Learning Solutions.

Warshaw, H. S. (2004). FAQs about Polyols. *Today's Dietitian*, 6:36-44.

WebWatch. (2008). Healthy Vegetarian Resources and Recipes. *Obesity Management*, 4(4): 209-212.

Xiao, C. W. (2008). Health effects of soy protein and isoflavones in humans. J ournal of Nutrition, 138:1244S-9S.

CHAPTER 4

Macronutrients Nutritional Requirement Applications

Esperanza J. Carcache de Blanco* **and Jay Mirtallo***

College of Pharmacy, The Ohio State University, Columbus, Ohio, USA

Abstract: Macronutrients are important components of human diet. The three most important macronutrients include carbohydrates, lipids, and proteins. Adequate consumption of the three major macronutrients has been associated with a good diet and good health. Analysis on the use of these macronutrients as part of the diet and the application of the concepts learned in chapter 3 will be presented in this chapter.

Keywords: AHA, breakfast, calories, carbohydrates, dinner, kilocalories, lipids, lunch, proteins, RDA.

INTRODUCTION

The aim of this chapter is to apply concepts learned in Chapter 3 regarding macronutrients such as CHOs, proteins, and lipids. For the purpose of performing calculations, Calories and kilocalories will be considered the same.

MACRONUTRIENT OVERVIEW

When provided in a diet, assessment of the macronutrient amount as it relates to the RDA and Healthy Diet Recommendations is a frequent function health care practitioners perform. Tables **1** and **2** below provide a summary of healthy recommendations for CHO, protein, and fat in the diet.

Table 1. Recommended Daily Allowances (RDA) for Carbohydrate and Protein.

Nutrient	Grams per day*	% Total Calories	Calorie Per Gram
Carbohydrate	130 180-330	45-65 60	4
Protein	0.8 per kg 50-80	10	4

*Based on 1200-2200 Calorie diet and body weight range from 62.5-100 kg.

***Corresponding authors Esperanza J. Carcache de Blanco and Jay Mirtallo:** College of Pharmacy, The Ohio State University, Columbus, OH 43210, USA; E-mails: carcache-de-blan.1@osu.edu; mirtallo.1@osu.edu

Table 2. Healthy Diet Recommendations for Lipids.

Nutrient	Grams per day	% Total Calories	Calorie Per Gram
Lipid, Total	44-78*	20-35	9
Saturated Fat	15.5	<7	
Trans Fat		<1	
Essential Fatty acids		5	
Maximum cholesterol	0.3		

*Based on a 2000 Calorie/day diet.

- The human body requires a constant source of energy (termed Calories in the U.S.) to maintain homeostasis

- When an imbalance in energy and protein occur, an increase or decrease in weight may result in changes in lean body mass and the health of an individual.

Label Overview

Based on the information in the labels below (Fig. **1**), respond to the following:

a. Mark the label that is used for food with a (F).

b. Mark the label used for dietary supplements with (DS).

c. Mention three different types of information found in each type of label.

d. What information makes these two types of labels different?

4.1. Carbohydrates

Carbohydrate Overview

- CHOs are primarily molecules of sugar.

- CHOs are the main fuel source of brain, nervous system, and red blood cells.

- CHOs provide an average of 4 kcal per gram.

- CHOs are readily available fuel in the form of blood glucose and glycogen stored in liver and muscles.

- Liver glycogen storage depletes in 18 hours if no carbohydrate is consumed.

- Recommendation: 45-65 % of calories from carbohydrates.

- Some types of CHOs promote health more than others.

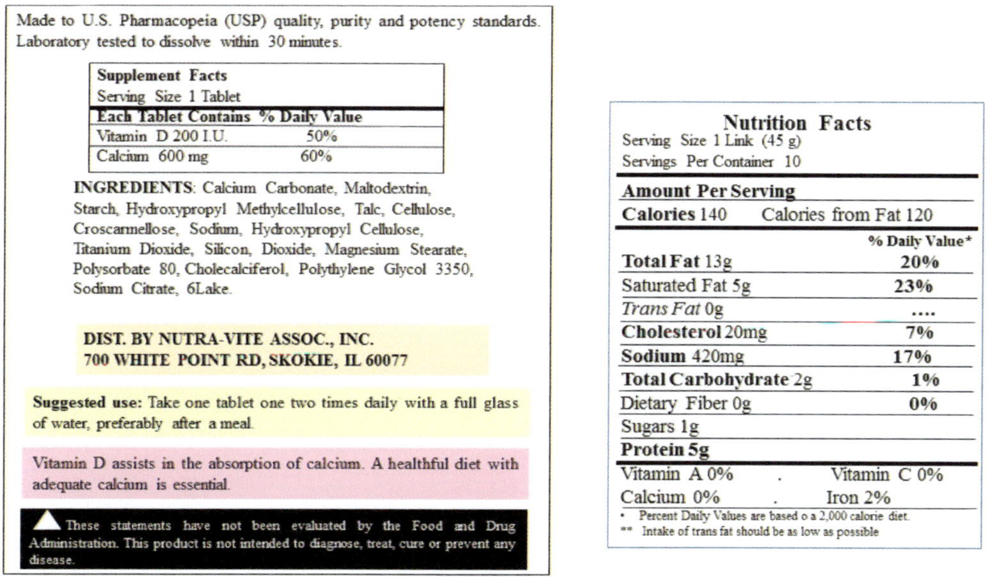

Fig. (1). Labels used in food and dietary supplements. Information on the label may not be accurate; it is used for practice purposes only.

Practice Session I

1. Nutrition label information.

Information provided in a food label states cereal serving size ¾ cup (30 g) and 17 servings per package. Total CHOs/serving 35 g, dietary fiber 1 g, sugar 20 g, other CHOs 13 g. Determine the following:

a. Number of calories from CHOs/serving.

b. Number of calories from CHOs/package.

c. Calculate the percentage of calories from CHOs in one serving *versus* the entire package.

d. Calculate the percentage of CHOs in one serving to the RDA in adults.

2. Look at Table **3** listing calories in common foods.

Table 3. Calories of common foods.

Food	Size	Calories**	Food	Size	Calories**
Apple	1 small (4 oz.)	80	Hamburger	1 (McDonald medium)	280
Asparagus	1 cup, boiled	36	Lettuce	1 cup	7
Banana	1 medium (5-6 oz.)	84-101	Mango	1 (8-9 oz.)	135-150
Bean curd	4 oz.	81	Milk, low-fat (1%)	1 cup	104
Beef, regular, cooked	1 slice (2 oz.)	120	Milk, low-fat (2%)	1 cup	121
Beer, regular	1 can or bottle	150	Milk, whole	1 cup	150
Bread, regular	1 slice (1 oz.)	75	Orange	1 (4-5 oz.)	71-88
Broccoli	1 cup	40	Orange Juice / Apple Cider	1 cup	115
Butter	1 tea spoon	100	Peach	1 (6 oz.)	38
Caesar salad	1 serving (3 cups)	360	Pear	1 (5 oz.)	100
Carrots	1 cup	45	Pineapple	1 cup	80
Cheeseburger	1 (McDonald medium)	360	Pizza	1 slice	180
Chicken, cooked	1 slice (2 oz.)	95	Pork, cooked	1 slice (2 oz.)	130
Chocolate	1 oz.	150	Potato (uncooked)	1 oz.	120
Coca-Cola Classic	1 cup	97	Rice, cooked	1 cup	225
Corn	1 cup, cooked	140	Sandwich	1 (6" Subway)	310
Cucumber	each	30-35	Shrimp, cooked	2 oz.	70
Diet Coke	1 cup	3	Strawberry	1 cup	53
Egg	large	79	Tomato	1 cup	29
Eggplant	1 cup, boiled	38	Watermelon	1 cup	45
Fish, Catfish, cooked	2 oz.	80	Yogurt, low-fat	1 cup	200
Grape	each	2	Yogurt, non-fat	1 cup	150

* 1 cup = ~250 milliliters, 1 teaspoon = ~5 milliliters, 1 ounce = ~28.35 grams; ** Values in this table may not be accurate; they are used for practice purposes only.

Complete the following:

a. Calories per gram of peaches, apples, and mangoes (use the table and the unit conversion provided).

b. Make the selection of your choice and explain briefly the reason of your choice.

3. The Basics of Pharmaconutrition profile states that its total calories requirement per day is 1800 kcal. Using the table listing calories in common foods, design a recipe that will cover the RDA of CHOs/day (CHO intake ranges from 45 to 65% of total calorie intake) distributed between breakfast, lunch, and dinner. Make smart choices such as including items rich in complex carbohydrates and fiber.

4.2. Proteins

Protein Overview

- Proteins are primarily molecules of C, H, N, and O.
- Limiting amino acids determine protein synthesis.
- Proteins are grouped as complete, incomplete, and complementary proteins.
- Recommendation: 0.8g/kg weight (10-15 % of calories from proteins).
- Proteins provide an average of 4 kcal per gram.
- High-protein diets can be harmful to some individuals.
- Food and Nutrition Board has upper range of 35% of calories from proteins.

Practice Session II

1. Using the information found on the Nutrition label (see Fig. **2**). Determine the following:

a. Number of calories from Proteins/serving.

b. Number of calories from Proteins/package.

c. Calculate the percentage of calories from proteins in one serving *versus* the entire package.

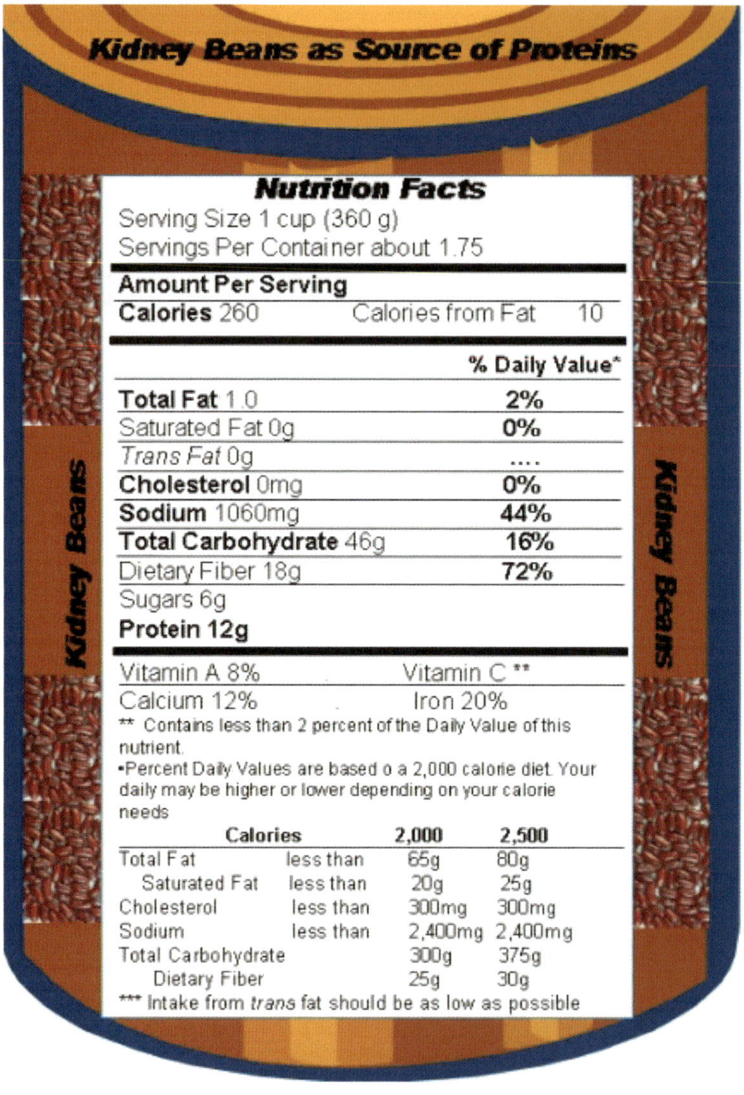

Fig. (2). Nutrition label. (The values used in this figure may not be accurate; they serve filling purposes only).

2. Look at Table **3**, listing calories in common foods. Complete the following:

a. Select three main sources of proteins for your diet.

b. Explain briefly the reason of your choice.

3. Use information from your personal profile to:

   a. Convert your personal weight from pounds to kg and *vice versa.*

   b. Calculate protein RDA.

4.3. Lipids

Lipid Overview

- Lipids are primarily molecules of C, H, and O
- Essential fatty acids are also lipids and play important roles in body function
- Some lipids are grouped in fatty acids, triglycerides, phospholipids, and sterols
- American Heart Association (AHA) recommendation: 30% of calories from fat for a 2100 kcal diet
- Lipids provide an average of 9 kcal per gram
- Essential fatty acid deficient diets can be harmful to some individuals

Practice Session III

1. Using the information found on a Nutrition label (see Fig. **3**), determine the following:

   a. Number of calories per link and % kcal from fat

   b. Number of calories per serving and % kcal from fat

   c. Number of calories from lipids per package

   d. Calculate the percentage of calories from lipids in one serving *versus* the entire package

   e. Calculate the percentage of lipids in one serving to the RDA in adults

2. Evaluate food products based on the macronutrients listed on the labels (see Fig. **4**).

Nutrition Facts	
Serving Size 1 link (45 g)	
Servings Per Container 10	
Amount Per Serving	
Calories 140	Calories from Fat 120
	% Daily Value*
Total Fat 13 g	**20%**
Saturated Fat 5 g	**23%**
Trans Fat 0 g	**
Cholesterol 20 mg	**7%**
Sodium 420 mg	**17%**
Total Carbohydrate 2 g	**1%**
Dietary Fiber 0 g	**0%**
Sugars 1 g	
Protein 5 g	
Vitamin A 0%	Vitamin C 0%
Calcium 0%	Iron 2%

* Percent Daily Values are based o a 2,000 calorie diet. Your daily may be higher or lower depending on your calorie needs

** Intake of trans fat should be as low as possible.

Ingredients

Pork, water, beef, salt, flavorings, corn syrup solids, dextrose, hydrolyzed soy and potato protein, sodium phosphates, extract of paprika, sodium erythorbate, sodium nitrite.

KEEP REFRIGERATED

Net Weight 16 OZ. (1LB) 454 g

Fig. (3). Nutrition facts label. Information on the label may not be accurate.

Label A

Nutrition Facts	
Serving Size	4 pieces (42 g)
Servings Per Container	6
Amount Per Serving 4 units	
Calories	180
Calories from Fat	50
	% Daily Value**
Total Fat 6 g	**9%**
Saturated Fat 0.5g	**3%**
Trans Fat 0g	**
Cholesterol 0mg	**0%**
Sodium 160mg	**7%**
Total Carbohydrate 29g	**10%**
Dietary Fiber 2g	**8%**
Sugars 11g	

Fig. (4). Contd.

Protein 4g		
Iron 6%		
Not a significant source of calcium, vitamin A and C.		
** Intake of *trans* fat should be as low as possible.		
**Percent Daily Values are based on a 2,000 calorie diet. Your daily values may be higher or lower depending on your calorie needs:		
Calories:	2,000	2,500
Total Fat Less than	65 g	80 g
Sat Fat Less than	20 g	25 g
Cholesterol Less than	300 mg	300 mg
Sodium Less than	2,400 mg	2,400 mg
Total Carbohydrates	300 g	375 g
Dietary Fiber	25 g	30 g

Ingredients: Wheat bran with other parts of wheat, corn syrup, folic acid, glycerin, iron, malt flavoring, niacinamide, pyridoxine hydrochloride (vitamin B6), raisins, riboflavin (vitamin B2), salt, sugar, thiamin hydrochloride (vitamin B1), vitamin A palmitate, vitamin B12, vitamin D, and zinc oxide.

Label B

Nutrition Facts		
Serving Size		4 units (38 g)
Servings Per Container		12
Amount Per Serving		
Calories		180
Calories from Fat		70
	% Daily Value**	
Total Fat 7 g		**11%**
Saturated Fat 2g		**10%**
Trans Fat 2g		**
Cholesterol 0mg		**0%**
Sodium 100mg		**4%**
Total Carbohydrate 26g		**9%**
Dietary Fiber 1g		**4%**
Sugars 12g		
Protein 2g		
Iron 2%		
-Calcium 0% -Vitamin A 0% -Vitamin C 0%		
** Intake of *trans* fat should be as low as possible.		
**Percent Daily Values are based on a 2,000 calorie diet. Your daily values may be higher or lower depending on your calorie needs:		
Calories:	2,000	2,500

Fig. (4). Contd.

Total Fat Less than	65 g	80 g
Sat Fat Less than	20 g	25 g
Cholesterol Less than	300 mg	300 mg
Sodium Less than	2,400 mg	2,400 mg
Total Carbohydrates	300 g	375 g
Dietary Fiber	25 g	30 g
Calories per gram: -Carbohydrate 4 -Fat 9 -Protein 4		

Ingredients: Wheat, Sugar, Caramel Color, Corn Syrup, Ferric Phosphate, Folic Acid (Folate), Honey, Niacinamide (Niacin), Partially Hydrogenated Soybean Oil, Pyridoxine Hydrochloride (Vitamin B6), Riboflavin, Salt, Thiamin Mononitrate, Vitamin A (Palmitate), Vitamin B12, Vitamin D, and Zinc Oxide

Fig. (4). Label examples (Label A and Label B).

Using the Labels A and B above, respond to the questions found in the box below.

i) Evaluate the products by comparing the nutrients reported in each label and complete the list below. Per serving, which label contains lower amount of the items in the list? Circle the best answer.			
Total Calories	(A)	(B)	No difference
Calories from fat	(A)	(B)	No difference
Cholesterol	(A)	(B)	No difference
Dietary Fiber	(A)	(B)	No difference
Iron	(A)	(B)	No difference
Protein	(A)	(B)	No difference
Saturated fat	(A)	(B)	No difference
Sodium	(A)	(B)	No difference
Sugars	(A)	(B)	No difference
Total Carbohydrates	(A)	(B)	No difference
Total fat	(A)	(B)	No difference
Trans Fat	(A)	(B)	No difference
ii) Which package listed more servings per container?			(A) (B) No difference
iii) Which of the two products would you choose for a balanced diet?			(A) (B) No difference
iv) What information on the labels contributed to your decision? Why? Provide an essay response.			

4.4. Dietary Assessment of Macronutrient Intake

Practice Session IV: Macronutrient Content of the Diet

A. An individual ingests 1000 calories, 60% of which are carbohydrates and 12% is protein.

Determine the amount of carbohydrate and protein that was ingested:

a. Carbohydrate grams

b. Protein grams

B. 2. An individual ingests a 750 calorie meal which contains 100 grams of Carbohydrate and 30 grams of Protein

Determine the percent of total calories provided by the meal for carbohydrate and protein

a. Carbohydrate %

b. Protein %

C. An individual ingests 1140 Calories, 44% of which is fat. Determine the amount of fat that was ingested.

a. Fat grams

D. An individual ingests a 940 Calorie meal which contains 40 Grams of fat. Determine the percent calories as fat provided by the meal.

a. Fat %

Practice Session V: Assessment of Macronutrient Daily Intake from a Diet History

A professional learns you are taking a nutrition class and expresses their interest in knowing the carbohydrate, protein and fat content of their diet. The person is a male and weighs 80 kg and is 6'0'' tall.

The nutritional intake of the individual is listed below:

Nutritional Intake

Breakfast: Low-fat Berry Smoothie and Blueberry Scone

Lunch: Garden Salad with Colonial Dressing, 1 cup of Bean soup, 2 Biscuits with margarine and Coca-Cola® with 2 refills.

Dinner: Cheese Ravioli with Marinara Sauce, 2 Breadsticks with garlic butter spread, 1 serving of Garden-Fresh Salad with dressing and Coca-Cola® with 2 refills.

Calculated Daily Nutrient Intake

1. Refer to Tables **4**, **5** and **6** for the nutritional content of the food items ingested for breakfast (Table **4**), lunch (Table **5**) and dinner (Table **6**). Determine the carbohydrate content in grams per day, CHO Calories per day and % total calories as carbohydrate. Also determine the protein intake in grams per day and grams per kg per day.

Meal	Carbohydrate Content			Protein Content	
	Grams	CHO Calories*	% Total	Grams	Grams/kg
Breakfast					
Lunch					
Dinner					
Total per Day					

*CHO = Carbohydrate.

2. Assess the daily nutritional intake as compared with normal requirements for this person's age and weight as it relates to carbohydrate intake, % of total Calories as carbohydrate and protein intake in grams per day and grams per kg per day.

	Carbohydrate Content			Protein Content	
	Grams	Calories	% Total	Grams	Grams/kg
RDA	180-330		45-65		0.8
Assessment					

3. Using the Tables **4**, **5** and **6**, identify the primary sources for simple and complex carbohydrates as well as protein ingested in the diet.

4. Refer to Tables **4**, **5** and **6** for the nutritional content of the food items ingested for breakfast (Table **4**), lunch (Table **5**) and dinner (Table **6**) to determine the content in Grams per day, Calories per day and % total Calories as fat. Also determine the type of fat; cholesterol, saturated and *trans* ingested.

Calculated Daily Nutrient Intake

Meal	Fat Content			Type of Fat Content, Grams		
	Grams	Calories	% Total	Cholesterol	Saturated Fat	Trans Fat
Breakfast						
Lunch						
Dinner						
Total per Day						

5. Assess the daily nutritional intake as compared with that recommended for a healthy diet for this person's age and weight as it relates to fat intake, % of total calories as fat and cholesterol, saturated fat and *trans* fat intake in grams per day or as percent of total calories.

	Fat Content			Type of Fat Content		
	Grams	Calories	% Total	Cholesterol	Saturated Fat	Trans Fat
Healthy Diet	44-78*		20-35	<300 mg	15.5 G or <7% of Total Calories	<1% of Total Calories
Total Daily Diet						
Assessment						

* Based on 2000 Calorie Diet.

Table 4. Nutrient Composition: Breakfast

Breakfast Item	Blueberry Scone	Low-Fat Berry Smoothie
Calories	300	365
Total Fat, g	11.2	1.7
Saturated Fat, g	2.01	1.2
Trans Fat, g	0	0
Cholesterol, mg	16	5
Sodium, mg	239	100
Total Carbohydrage, g	46	80
Dietary Fiber , g	1.3	1.9

Table 4: contd….

Sugars, g	26.4	70
Protein, g	3	5
Vitamin A , %DV	62	3
Vitamin C , %DV	3	220
Calcium, %DV	3	27
Iron, %DV	9	3
Caffeine, mg	0	0
Vitamin B_6,, %DV		180
Vitamin B_{12}, %DV		120

%DV = percent of daily value

Table 5. Nutrient Composition: Lunch

Lunch Item	**Garden Salad**	**Colonial Dressing**	**Bean Soup**	**Biscuit (each)**	**Soda**
Calories	75	245	110	240	110
Total Fat, g	5	21	2	10	0
Saturated Fat, g	3	2.5	1	6	0
Trans Fat, g	0	0	0	0	0
Cholesterol, mg	0	0	4	0	0
Sodium, mg	125	210	715	790	0
Total Carbohydrage, g	9	11	15	30	30
Dietary Fiber , g	2	0	6	1.5	0
Sugars, g	3	11	0	3	28
Protein, g	5	0	6	5	0
Vitamin A , %DV	45	0	8	5	0
Vitamin C , %DV	15	0	4	0	0
Calcium, %DV	10	0	5	8	0
Iron, %DV	4	0	12	10	0

%DV = percent of daily value

Table 6. Nutrient Composition: Dinner

Dinner Item	Garden Salad	Cheese Ravioli	Breadstick (each)	Soda
Calories	160	570	150	110
Total Fat, g	11	24	9	0
Saturated Fat, g	2	12	1	0
Trans Fat, g	0	1	0	0
Cholesterol, mg	0	5	0	0
Sodium, mg	750	750	450	0
Total Carbohydrage, g	12	12	27	30
Dietary Fiber , g	2.5	3	1	0
Protein, g	2	2.5	4	0

Practice Session VI: SuperTracker Assessment of Personal Diet

The purpose of this exercise is that you use your personal diet to practice nutritional assessment. In this way, you will be more aware of your nutritional status, and you will also know how to help a patient assess and modify his (her) diet.

The exercise will focus on the nutritional aspects of a one day food intake record and of a seven day record of snacks. You will need to calculate all nutritional values of your one day record meals including snacks to answer the questions in this section.

Diet Record and Analysis Using SuperTracker

1. Use SupperTracker from USDA (http://www.choosemyplate.gov/supertracker-tools/supertracker.html) as shown in Fig. **5**.
2. Create your profile (upper right corner of screen):
   - Personalize your profile so the caloric and nutritional goals correspond to your height, weight, and activity level.
   - Register to save your profile. The use of this USDA tool is free.
   - Submit.
3. Sign in

- Do not set goals or use My Coach Center; if you would like to continue to use this program after the project, you can set goals at that time

Food Intake Record

Use SuperTracker to track all the food and beverages you consume over 24 hours (you can choose any day for the assignment). Include all meals and snacks; be honest in recording your serving size, and don't forget to include that cookie you had with lunch. This is an informative exercise for you, so you are more aware of the quality and quantity of your personal daily consumption.

Be careful to use precise measures like cups or ounces for your food records to be able to calculate all nutritional values.

4. Type the name of the product (s), select from the list of this product options, hit go, select the time of the day meal under food details (breakfast, snack, *etc.*) and the correct unit such as ounces, cups, etc

5. Click add and do the same process for the next selection

Snacks. Next, you will need to record all snacks consumed in one week (7 days), calculate nutritional/caloric values, and the mean for one day. Add this average information to your one day record.

Activities. Also, keep a record of all activities of the same day, including a brief description and the time spent. Once you have chosen the day and kept the record, calculate the nutritional/caloric values of every one of the products you consumed. This includes caloric content determination, RDA calculation, *etc.* The data collected for your assignment will be used to analyze the Pharmaconutritional factors of your personal food intake.

6. Once you have completed including all your food items as well as your snacks and your physical activities you can start reviewing the reports generated from your personal data (Fig. **5**) and taking notes of your findings.

7. Answer the questions below using your personal data

<u>SuperTracker Questions.</u> Respond to the questions below using your recorded data and for all but question #1a, you can use a 3% limit for categorizations (for instance, you can be 3% over or under your ideal body weight and you can still say normal). For question 1b, please use only 1% limit.

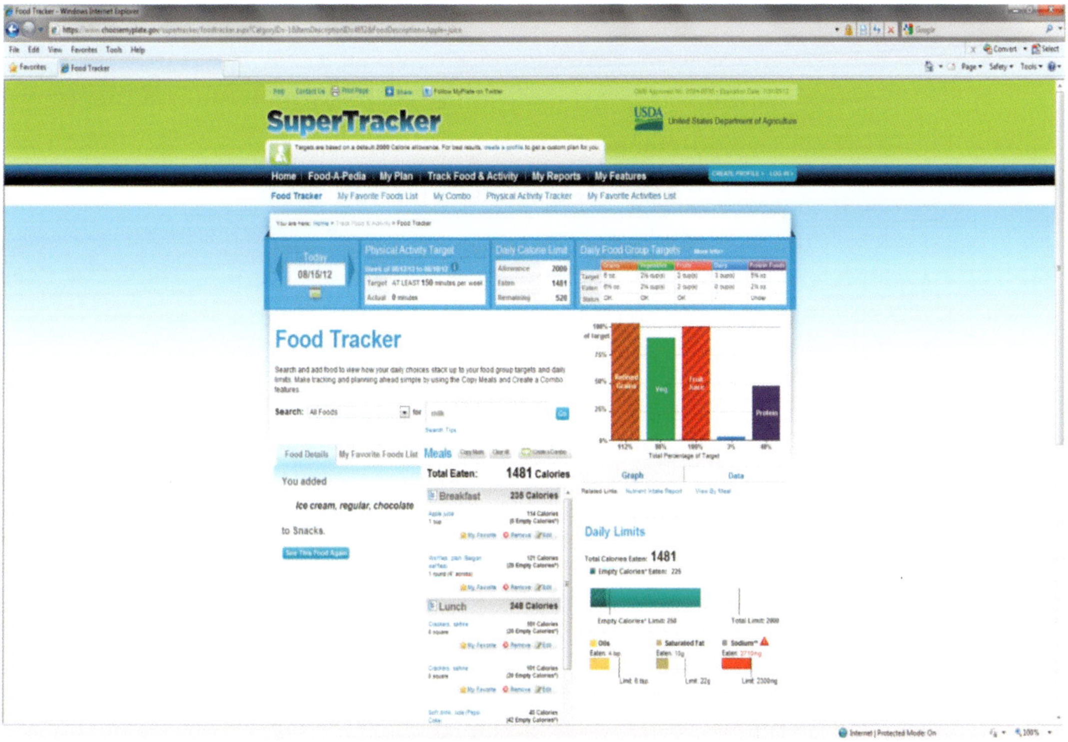

Fig. (5). Food Tracker Website from USDA.

1. Look at your report under Calorie and Fat to note how many grams of fat you ate.

   a. What % of your total calorie intake did the grams of fat you consumed represent?

   b. Now, look at the American Heart Association's Recommendation (AHA suggests 30% of Calories as fat Calories). How does your % Calories from fat compare to AHA recommendations? Please circle or underline the best answer for your case.

   * Less than Equal to Greater than

c. Is your 7-day (snack) percent Calories from fat significantly higher or lower than your 24 hour data? Does this percent exceed the AHA recommendation?

d. How might you alter your snacking habits?

2. Have you looked at your BMI? You can calculate it by clicking on "BMI calculator" found on the left column of SuperTracker. Based on your BMI, circle or underline what best describes your body weight for your height (you can look for the normal range on the box Weight Status next to your BMI).

   *Underweight Normal Overweight Obese

3. Now, look at your caloric intake.

3a. How many Calories (Kcals) did you consume on the day you recorded?

   *

3b. How many Calories did you use?

   *

3c. What would happen to your weight at this rate? (Circle or underline one)

   *Lose weight Maintain the same weight Gain weight

CONCLUDING REMARKS

This chapter has summarized and applied concepts related to macronutrients consumed as part of the diet. After completing the exercises above, the reader should have understood importance of macronutrients as part of a good diet and applied concepts to be able to design a healthy diet.

CONFLICT OF INTEREST

The authors confirm that this chapter contents have no conflict of interest.

ACKNOWLEDGEMENTS

The authors would like to thank you to Michelle OgavaIgual for preparing the graphics on Figs. **1** and **2**.

Nutrition: An Approach to Good Health and Disease Management

CHAPTER 5

Micronutrients

Roshamur C. Forestrania, Michelle OgavaIgual and Esperanza J. Carcache de Blanco*

College of Pharmacy, The Ohio State University, Columbus, Ohio, USA

Abstract: The human body is a complex system that requires multiple nutrients to function properly. Most of the micronutrient components are not energy-yielding substances and include vitamins, minerals, and water. This chapter focuses on studying the importance of these micronutrients as key components in a balanced and healthy diet. They are indispensable in good health and the human body uses them to perform its functions.

Keywords: Biotin, calcium, copper, cyanocobalamin, folate, hydrosoluble vitamins, iodide, iron, liposoluble vitamins, macrominerals, magnesium, manganese, molybdenum, niacin, pantothenic acid, potassium, riboflavin, sodium, thiamine, trace minerals, vitamin A, vitamin C, vitamin D, vitamin E, vitamin K, water, water, zinc.

INTRODUCTION

Micronutrients in diet are directly correlated to nutrition and health. The human body needs multiple nutrients and some of them are required in small quantities. These micronutrients do not provide energy, but are required in many metabolic processes (Wardlaw and Smith, 2011). The main micronutrients used by the human body include vitamins, minerals, and water. Vitamins are divided into hydro- and lipo-soluble depending on the chemical properties (Graham Solomons *et al.*, 2013, Lemke and Williams, 2008). Minerals are organized in major and trace minerals depending on the amount needed by the body (Lemke and Williams, 2008, Wardlaw and Smith, 2011). Water is classified in tap, filtered, mineral, and demineralized water (Wardlaw and Smith, 2011). The main content of this chapter will focus on the description of these micronutrients as part of nutrition and health and how the body uses them in different metabolic processes.

***Corresponding author Esperanza J. Carcache de Blanco:** College of Pharmacy, The Ohio State University, Columbus, OH 43210, USA; E-mail: carcache-de-blan.1@osu.edu

Esperanza J. Carcache de Blanco and Jay Mirtallo (Eds)

MICRONUTRIENTS

VITAMINS

Vitamins are essential organic compounds needed in the diet in small amounts for normal growth, function, and maintenance of the body. The inclusion criteria for vitamins is based on a) the body is unable to produce enough of the vitamin to preserve health, and b) lack of these products or their precursors from the diet for a defined period generates symptoms of deficiency that can be resolved if resupplied (Wardlaw and Smith, 2011, American Dietetic Association, 2005). Vitamins are divided into two main groups, liposoluble (A, D, E, and K) and hydrosoluble vitamins (B group and C) (Lemke and Williams, 2008, Graham Solomons *et al.*, 2013). Fat-soluble vitamins are not readily excreted from the body; hence, they can accumulate and cause toxic effects. Excess quantities of the hydrosoluble vitamins are excreted through the urine, requiring a constant supply of such vitamins in the diet. Vitamins do not yield energy to the body, but they are part of energy-yielding reactions (Wardlaw and Smith, 2011).

There are several factors that can destroy vitamins, including heat (cooking in water or excessive cooking) and improper storage (exposure to air, light, and pH changes). To best preserve vitamins, fruits and vegetables are often frozen directly after harvesting (Wardlaw and Smith, 2011).

RECOMMENDATIONS

The Recommended Dietary Allowance (RDA) for vitamins reflects the required daily intake of each vitamin for most individuals (Wardlaw and Smith, 2011, Association, 2005, American Dietetic Association, 2005). Hence, the following should apply.

- The RDA for vitamins should be made a goal for each person.
- Amount of vitamin each individual needs depend on age and gender.
- Other factors can affect RDA values for certain individuals, such as pregnancy, breast-feeding, and illnesses that may increase the amount needed.

LIPOSOLUBLE VITAMINS

Fat-soluble vitamins are typically deposited in the liver and fatty tissue. People with medical conditions that interfere with normal digestion or fat absorption may develop deficiencies of these vitamins (Wardlaw and Smith, 2011).

VITAMIN A

Vitamin A is a fat-soluble vitamin (Fig. **1**) (Lemke and Williams, 2008). It is essential for the proper development and functioning of eyes, immune system, skin, and many other parts of the body. Lack of enough vitamin A increases the risk of infectious diseases and vision problems such as night blindness. On the contrary, too much vitamin A can develop toxicity symptoms (Wardlaw and Smith, 2011). The RDA for vitamin A is 700-900 mcg of retinol activity equivalents (RAEs) while the daily value used in food and supplement labels is 1000 mcg (5000 UI) (Wardlaw and Smith, 2011, American Dietetic Association, 2005, Food and Nutrition Board, 2001, Food and Nutrition Board, 2000).

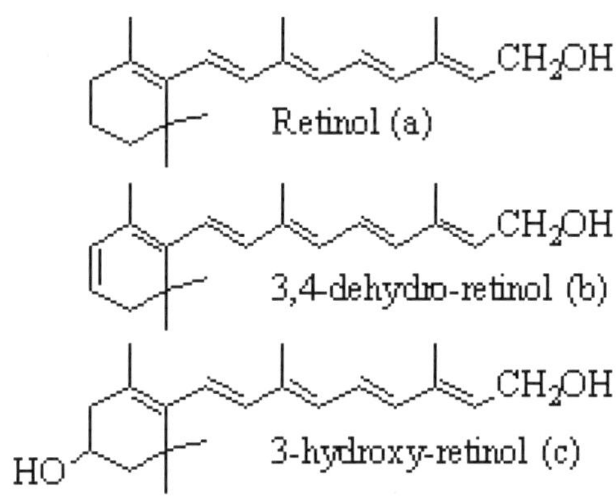

Fig. (1). Structures of (a) vitamin A_1, (b) vitamin A_2, and (c) vitamin A_3 (Graham Solomons *et al.*, 2013, Lemke and Williams, 2008).

FUNCTION

Vitamin A is known as retinol because of its relation with pigments in the retina of the eye. This vitamin aids in the development and maintenance of healthy skin, teeth, skeletal and soft tissue, mucus, and membranes. Retinol is considered an active form of vitamin A. Vitamin A plays an important role in light-dark vision. It also contributes with the production of mucus by the cells lining the cornea of the eye. Overall, vitamin A promotes good vision. Vitamin A also sustains the health of epithelial cells found in the lungs, eyes, intestines, skin, stomach, *etc.*

Moreover, vitamin A participates in growth and development. It affects gene expression by binding to receptors on DNA to increase synthesis of proteins. It may also be required for breast-feeding and reproduction. It is found in animal liver, whole milk, and some fortified foods (Lemke and Williams, 2008, Wardlaw and Smith, 2011).

Carotenoids are dark-colored dyes (pigments) found in and responsible for the color of certain plant foods that can be converted into a form of vitamin A. More than 500 known carotenoids have been reported (Lemke and Williams, 2008, Graham Solomons *et al.*, 2013). These substances have been found to play a role in the prevention of certain diseases such as cardiovascular diseases, possibly linked to their antioxidant capacity. Beta-carotene is an important carotenoid and a very potent antioxidant. Antioxidants protect cells from damage caused by substances called free radicals that are believed to contribute to the development of certain chronic diseases and that play key roles in the aging processes. Furthermore, regular consumption of carotenoids has been correlated to decreased risk of lung and oral cancers, in population studies. Research studies on dietary carotenoids, particularly on lycopene, have been found to protect against prostate cancer (Wardlaw and Smith, 2011, Voutilainen *et al.*, 2006).

FOOD SOURCES

Vitamin A can be found in animal sources, such as cheese, cream, eggs, fortified milk, kidney, liver, meat, cod, and halibut fish oil. However, most of these sources are high in saturated fat and cholesterol, except skim milk, particularly if it has been fortified with Vitamin A (Wardlaw and Smith, 2011, Lichtenstein and Russell, 2005).

Food sources of carotenoids such as beta-carotene have been associated with reduced risk of many chronic and infectious diseases. Sources of beta-carotene include:

- Bright yellow fruits such as apricots, cantaloupe, orange, and pink grapefruit.
- Vegetables such as carrots, pumpkin, sweet potatoes, and winter squash.
- Additional sources include broccoli, spinach, and most dark green, leafy vegetables.

Natural vegetable sources (unprocessed) of beta-carotene are considered as fat- and cholesterol-free. If a source (fruit or vegetable) is rich in carotenoids, the more intense the color is, the higher the beta-carotene content is. Different sources of vitamin A from four different categories (Table **1** for main sources) include Acorn squash (122 mcg RAE covers 14% male RDA and 18% female RDA), apricots (46 mcg RAE covers 5% male RDA and 7% female RDA), baby carrots (75 mcg RAE cover 8% male RDA and 11% female RDA), broccoli (138 mcg RAE covers 15% male RDA and 20% female RDA), Cheddar cheese (78 mcg RAE covers 9% male RDA and 11% female RDA), cooked kale (206 mcg RAE covers 23% male RDA and 29% female RDA), peach (26 mcg RAE covers 3% male RDA and 4% female RDA), Romaine lettuce (72 mcg RAE covers 8% male RDA and 10% female RDA), scallions (32 mcg RAE covers 4% male RDA and 5% female RDA), and spinach (247 mcg RAE covers 28% male RDA and 36% female RDA) (Wardlaw and Smith, 2011).

Table 1. Sources of Vitamin A (USDA, 2016).

Product	Vitamin A (mcg RAE*)	%RDA Male**	%RDA Female**	Category
Sweet Potato, 1 cup	2581	285%	369%	Vegetables
Mango, 2	362	41%	51%	Fruits
Nonfat milk, 1 cup	5	0.6%	0.1%	Dairy
Hard margarine, ½ tsp	19	2%	3%	Oils
RDA	700-900	100%	100%	

*Retinol activity equivalents; **Daily value = 1000 mcg; Adult RDA: Male 900 mcg and Female 700 mcg.

Over 50% of vitamin A comes from preformed vitamin A in a typical North American diet while provitamin A is predominantly consumed as part of the diet in countries around the world (Wardlaw and Smith, 2011).

SIDE EFFECTS AND TOXICITY

Vitamin A toxicity is the most frequently observed fat-soluble vitamin toxicity. The upper level of vitamin A for adult men and women is 3000 mcg (3000 RAE or 10,000 IU) per day. Taking several hundred thousand IUs of vitamin A can cause acute vitamin A poisoning in adults. Adults who regularly take more than 25,000 IU a day can develop symptoms of chronic vitamin A poisoning. Babies and children can become sick after taking even smaller doses of vitamin A or vitamin A-containing products (such as retinol found in skin creams) because they are more sensitive to vitamin A. Large doses of vitamin A have also been associated birth defects. Hence, women of childbearing age have been recommended to limit vitamin A consumption to 100 % of the daily limit (1000 mcg or 5000 IU) (Wardlaw and Smith, 2011).

Large amounts of beta-carotene usually do not result in sickness, but can turn the skin yellow or orange. The skin color will turn back to normal once the intake of beta-carotene is reduced (Wardlaw and Smith, 2011).

VITAMIN D

Vitamin D is a steroidal vitamin. It belongs to a group of fat-soluble pro-hormones that participates in the absorption and metabolism of calcium and phosphorous. Inadequate calcium and phosphorous intake and deposition can lead to the disease called rickets in children. In adults, a disease similar to rickets is called osteomalacia and it results from inadequate calcium absorption in the intestine and poor management of calcium by the kidneys. People who are exposed to normal quantities of sunlight do not require vitamin D supplements. Sunlight promotes sufficient vitamin D synthesis in the skin (Fig. **2**). However, individuals with limited sun exposure may develop osteomalacia if diet is not supplemented. The adequate intake for vitamin D is 5 mcg per day (200 IU/ day) for individuals under 51 years old and two to three times higher for older adults. The daily value used on food and supplements is 10 mcg (400 IU) (Wardlaw and Smith, 2011, American Dietetic Association, 2005, Food and Nutrition Board, 1997, Nield *et al.*, 2006).

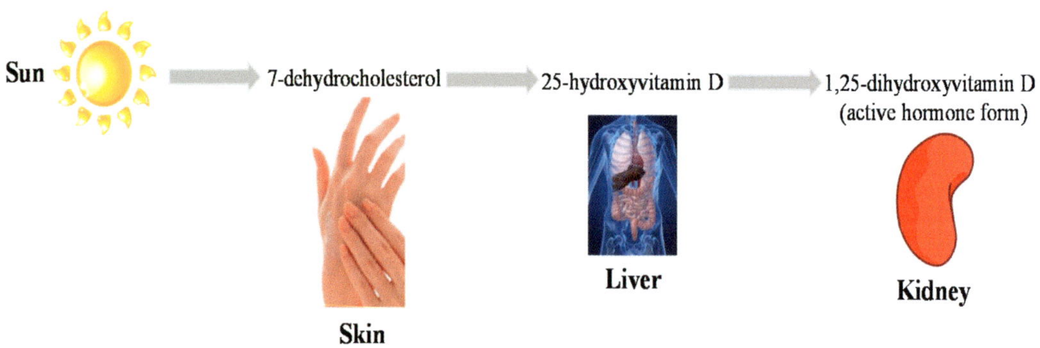

Fig. (2). Vitamin D synthesis.

In brief, 7-dehydrocholesterol found in the skin is converted to the prohormone vitamin D in the presence of ultraviolet B rays for the sunlight. This prohormone is then transformed in the liver and kidneys to the active form of vitamin D. The amount of sun exposure needed to produce enough vitamin D to reach the Adequate Intake level set for this vitamin depends on many factors such as the individuals' age, location, skin color, season, and time of day (Wardlaw and Smith, 2011).

Five forms of vitamin D are known. Vitamins D_2 and D_3 are the major forms of this vitamin in humans (Fig. **3**) (Wardlaw and Smith, 2011). They are known together as *calciferol.*

1) **Vitamin D_1**, ergocalciferol (lumisterol).

2) **Vitamin D_2**, made from ergosterol.

3) **Vitamin D_3**, made from 7-dehydrocholesterol and known as cholecalciferol.

4) **Vitamin D_4**, 22-dihydroergocalciferol.

5) **Vitamin D_5**, made from 7-dehydrositosterol and known as sitocalciferol.

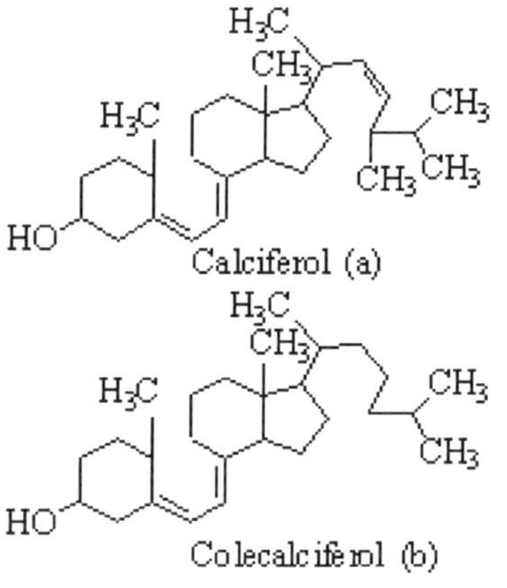

Fig. (3). Structures of vitamin D_2 (a) and vitamin D_3 (b) (Wardlaw and Smith, 2011, Lemke and Williams, 2008).

In response to sunlight (UV radiation), ergocalciferol is produced by invertebrates, fungus and plants. Vertebrates including humans do not produce vitamin D_2. The function of vitamin D_2 in invertebrates is unclear, but it is known that ergosterol absorbs UV radiation, which can damage DNA, RNA and proteins. Consequently, many scientists believe that ergosterol may protect organisms from sunlight damage by serving as a sunscreen (Wardlaw and Smith, 2011).

Cholecalciferol is made from 7-dehydrocholesterol on the skin, by reaction with UV light at 270-300 nm wavelengths. The highest level of production of vitamin D_3 occurs when the UV index is greater than 3 (between 295-297 nm), such as every day in the tropics. An UV index of more than 3 also occurs every day during some of spring, all of summer, and parts of autumn in temperate areas. It almost never occurs near the arctic circles. To produce adequate amounts of vitamin D_3, humans need ten to fifteen minutes of sun exposure with an UV index greater than 3 on the arms, back, face, and hands without sunscreen, at least twice a week. Longer exposure to sunlight results in production of extra vitamin that is degraded as fast as it is generated (Wardlaw and Smith, 2011).

FUNCTION

- Vitamin D is essential for the absorption and metabolism of Ca and P. Both Ca and P have various functions, particularly the maintenance of healthy bones by working together with hormones (*e.g.*, parathyroid hormone) and supplying appropriate amounts of calcium to the cells (Edible Science, 2015).

- It is also an immune system regulator and contributes to skin cell development, muscle and gum health, and regulation of blood pressure. "It may be an important way to arm the immune system against disorders like the common cold", report scientists in Science Daily from the University of Colorado Denver School of Medicine, Massachusetts General Hospital and Children's Hospital Boston. "A form of vitamin D could be one of our body's main protections against damage from low levels of radiation", say radiological experts from the New York City Department of Health and Mental Hygiene (Science Daily, 2009).

- Vitamin D may reduce the risk of developing multiple sclerosis. Near the tropics, where there is much more sunlight, multiple sclerosis is much less common according to Dennis Bourdette, chairman of the Department of Neurology and director of the Multiple Sclerosis and Neuroimmunology Center at Oregon Health and Science University, USA (Edible Science, 2015, Holick, 2004).

- In a study with 3000 European men, ages between 40 and 79, vitamin D may have a key role in helping the brain to keep working well later in life (Edible Science, 2015).

- Vitamin D is probably linked to controlling body weight, according to research pursued at the Medical College of Georgia, USA (Edible Science, 2015, Ross *et al.*, 2011).

- After monitoring 616 children in Costa Rica, researchers from Harvard Medical School found that vitamin D reduced the severity and frequency of asthma symptoms as well as the prospect of hospitalizations due to asthma crisis (Edible Science, 2015, Holick, 2004).

- Vitamin D has been shown to decrease the risk of chronic diseases such as rheumatoid arthritis in women (Edible Science, 2015, Holick, 2004).

- According to a study by Cancer Treatment Centers of America, vitamin D deficiency was widespread in cancer patients irrespective of nutritional status. Other studies have shown that adequate level intake of vitamin D significantly lower risk of developing cancer (Garland *et al.*, 2007, Ross *et al.*, 2011).

FOOD SOURCES

Salmon, mackerel and tuna, as well as fish liver oils are considered to be the best sources of vitamin D, particularly Vitamin D_3. It is also present in beef liver, cheese, and egg yolks (Wardlaw and Smith, 2011). Mushrooms on the other hand are considered as sources of vitamin D_2. In western diet, most vitamin D comes from fortified foods, where vitamin D is artificially added. Milk in the United States is fortified with 100 IU/cup of vitamin D. Different sources of vitamin D from four different categories (Table **2** for main sources) include baked bluefish (0.3 mcg corresponds to 11 IU and 6% RDA), canned tuna (1.1 mcg corresponds to 45 IU and 23% RDA), cooked egg yolk (0.6 mcg corresponds to 25 IU and 13% RDA), Italian pork sausage (0.4 mcg corresponds to 15 IU and 7% RDA), nonfat milk (2.5 mcg corresponds to 98 IU and 49% RDA), sardines (3.4 mcg corresponds to 136 IU and 68% RDA), soy milk (1.0 mcg corresponds to 40 IU and 20% RDA), and Special K cereal (0.3 mcg corresponds to 10 IU and 5% RDA), (Wardlaw and Smith, 2011).

Table 2. Sources of Vitamin D (USDA, 2016).

Product	Vitamin D (µg)	Vitamin D (IU)**	%RDA*	Category
Baked Salmon, 1 ounce	1.4	55	10%	Meat and Beans
Milk Non-fat, 1 cup	2.9	116	19%	Dairy
American Cheese, 1 ounce	0.2	6	2%	Oils
Raisin Bran Cereal, ¼ cup	0.6	25	4%	Grains
RDA	15	600	100%	

*Daily value and RDA for Adult Male and Female = 15 µg; **IU = International Units.

VITAMIN D AND NUTRITION

Human lifestyles have changed over years. In the past, societies worldwide wore more clothing than in current times, reducing skin exposure to sunlight. Modifications in the history of costume have caused a substantial variation in natural production of vitamin D and consequent diseases. Some countries reacted to these variations by using synthetic vitamins D_2 and D_3 to fortify some foods; examples of fortified products include bread, breakfast cereals, margarine, pastries, oil spreads, milk and other dairy products. Initially, some scientists criticized the modifications in the intake of vitamin D and suggested that doses used in nutritional fortification and recommended supplementation were not enough to cover the shortfall. Complaints were disregarded, and sometimes scientists were ridiculed. However, over the last few years studies suggest that these scientists may have been right since job culture has moved toward office related activities with no access to sunlight and not very many foods contain vitamin D. On the other hand, too much vitamin D can also cause health issues. Hence, the upper level for vitamin D is 50 mcg per day (200 IU/day) based on the risk of over absorption of calcium that may cause calcium deposits in the kidneys and other organs (Wardlaw and Smith, 2011, Holick, 2007).

VITAMIN E

Vitamin E is also a fat-soluble vitamin (Fig. **4**) that is needed for the proper function of many organs in the body. The RDA if vitamin E in the form of alpha-tocopherol is 15 mg per day for adults. Fifteen milligrams is equivalent to 22 IU of a natural source and 33 IU of a synthetic source. The average consumption of vitamin E by North Americans is one-third below the recommended value. The daily value used on food and supplements labels to express vitamin E content is 30 IU. Over $1 billion is spent every year on this vitamin by North Americans (Wardlaw and Smith, 2011, Food and Nutrition Board, 2000).

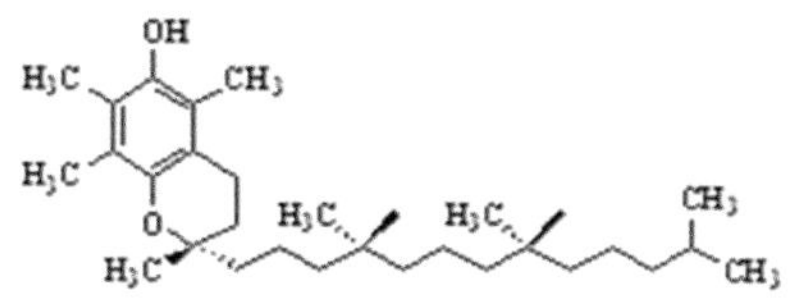

Fig. (4). Structure of active form of vitamin E (Wardlaw and Smith, 2011, Lemke and Williams, 2008).

The chemical structure of the isoform varies depending of the source of vitamin E. Natural sources contain d isoform of vitamin E while dl form of the isomer is found in the synthetic version of vitamin E. One IU of vitamin E from natural sources equals to 0.67 mg since the natural form is more potent than the synthetic form of vitamin E.

FUNCTION

Vitamin E is an antioxidant that guards body tissues from harm caused by free radicals. Free radicals arc highly reactive species that can injury cells, tissues, and organs. Free radicals are also suggested to perform a role in certain conditions linked to aging. Vitamin E participates in the formation of erythrocytes and aids the body in the use of Vitamin K. Vitamin E also aids broaden blood vessels and prevent blood from clotting. The body also requires vitamin E to develop a strong immune system against viruses and bacteria. Cells use vitamin E to interrelate with each other. Vitamin E participates in many other important functions including prevention of cell membranes to breakdown. Oxidizing agents can attack unsaturated fatty acids found on cell membranes and vitamin E can neutralize these agents, protecting cell membrane from damage and avoiding hemolysis in red blood cells. Studies have also shown that male smokers with high levels of vitamin E reduce the risk of dying from lung cancer, prostate cancer, respiratory diseases, and stroke (Wardlaw and Smith, 2011).

FOOD SOURCES

The best way to achieve the daily requirement of vitamin E is through food sources (Table 3) (Wardlaw and Smith, 2011). Vitamin E is found in the following foods:

- Fortified products
- Green leafy vegetables
- Nuts
- Seeds
- Vegetable oils

Different sources of vitamin E from four different categories (Table **3** for main sources) include fortified almonds (4.5 mg corresponds to 6.8 IU and 30% RDA), Bran cereal (7.5 mg corresponds to 11.2 IU and 50% RDA), Canola oil (2.9 mg corresponds to 4.3 IU and 19% RDA), chunky peanut butter (1.2 mg corresponds to 1.8 IU and 8% RDA), dry-roasted almonds (7.5 mg corresponds to 11.1 IU and 50% RDA), Italian dressing (1.6 mg corresponds to 2.3 IU and 11% RDA), mango (2.3 mg corresponds to 3.5 IU and 15% RDA), mayonnaise (3.0 mg corresponds to 4.5 IU and 20% RDA),oil-roasted Sunflower seeds (3.4 mg corresponds to 5 IU and 23% RDA), peanuts (2.1 mcg corresponds to 3.1 IU and 14% RDA), and Safflower oil (5.9 mg corresponds to 8.7 IU and 39% RDA) (Wardlaw and Smith, 2011).

Table 3. Vitamin E food sources (USDA, 2016).

Product	Vitamin E (mg)	Vitamin E (IU)*	%RDA**	Category
Dry-roasted Sunflower Seeds, 1 ounce	7.4	11.0	49%	Meat and Beans
Sunflower Oil, 1 tablespoon	5.6	8.3	37%	Oils
Avocado, 1 unit	2.7	4.0	18%	Fruits
Wheat Germ, 1 ounce	0.16	0.24	1%	Grains
RDA	15	22.33	100%	

*IU = International Units; **Daily value = 30 IU and RDA for Adult Male and Female = 15 mg.

SIDE EFFECTS AND TOXICITY

Adequate intake of vitamin E found in foods is not risky or harmful. High intake or high doses of vitamin E, however, might increase the risk for spread bleeding and serious bleeding in the brain, or stroke. According to the literature, high levels of vitamin E may also increase the risk of birth defects. Amount of vitamin E can be calculated *via* using the following equation: [(source amount in mg)/(conversion factor for the source of vitamin]/ number of isomer types. The upper level of vitamin E as alpha-tocopherol is 1000 mg per day based on the interference of this vitamin with vitamin K's role in the clotting mechanism, which leads to hemorrhage. To calculate the amount of vitamin E in 1000 mg do as follow [1500 IU from natural sources (*d* isomer =1000/0.67) and 1100 IU from synthetic source (*d* and *l* isomer = 1000/0.45/2)] (Wardlaw and Smith, 2011).

VITAMIN K

Vitamin K is a liposoluble vitamin (Fig. **5**) (Wardlaw and Smith, 2011). It is a necessary participant in the production of proteins that mediate both coagulation and anticoagulation. The three basic forms of Vitamin K are K1 (phylloquinone), K2 (menaquinone), and K3 (menadione). The adequate intake for adults of vitamin K is 90 to 120 mcg per day. The daily value used on food and supplements to express vitamin K content is 80 mcg (Wardlaw and Smith, 2011, Food and Nutrition Board, 2001).

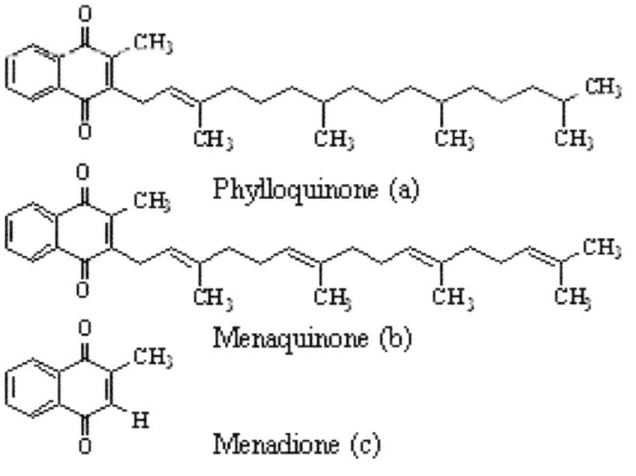

Fig. (5). Structure of vitamin K1 (a), K2 (b), and K3 (c) (Wardlaw and Smith, 2011, Lemke and Williams, 2008).

FUNCTION

Vitamin K is known as the clotting vitamin, because lack of vitamin K could cause that blood would not clot. Some studies also suggest that vitamin K helps maintaining strong bones in the elderly as it activates proteins found in bone, muscle, and kidneys to support calcium binding in these organs. Other studies have linked poor vitamin K to increase in hip fractures (Wardlaw and Smith, 2011).

FOOD SOURCES

The best way to reach the daily requirement of vitamin K is through adequate food supply (Table **4**). It is also made in the human body by the bacteria that line the gastrointestinal tract (Wardlaw and Smith, 2011). Vitamin K is resistant to cooking loss and can be found in the following products:

- Green leafy vegetables.
- Cereals, eggs, fish, liver, and meat.
- Other vegetables.

Different sources of vitamin K from two different categories (Table **4** for main sources) include Canola oil (17 mcg covers to 14% AI males and 19% AI female), raw cabbage (42 mcg covers to 35% AI males and 47% AI female), cooked asparagus (144 mcg covers to 120% AI males and 160% AI female), cooked broccoli (220 mcg covers to 184% AI males and 244% AI female), cooked brussel sprouts (300 mcg covers to 250% AI males and 334% AI female), cooked cauliflower (20 mcg covers to 17% AI males and 22% AI female), cooked green beans (98 mcg covers to 82% AI males and 108% AI female), cooked spinach (480 mcg covers to 400% AI males and 533% AI female), cooked turnip greens (520 mcg covers to 433% AI males and 578% AI female), green peas (52 mcg covers to 44% AI males and 58% AI female), loose leaf lettuce (97 mcg covers to 81% AI males and 108% AI female), raw spinach (144 mcg covers to 120% AI males and 160% AI female), and Sauerkraut (60 mcg covers to 50% AI males and 66% AI female) (Wardlaw and Smith, 2011).

Table 4. Vitamin K food sources (USDA, 2016).

Product	Vitamin K (µg)	Adult Male (% AI)*	Adult Female (%AI)*	Category
Cooked Kale, 1 cup	113	94%	1178%	Vegetables
Soybean Oil, 1 tablespoon	25	21%	28%	Oils
RDA**	90-120	100%	100%	

*AI = Adequate Intake; *Male AI = 120 µg and Female AI = 90 µg; **Daily value = 80 µg.

SIDE EFFECTS

Vitamin K deficiency occurs when the body cannot appropriately absorb it from the intestinal tract; hence, it is very unusual. It. Vitamin K deficiency can also be observed in some individuals with long-term antibiotic treatment. Deficient individuals are more prompt to have bruising and bleeding. Individuals taking blood thinning drugs (such as anticoagulant/antiplatelet drugs) should pay special attention to food rich in vitamin K because vitamin K or foods rich in vitamin K can interfere with the effect of these drugs. For these individuals, it is especially important to maintain steady levels of vitamin K in blood from day to day. The health care provider could be a good source of guidance on how much vitamin K containing foods an individual on blood thinning drugs should consume. No upper level has been set for vitamin K as it poses no risk of toxicity when administered orally (Wardlaw and Smith, 2011, American Dietetic Association, 2005).

HYDROSOLUBLE VITAMINS

Water-soluble vitamins are freely eliminated from the body through the urine or stool. They are lost during food processing and separation as well since they dissolve in water (Wardlaw and Smith, 2011).

VITAMIN B FAMILY

The vitamins from the B complex play key roles in metabolism and function as coenzymes to contribute to enzyme activity (Fig. **6**). They are also considered as interdependent as they participate in the same processes. They are often found in the same food, suggesting that lack of one of them may mean other vitamins from this group are also low. Symptoms of deficiency of these vitamins occur in the brain, nervous system, skin, and GI tract. Vitamin-like compounds are also synthesized by the body and include carnitine, inositol, taurine, and lipoic acid. Carnitine is a vitamin-like compound that is needed to transport fatty acids into the mitochondria. Inositol is also a vitamin-like substance that is found as part of cell membranes while taurine is found as part of bile acids. Lipoic acid acts as an antioxidant and participates in the metabolism of carbohydrates (Wardlaw and Smith, 2011, American Dietetic Association, 2005, Food and Nutrition Board, 1998).

Whole grains are good sources of these vitamins. However, milling the grains lead to losses of both vitamins and minerals since seeds are crushed and the germ, bran, and husk layers are discarded, leaving only the starch containing endosperm. Hence, US products made from milled grains are enriched with four B vitamins (thiamin, riboflavin, niacin, and folic acid) as well as with the mineral iron.

Vitamin B complexes, found as supplements, contain several vitamin-B products including thiamine (vitamin B1), riboflavin (vitamin B2), niacin/niacinamide

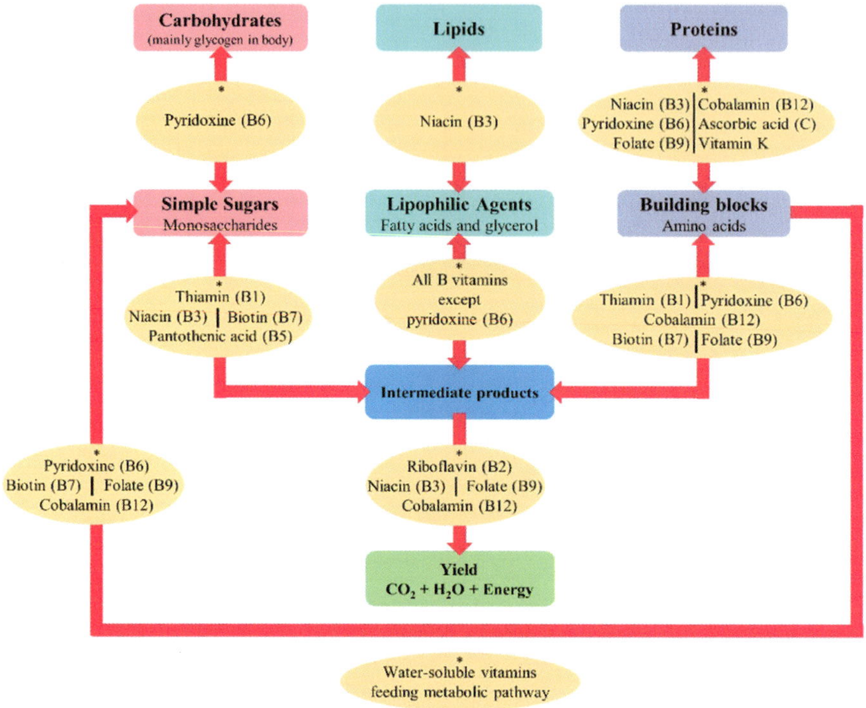

Fig. (6). Hydrosoluble vitamins participate in the metabolism of energy-yielding nutrients (Wardlaw and Smith, 2011)

(vitamin B3), pantothenic acid (vitamin B5), pyridoxine (vitamin B6), cyanocobalamin (vitamin B12), and folic acid. However, some dietary supplements do not contain all B vitamins and some may include other vitamin B like nutrients, such as biotin, para-aminobenzoic acid (PABA), choline bitartrate, carnitine, and inositol (Wardlaw and Smith, 2011, Food and Nutrition Board, 1998).

THIAMINE

Thiamine is also called vitamin B1 (Fig. **7**). Thiamine is a coenzyme that participates in reactions resulting in the loss of a carbon dioxide from the molecule. This reaction helps release energy by breaking down carbohydrates and amino acids for energy needs. The RDA for thiamine is 1.1 to 1.2 mg per day. The daily value used to express the thiamine content in food and supplements is 1.5 mg (Wardlaw and Smith, 2011, Food and Nutrition Board, 1998).

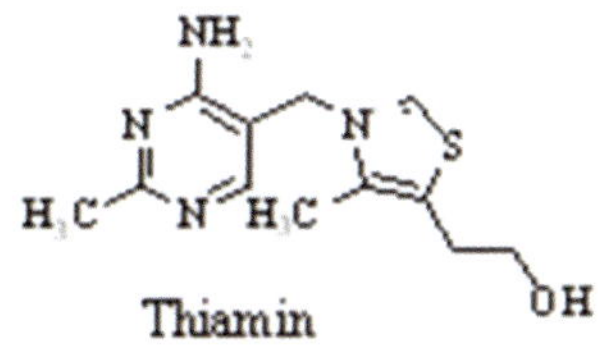

Fig. (7). Structure of vitamin B1, thiamin (Wardlaw and Smith, 2011, Lemke and Williams, 2008).

FOOD SOURCES

Vitamin B1 is found in many dietary products including beans, cereal grains, meat, nuts, and yeast. It is frequently used by the human body together with other B vitamins, and found in combination with many vitamin B complex products. Different sources of thiamin from five different categories (Table **5** for main sources) include baked beans (0.2 mg covers to 17% RDA males and 18% RDA female), Canadian bacon (0.25 mg covers to 21% RDA males and 23% RDA female), cooked green peas (0.2 mg covers to 17% RDA males and 18% RDA female), corn (0.2 mg covers to 17% RDA males and 18% RDA female), flour tortilla (0.4 mg covers to 33% RDA males and 36% RDA female), fresh orange juice (0.2 mg covers to 17% RDA males and 18% RDA female), ham lunch meat (0.2 mg covers to 13% RDA males and 14% RDA female), Navy beans (0.2 mg covers to 17% RDA males and 18% RDA female), and pork chops (0.15 mg covers to 13% RDA males and 14% RDA female) (Wardlaw and Smith, 2011).

Table 5. Thiamin food sources (USDA, 2016).

Product	Thiamin (mg)	Male* (% RDA)	Female* (% RDA)	Category
Canned lean ham, 1 ounce	0.2	17%	18%	Meat and Beans
Wheat germ, 1 cup	2.1	175%	190%	Grains
Acorn squash, 1cup	0.2	17%	18%	Vegetables
Soy milk, 8 ounces	0.4	33%	36%	Dairy
Watermelon, 1 cup	0.05	4%	5%	Fruits
RDA	1.1-1.2	100%	100%	

*RDA = adult male 1.2 mg and female 1.1 mg; Daily value = 1.5 mg.

FUNCTION AND USES

Thiamine is needed by the body to properly metabolize carbohydrates. High consumption of dietary thiamine from food or vitamin B1 as dietary supplement is taken for conditions associated with syndromes of thiamine deficiency, including beriberi and inflammation of the nerves outside the brain (peripheral neuritis) or pellagra, a vitamin-deficiency disease (Wardlaw and Smith, 2011). Thiamine may be useful in digestive problems such as ongoing diarrhea, poor appetite, and ulcerative colitis. Thiamine may also be useful for AIDS, alcoholism, aging, cancer sores, diabetic pain, heart disease, a type of brain damage called cerebellar syndrome, vision problems such as cataracts and glaucoma, motion sickness, for boosting the immune system, and improving athletic performance. Additional potential uses reported include the use in prevention of cervical cancer and in patients with type 2 diabetes the use in preventing the progression of kidney disease (Wardlaw and Smith, 2011). Some individuals take thiamine for enhancing learning abilities; increasing energy; fighting stress; maintaining a positive mental attitude; and preventing memory loss, including Alzheimer's disease. In some countries, thiamine shots are prescribed for a memory disorder called Wernicke's encephalopathy syndrome. Additional syndromes of thiamine deficiency can be observed in critically ill people, alcohol withdrawal, and coma. A diet rich in processed food can create thiamine deficiency; hence enriched food can overcome this issue. Excess of this vitamin is rapidly eliminated through the urine; no upper level has been set for thiamine (Wardlaw and Smith, 2011, American Dietetic Association, 2005).

RIBOFLAVIN

Riboflavin is a vitamin B type and is also known as vitamin B2 (Fig. **8**). It is a hydrosoluble vitamin, which means it is not stored in the body. This vitamin must be replenished every day. The RDA is 1.1 to 1.3 mg per day. The daily value used in food and dietary supplement labels is 1.7 mg (Wardlaw and Smith, 2011, Food and Nutrition Board, 1998).

FUNCTION

Riboflavin (vitamin B2) works with the other B complex vitamins. The riboflavin coenzyme participates in energy-yielding reactions of cells that generate energy using pathways requiring oxygen. It is important for body growth and red blood cell production and aids in releasing energy from fatty acids and carbohydrates (Wardlaw and Smith, 2011).

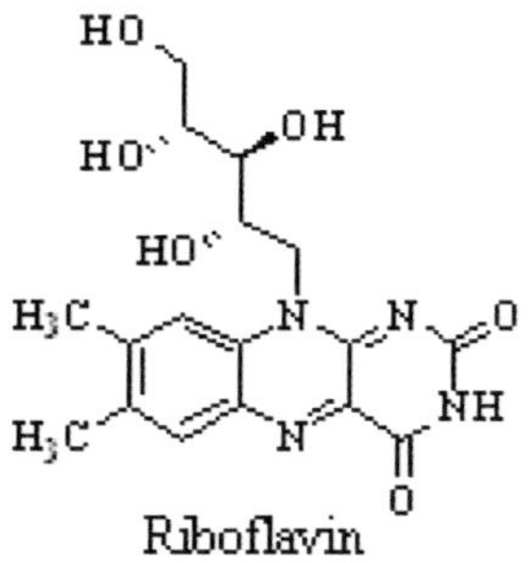

Fig. (8). Structure of vitamin B2, riboflavin (Wardlaw and Smith, 2011, Lemke and Williams, 2008).

FOOD SOURCES

Riboflavin is found in many vegetables and some animal sources (Table **6**). The following products can be good sources of vitamin B2 in the diet: dairy products, green leafy vegetables, lean meats, legumes, and nuts. Breads and cereals are regularly fortified with this vitamin. Riboflavin is chemically degraded when exposed to light; hence, riboflavin rich foods should be stored in glass containers that protect this vitamin from to light. Because riboflavin is a hydrosoluble vitamin, excess amounts leave the body through the urine. There is no known report on poisoning by riboflavin; hence, no upper level has been set (Wardlaw and Smith, 2011). Different other sources of riboflavin from four different categories (Table **6** for main sources) include boiled egg (0.3 mg covers to 23% RDA males and 27% RDA female), buttermilk (0.4 mg covers to 31% RDA males and 36% RDA female), cooked spinach (0.4 mg covers to 31% RDA males and 36% RDA female), Feta cheese (0.2 mg covers to 15% RDA males and 18% RDA female), lean ham (0.1 mg covers to 5% RDA males and 6% RDA female), 1% milk (0.4 mg covers to 31% RDA males and 36% RDA female), Sirloin steak (0.1 mg covers to 8% RDA males and 9% RDA female), steamed oysters (0.11 mg covers to 8.5% RDA males and 10% RDA female), and tortilla (0.2 mg covers to 15% RDA males and 18% RDA female) (Wardlaw and Smith, 2011).

GROUPS AT RISK

Pregnant women or breast-feeding women need higher intake of riboflavin. Because of poor-diet, people with alcoholism are at risk of riboflavin deficiency (Wardlaw and Smith, 2011, American Dietetic Association, 2005).

Table 6. Riboflavin food sources (USDA, 2016).

Product	Riboflavin (mg)	Male* (% RDA)	Female* (% RDA)	Category
Multigrain oat cereal, 1 cup	0.14	11%	13%	Grains
Fried beef liver, 1 slice	2.0	154%	182%	Meat and Beans
Plain yogurt, 1cup	0.35	27%	32%	Dairy
Raw mushroom, 1 unit	0.1	8%	9%	Vegetables
RDA	1.3 &1.1	100%	100%	

*RDA = adult male 1.3 mg and female 1.1 mg; Daily value = 1.7 mg.

RIBOFLAVIN DEFICIENCY

Deficiency of riboflavin is uncommon in the United States because this vitamin is abundant in the food supply. Symptoms of severe deficiency of riboflavin include: anemia, inflammation of the mouth and tongue, mouth or lip sores, cheilosis, sore throat, skin disorders, and swelling of mucus membranes, and confusion (Wardlaw and Smith, 2011).

NIACIN

Niacin is also called vitamin B3 (Fig. **9**). The RDA for niacin in adults is 14-16 mg per day and is expressed as niacin equivalents (NE). The daily value used to express niacin content in food and dietary supplement labels is 20 mg. The upper level for this vitamin is 35 mg per day in the form of nicotinic acid (Wardlaw and Smith, 2011, Food and Nutrition Board, 1998).

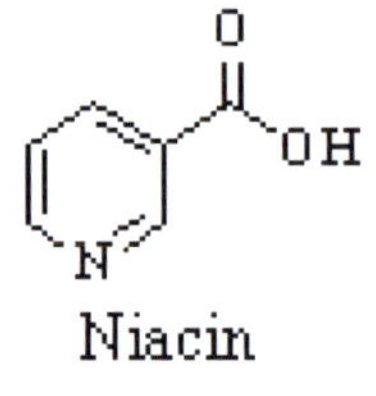

Fig. (9). Structure of vitamin B3, niacin (Wardlaw and Smith, 2011, Lemke and Williams, 2008).

FOOD SOURCES

Vitamin B3 is found in many foods including beans, cereal grains, eggs, fish, green vegetables, meat, milk, and yeast. Niacin and niacinamide are also found in many vitamin B complex supplements in combination with other B vitamins. Different sources of niacin from three different categories (Table **7** for main sources) include baked cod (0.7 mg covers to 4% RDA males and 5% RDA female), baked salmon (3 mg covers to 18% RDA males and 20% RDA female), broiled halibut (0.5 mg covers to 3% RDA males and 4% RDA female), chunky peanut butter (2.2 mg covers to 14% RDA males and 16% RDA female), fried beef liver (4.1 mg covers to 26% RDA males and 29% RDA female), ground beef

Table 7. Niacin food sources (USDA, 2016).

Product	Niacin (mg)	Male (% RDA)*	Female (% RDA)*	Category
Tuna, 1 ounce	2.5	16%	18%	Meat and Beans
Raw mushrooms, 1 unit	1.0	6%	7%	Vegetables
Raisin Nut Bran cereal, 1 cup	6.7	42%	48%	Grains
RDA	14-16	100%	100%	

*RDA = adult male 16 mg and female 14 mg; Daily value = 1.5 mg.

(1.5 mg covers to 10% RDA males and 12% RDA female), lean steak (1.1 mg covers to 7% RDA males and 8% RDA female), peanuts (9.9 mg covers to 62% RDA males and 71% RDA female), potato (2.1 mg covers to 13% RDA males and 15% RDA female), roasted chicken (3.4 mg covers to 21% RDA males and 24% RDA female), tortilla (2.6 mg covers to 16% RDA males and 19% RDA female), and turkey lunch meat (1.8 mg covers to 11% RDA males and 13% RDA female) (Wardlaw and Smith, 2011)

FUNCTION AND USES

Niacinamide can be biosynthesized in the body from niacin for proper body functioning. Niacin and niacinamide are required for the proper metabolism of fats and sugars and to preserve healthy cells. The coenzyme forms participate in many of the cellular metabolic pathways, particularly when energy is being released from the energy nutrients and used by the cells. In the synthesis of fatty acids, for instance, a niacin coenzyme is used; hence, niacin is frequently taken by individuals with high cholesterol. Other individuals also take niacin along with other treatments for issues related to circulation, dizziness, headache, migraine and diarrhea associated with cholera. Niacin is sometimes taken by people who take illegal drugs to prevent positive drug screens. Niacinamide is used for treating diabetes and for bullous pemphigoid and granuloma annulare. Niacinamide is used for preventing symptoms related to disorders such as pellagra. Vitamin B3, niacin, is also used in alcohol dependence, Alzheimer's disease and age-related loss of thinking skills, chronic brain syndrome, depression, hallucinations due to drugs, motion sickness, schizophrenia, and fluid collection (edema) (Wardlaw and Smith, 2011, American Dietetic Association, 2005).

Some individuals use niacin or niacinamide for acne, arthritis, attention deficit-hyperactivity disorder (ADHD), improving circulation, improving digestion, improving orgasm, leprosy, lowering blood pressure, memory loss, preventing premenstrual headache, preventing cataracts, promoting relaxation, protecting against toxins and pollutants, and reducing the effects of aging. Niacinamide is also applied to the skin for acne vulgaris, an inflammatory disease (Wardlaw and Smith, 2011).

GROUPS AT RISK

Niacin deficiency is observed in people with rare disorders of tryptophan metabolism and those with alcoholism (Wardlaw and Smith, 2011).

NIACIN DEFICIENCY

Due to use of niacin coenzymes in almost every cellular metabolic pathway, deficiency of this vitamin causes widespread symptoms. The disease deficiency associated to niacin is called Pellagra. Pellagra has reached epidemic levels in the United States in the past (Wardlaw and Smith, 2011).

VITAMIN B6

It is known as pyridoxine and exists in three chemical forms (Fig. **10**).Vitamin B6 is also a hydrosoluble vitamin. The body does not store it and excess intake of the vitamin leave the body through the urine. That means there is a need of constant supply of this vitamin in the diet. The RDA for adults is 1.3-1.7 mg per day. The daily value use to express vitamin B6 in food and dietary supplement labels is 2 mg (Wardlaw and Smith, 2011, American Dietetic Association, 2005, Food and Nutrition Board, 1998).

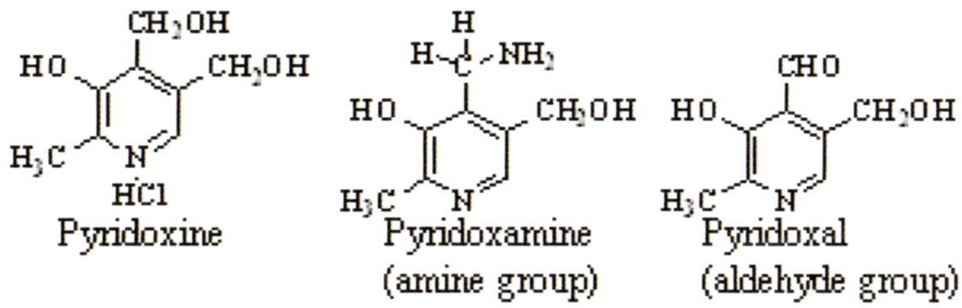

Fig. (10). Structure of vitamin B6 (pyridoxine, pyridoxamine, pyridoxal) (Wardlaw and Smith, 2011, Lemke and Williams, 2008).

FOOD SOURCES

Vitamin B6 is found in many natural sources including: banana, legumes (dried beans), meat, nuts, poultry, and whole grains. Fortified breads and cereals may also be enriched with vitamin B6. Different sources of vitamin B6 from four different categories (Table **8** for main sources) include Acorn squash (0.5 mg covers to 38% RDA), avocado (0.6 mg covers to 46% RDA), cooked spinach (0.4 mg covers to 30% RDA), fried beef liver (0.4 mg covers to 31% RDA), lean ham (0.4 mg covers to 31% RDA), roasted chicken breast (0.16 mg covers to 13% RDA), roasted turkey lunch meat (0.13 mg covers to 10% RDA), sirloin steak (0.13 mg covers to 10% RDA), sunflower seeds (0.3 mg covers to 23% RDA), and water melon (0.3 mg covers to 23% RDA) (Wardlaw and Smith, 2011).

Table 8. Vitamin B-6 food sources (USDA, 2016).

Product	Vitamin B6 (mg)	% RDA*	Category
Atlantic Salmon, 1 ounce	0.2	15%	Meat and Beans
Baked potato, 1 medium	0.5	36%	Vegetables
Banana, 1 unit	0.6	46%	Fruits
Special K cereal, 1 cup	2.0	153%	Grains
RDA	1.3	100%	

*RDA = adult male and female 1.3 mg; Daily value = 2 mg.

FUNCTION

Vitamin B6 participates in many metabolic reactions and helps the body in: the synthesis of white blood cells (play role in immune system to combat many diseases), maintaining normal nerve function, and making hemoglobin (carries oxygen in the red blood cells). The more protein is consumed in the diet, the more vitamin B6 is needed as vitamin B6 removes the nitrogen group from certain amino acids and makes them available to other amino acids. It also plays a role in homocysteine metabolism. Vitamin B6 deficiency can cause a type of anemia (Wardlaw and Smith, 2011).

GROUPS AT RISK

Vitamin B6 deficiency is observed in people with alcoholism since the coenzyme form of vitamin B6 is displaced by a metabolite formed in alcohol metabolism and left at risk of being destroyed or eliminated. The liver tissue of people with hepatitis and cirrhosis also has impaired metabolism of vitamin B6 (Wardlaw and Smith, 2011, American Dietetic Association, 2005).

VITAMIN B6 DEFICIENCY, ADVERSE EFFECTS, AND TOXICITY

Vitamin B6 deficiency is uncommon in the United States, but deficiency can occur and this anomaly can cause: confusion, depression, irritability, mouth and tongue sores. Large doses of vitamin B6, however, can cause: difficulty coordinating movement, numbness, sensory changes, and nerve damage. The upper safe level of vitamin B6 is 100 mg per day (Wardlaw and Smith, 2011, Food and Nutrition Board, 1998).

VITAMIN B12

Vitamin B12 is a water-soluble vitamin that contains cobalt (Fig. **11**). The body can store vitamin B12 in the liver for years but only about 50% of the vitamin B12 provided in the diet is absorbed. The RDA of vitamin B12 is 2.4 mcg per day for adults. The daily value used in food and supplement labels to represent vitamin B12 is 6 mcg. However, vitamin B12 is non-toxic and no upper level has been set (Wardlaw and Smith, 2011, Food and Nutrition Board, 1998).

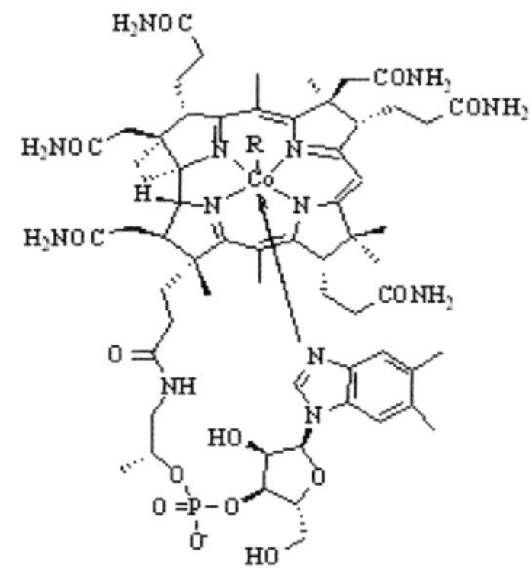

Fig. (11). Structure of vitamin B12, cyanocobalamin (Wardlaw and Smith, 2011, Lemke and Williams, 2008).

Vitamin B12 represents a family of compounds that is synthesized by bacteria, fungi, and other lower organisms (Wardlaw and Smith, 2011).

FUNCTION

Vitamin B12, like the other B vitamins, is essential in the metabolic process and in a variety of cellular processes. It aids in the formation of red blood cells and in the preservation of the central nervous system functions. It converts folate coenzymes to the active forms needed for metabolic reactions, including DNA synthesis. It also maintains myelin sheaths that insulate neurons as well as participates in homocysteine metabolism (Wardlaw and Smith, 2011).

FOOD SOURCES

Vitamin B12 is found in many natural sources (Table **9**), including: eggs, fortified foods, meat, dairy, organ meats (liver and kidney), poultry, and shellfish (Wardlaw and Smith, 2011). Different other sources of vitamin B12 from three different categories (Table **9** for main sources) include 1% milk (0.9 mcg covers to 38% RDA), beef hotdog (0.5 mcg covers to 21% RDA), boiled egg (0.6 mcg covers to 25% RDA), boiled oysters (7.2 mcg covers to 300% RDA), ham lunch meat (0.2 mcg covers to 8.5% RDA), lean ham (0.2 mcg covers to 8% RDA), lobsters (0.9 mcg covers to 38% RDA), pot roast (0.8 mcg covers to 35% RDA), shrimp (0.3 mcg covers to 14% RDA), and soy milk (0.8 mcg covers to 33% RDA) (Wardlaw and Smith, 2011).

Table 9. Vitamin B12 food sources (USDA, 2016).

Product	Vitamin B12 (mcg)	% RDA*	Category
Raw clams, 1 ounce	3.2	133%	Meat and Beans
Plain yogurt, 1 cup	0.9	38%	Dairy
Corn Flakes cereal, 1 cup	1.4	58%	Grains
RDA	2.4	100%	

*RDA = adult male and female 2.4 μg; Daily value = 6 μg.

GROUPS AT RISK

Women who are pregnant or breast-feeding require higher amounts of this vitamin as well as individuals over age 50 that lose the ability to absorb vitamin B12 from foods. Strict vegetarians or vegans that exclude eggs or dairy products may need vitamin B12 supplements since vegan diets supply little vitamin B12. Additionally, strict vegetarian or vegans that breastfeed their infants put their infants at risk of vitamin B12 deficiency, anemia, and long-term nervous system problems. Moreover, those who have experienced surgery in the gastrointestinal tract (*e.g.*, weight loss surgery) lose the ability to absorb vitamin B12. Individuals with digestive disorders (*e.g.*, celiac disease or Crohn's disease) may not absorb sufficient amounts of this vitamin (Wardlaw and Smith, 2011, American Dietetic Association, 2005, Andrès *et al.*, 2005).

VITAMIN B12 DEFICIENCY

A lack of this vitamin occurs when the intake is not enough or the body is unable to absorb appropriate amounts of vitamin needed. Symptoms associated to inadequate amounts of B12 include: anemia, loss of balance, numbness or tingling in the arms and legs, and weakness. Vitamin B12 deficiency can cause nerve destruction after about 20 years of consuming a diet free of this vitamin. Because of its role in nerve destruction, vitamin B12 deficiency causes pernicious anemia. Additionally, body reactions needing folate active forms do not take place without vitamin B12; hence, deficiency of this vitamin can result in symptoms of folate deficiency (Wardlaw and Smith, 2011).

PANTOTHENIC ACID

It is also called vitamin B5 (Fig. **12**). The adequate intake of pantothenic acid for adults is 5 mg per day. The daily value used to express the content of pantothenic acid in food and dietary supplement labels is 10 mg. Since no toxicity is known for pantothenic acid, no upper level has been set (Wardlaw and Smith, 2011, Food and Nutrition Board, 1998).

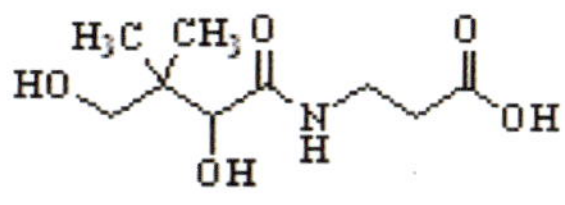

Fig. (12). Structure of vitamin B5, pantothenic acid (Wardlaw and Smith, 2011, Lemke and Williams, 2008).

FOOD SOURCES

It is extensively found in both plants and animals including cereal grains, eggs, legumes, meat, milk, and vegetables. Different sources of pantothenic acid from four different categories (Table **10** for main sources) include Acorn squash (1.2 mg covers to 24% AI), baked potato (0.7 mg covers to 14% AI), broccoli (0.8 mg covers to 16% AI), cooked egg yolk (0.6 mg covers to 12% AI), fried beef liver (1.7 mg covers to 34% AI), legumes (0.7 mg covers to 14% AI), Luna bar (9.9 mg covers to 198% AI), 1% milk (0.9 mg covers to 18% AI), peanuts (1.0 mg covers to 20% AI), roasted chicken breast (0.3 mg covers to 5% AI), and sunflower seeds (2.3 mg covers to 46% AI) (Wardlaw and Smith, 2011).

Table 10. Pantothenic acid food sources (USDA, 2016).

Product	Pantothenic acid (mg)	% AI*	Category
Cereal, 1 cup	0.2	4%	Grains
Power bar, 1	10.0	200%	Meat and Beans
Raw mushrooms, 100 g	2.0	40%	Vegetables
Plain yogurt, 100 g	0.4	8%	Dairy
AI	5	100%	

*AI = Adequate Intake for adult male and female 5 mg; Daily value = 10 mg.

FUNCTION AND USES

Pantothenic acid is vital for the body to properly use carbohydrates, proteins, and lipids and for healthy skin. Pantothenic acid is commonly used in a multitude of health related conditions even though there is no scientific evidence of the potential benefit of pantothenic acid on these types of applications. Some individuals take pantothenic acid as supplement for acne, alcoholism, allergies, asthma, attention deficit-hyperactivity disorder (ADHD), autism, baldness, burning feet syndrome, celiac disease, colitis, conjunctivitis, convulsions, carpal tunnel syndrome, cystitis, heart failure, respiratory disorders, treatment of dietary deficiencies, and tongue infections, such as yeast infections. Other individuals take pantothenic acid by mouth for skin related conditions including dandruff and other issues such as depression, diabetic nerve pain, enhancing immune function, improving athletic performance, headache, dizziness, hypoglycemia, insomnia, irritability, hypotension, multiple sclerosis, muscular dystrophy, muscular cramps in the legs associated with pregnancy or alcoholism, neuralgia, and obesity. Pantothenic acid is also taken orally for benign prostate hyperplasia, osteoarthritis / rheumatoid arthritis, Parkinson's disease, premenstrual syndrome, protection against mental and physical stress and anxiety, reducing adverse effects of thyroid therapy in congenital hypothyroidism, reducing signs of aging, reducing susceptibility to colds and other infections, retarded growth, shingles, stimulating adrenal glands, chronic fatigue syndrome, minimizing symptoms of salicylate toxicity, combating streptomycin neurotoxicity, and wound healing. People apply topically to the skin a product that contains pantothenic acid, dexpanthenol, for itching, promoting healing of mild eczemas and other skin conditions, insect stings, bites, poison ivy, diaper rash, and acne. In some cases, it has also been applied to prevent skin reactions to radiation therapy (Wardlaw and Smith, 2011, American Dietetic Association, 2005).

GROUPS AT RISK

Deficiency might occur in people with alcoholism that have a nutrient-deficient diet (Wardlaw and Smith, 2011).

BIOTIN

Adequate Intake of biotin for adults is 30 mg per day (Fig. **13**). The daily value used in food and dietary supplements to express biotin content is 30 mcg. Biotin is considered non-toxic; hence, no Upper limit has been set (Wardlaw and Smith, 2011, Food and Nutrition Board, 1998).

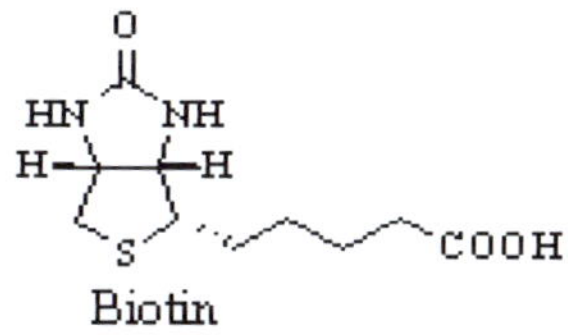

Fig. (13). Structure of Biotin (Wardlaw and Smith, 2011, Lemke and Williams, 2008).

FOOD SOURCES

Biotin is a vitamin that is found in small quantities in a variety of foods. The current dietary pattern in North America provides 40-600 mcg of biotin per day. Different sources of biotin from four different categories (Table **11** for main sources) include American cheese (0.7 mcg covers to 3% AI), boiled egg (9.3 mcg covers to 31% AI), Cheddar cheese (0.9 mcg covers to 3% AI), cooked egg yolk (8.1 mcg covers to 27% AI), cooked lamb liver (11.6 mcg covers to 39% AI), egg noodles (4.0 mcg covers to 13% AI), nonfat milk (4.9 mcg covers to 16% AI), roasted peanut (1.3 mcg covers to 4.4% AI), salmon (1.4 mcg covers to 5% AI), Swiss cheese (1.1 mcg covers to 4% AI), and wheat bran (6.4 mcg covers to 21% AI) (Wardlaw and Smith, 2011).

Table 11. Biotin food sources (Staggs *et al.*, 2004).

Product	Biotin (μg)	% AI*	Category
Peanut, 1 s	5.0	17%	Meat and Beans
Yogurt, 1 s	0.1	0.3%	Dairy
Frosted flakes, 1 s	0.04	0.1%	Grains
Raw cauliflower, 1 s	0.05	0.1%	Vegetables
AI	30.0	100%	

*AI = Adequate Intake for adult male and female 30 μg; Daily value = 30 μg.

FUNCTION AND USES

Biotin is a key component of the body enzymes that metabolize certain substances like fats, carbohydrates, and others. There is not a good laboratory test to detect biotin deficiency and there is not enough scientific evidence to support all its uses.

Symptoms that identify deficiency of biotin include thinning of the hair (frequently with loss of hair color) and red scaly rash around the eyes, nose, and mouth. Biotin is taken orally for preventing and treating deficiency connected with pregnancy, tube feeding in long-term illnesses, malnutrition, and rapid weight loss. It is also used orally for brittle nails, diabetes, skin rash in infants (seborrheic dermatitis), and mild depression (Wardlaw and Smith, 2011, American Dietetic Assocaition, 2005).

FOLATE

The synthetic chemical form of folate is folic acid (Fig. **14**). Natural folate contains extra units of glutamic acid that need to be removed before absorption, making folic acid more readily absorbed (1.7 times greater). The RDA of folate is 400 mcg per day for adults. Dietary recommendations are based on dietary folate equivalents (DFE) that includes both natural folate and synthetic folic acid added to foods (Wardlaw and Smith, 2011, Food and Nutrition Board, 1998).

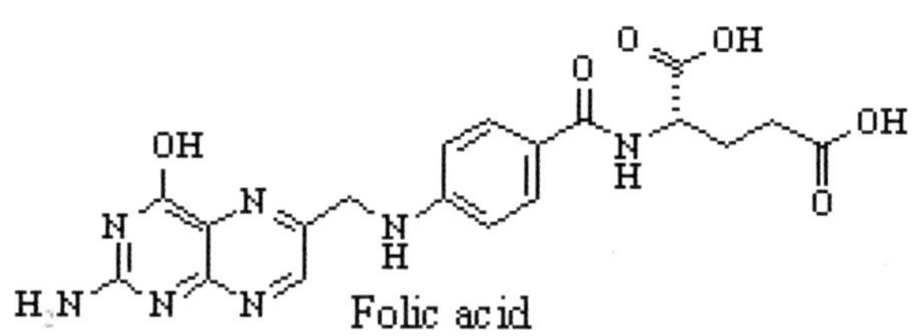

Fig. (14). Structure of folic acid (Wardlaw and Smith, 2011, Lemke and Williams, 2008).

FOOD SOURCES

Rich sources of folate include dried beans, green leafy vegetables, organ meats, sprouts, and orange juice. Steaming, stir-frying, or microwaving are good approaches to avoid destruction of folate by heat. Different sources of folate from four different categories (Table **12** for main sources) include black-eyed peas (179 mcg covers to 45% RDA), cooked beets (68 mcg covers to 17% RDA), cooked broccoli (78 mcg covers to 20% RDA), cooked spinach (262 mcg covers to 66% RDA), cooked turnips (85 mcg covers to 21% RDA), Kidney beans (65 mcg covers to 16% RDA), Romaine lettuce (142 mcg covers to 23% RDA), Sunflower seeds (76 mcg covers to 19% RDA), and tortilla (89 mcg covers to 22% RDA) (Wardlaw and Smith, 2011).

Table 12. Folate food sources (USDA, 2016).

Product	Folate (mcg)	% RDA*	Category
Asparagus, 1 cup	70	18%	Vegetables
Cooked lentils, 1 cup	358	90%	Meat and Beans
Great Grains cereal, 1 cup	332	83%	Grains
Fresh orange juice, 1 cup	74	19%	Fruits
RDA	400	100%	

*RDA = adult male and female 400 μg; Daily value = 400 μg.

FUNCTION AND USES

Folate coenzymes help form DNA and supply or accept single carbon atoms. Research has found a link between folate and cancer prevention (Wardlaw and Smith, 2011).

GROUPS AT RISK

Deficiency might occur in pregnant women. To accommodate the increased demand of cell division and DNA synthesis, pregnant women need extra folate with a total of 600 mcg per day. There is also risk of deficiency in older people due to inadequate folate intake and decreased absorption as well as in people with alcoholism due to poor intake and absorption (Wardlaw and Smith, 2011).

FOLATE DEFICIENCY AND TOXICITY

Maternal deficiency has been linked to neural tube defects in the fetus such as spina bifida and anencephaly. The upper limit for the synthetic form of folate is 1 mg per day. Large amounts of folate consumption can hide the signs of vitamin B12 deficiency (Wardlaw and Smith, 2011, American Dietetic Association, 2005, De Wals *et al*., 2007).

CHOLINE

Choline is not included as an "official" B-vitamin (Fig. **15**). It is a chemical with similarity to the B-vitamins, and is often found together with B-complex vitamins. It is found as part of acetylcholine and of phospholipids. Although the complete mechanism of action, particularly how it interrelates with other nutrients, is not entirely understood, it seems to work together with folate and the amino acid called methionine. The adequate intake of choline is 425-550 mg per day for adults (Wardlaw and Smith, 2011, Food and Nutrition Board, 1998).

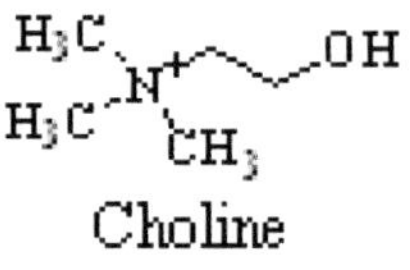

Fig. (15). Structure of choline (Wardlaw and Smith, 2011, Lemke and Williams, 2008).

FUNCTION

Choline participates in various body processes, including in the formation of cell membrane structures, protection of the liver from fat accumulation, and as precursor molecule for the neurotransmitter acetylcholine. Choline has been shown to have a protective role of the liver in preventing certain types of damage, and reversing impairment already occurred in the liver. The rapid development of fetuses and infants demands for great requirement for choline in early life. Choline started to draw more attention from nutrition researchers when it was found that mothers who did not consume enough choline in the diet have fetal rats with less brain development and poorer memories after birth than those whose mothers had an adequate intake of choline. In recent years, research has shown that adequate intake of choline may be useful in both brain development of fetuses and infants, and in preventing memory loss associated with aging (Wardlaw and Smith, 2011, American Dietetic Assocaition, 2005).

FOOD SOURCES OF CHOLINE

Most foods contain small amounts of choline, but some individuals may have to be careful in their diets, particularly if the diet does not include whole eggs. Below are some examples of foods that are particularly high in choline (taken from the USDA's Database for choline in foods*). This is in addition to the list found in Table **13** that shows different sources of choline from three different categories (Wardlaw and Smith, 2011).

- Beef liver* - when pan-fried - 100 grams (about 3.5 oz) - 418 mg choline
- Cauliflower* - 3/4 C if cooked (1" pieces) - 62 mg choline

- Navy beans* - 1/2 C if cooked - 48 mg choline
- Tofu* - 100 grams of cooked (about 3.5 oz) - 28 mg choline
- Almonds* - if sliced - 1/2 cup - 26 mg choline

Other sources include beef (12 mg covers to 2% AI male and 3% AI female), chicken (19 mg covers to 3% AI male and 4% AI female), cod (23 mg covers to 4% AI male and 5% AI female), Cotagge cheese (20 mg covers to 4% AI male and 5% AI female), peanut butter (10 mg covers to 2% AI male and 3% AI female), and yogurt (31 mg covers to 6% AI male and 7% AI female) (Wardlaw and Smith, 2011).

Table 13. Choline food sources (USDA, 2016).

Product	Choline (mg)	Male (% AI)	Female (% AI)	Category
Egg, 100 g	250	45%	59%	Meat and Beans
Fat Free Milk, 100 g	16	3%	4%	Dairy
Wheat germ toasted, 100 g	180	33%	42%	Oils
AI	425-550	100%	100%	

*AI = adult male 550 mg and female 425 mg; Daily value = 60 mg.

CHOLINE LIMITS AND ADVERSE EFFECTS

The Tolerable Upper Intake level for adults has been set at 3.5 grams (3500 mg) per day. Above this level, potential adverse effects include diarrhea, fishy body odor, and low blood pressure (Wardlaw and Smith, 2011).

VITAMIN C

Vitamin C is a water-soluble vitamin, also known as ascorbic acid (Fig. **16**) that does not belong to the B vitamin group. It is synthesized in most animals from glucose. The RDA of vitamin C is 75-90 mg per day for adults. The daily value used on food and dietary supplement labels to express vitamin C content is 60 mg (Wardlaw and Smith, 2011, Food and Nutrition Board, 2000).

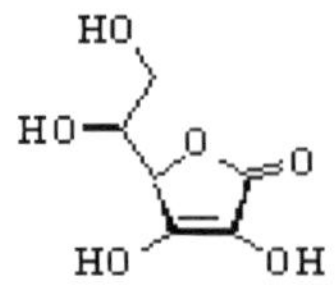

Fig. (16). Structure of vitamin C, ascorbic acid (Wardlaw and Smith, 2011, Lemke and Williams, 2008).

FUNCTION AND USES

Vitamin C is required for growth and development. Vitamin C is needed for tissue repair in all parts of the body. It has been associated with four major body functions including collagen synthesis, iron absorption, immune function, and as antioxidant (Wardlaw and Smith, 2011, Medline Plus, 2015). It is used to:

- Form collagen, an important protein used to make skin, tendons, ligaments, and blood vessels;
- Heal wounds and form scar tissue;
- Repair and maintain cartilage, bones, and teeth.

Vitamin C is an important antioxidant that may block some of the injury caused by free radicals. It may reduce in the stomach the formation of nitrosamines involved in cancer. This has been supported by some population studies, suggesting vitamin C has cancer chemopreventive properties. Vitamin C rich products have also been reported to be able to enhance iron absorption. Moreover, vitamin C is considered to be vital for immune system functions (Wardlaw and Smith, 2011, Medline Plus, 2015).

For many years, vitamin C has been used as a popular remedy for the common cold, but according to the literature (Medline Plus, 2015, American Dietetic Association, 2005):

- foods containing large amounts of vitamin C or the intake of vitamin C supplements do not decrease the risk of common cold;
- taking vitamin C supplements regularly might slightly shorten the time of colds or to some extent reduce intensity of symptoms; and

- taking vitamin C supplement after a cold starts does not seem to reduce symptoms or shorten the time.

FOOD SOURCES

All fruits and vegetables contain some quantities of vitamin C. Vitamin-C rich fruits include: cantaloupe, blueberries, cranberries, orange and other citrus fruits, mango, papaya, raspberries, and watermelon. Vitamin-C rich vegetables include: cabbage, turnip greens, and other leafy greens, and winter squash. Overall, the best food sources of vitamin C are uncooked or raw fruits and vegetables (Wardlaw and Smith, 2011, Medline Plus, 2015). Different sources of vitamin C from two different categories (Table **14** for main sources) include cooked broccoli (33 mg covers to 37% RDA male and 44% RDA female), cooked spinach (9 mg covers to 10% RDA male and 12% RDA female), grapefruit juice (80 mg covers to 89% RDA male and 107% RDA female), green pepper rings (9 mg covers to 10% RDA male and 12% RDA female), kale (27 mg covers to 30% RDA male and 36% RDA female), kiwi fruit (57 mg covers to 63% RDA male and 76% RDA female), pineapple chunks (12 mg covers to 13% RDA male and 16% RDA female), raw cauliflower (23 mg covers to 26% RDA male and 31% RDA female), red peppers (71 mg covers to 79% RDA male and 95% RDA female), strawberries (94 mg covers to 104% RDA male and 125% RDA female), and sweet potato (17 mg covers to 19% RDA male and 23% RDA female) (Wardlaw and Smith, 2011).

Table 14. Vitamin C food sources (USDA, 2016).

Product	Vitamin C (mg)	Male* (% RDA)	Female* (% RDA)	Category
Orange, 1 unit	68	76%	91%	Fruits
Baked potato, 1 medium	20	22%	27%	Vegetable
Cooked Brussels sprouts, 1 cup	97	108%	129%	Vegetable
Tomato juice, 1 cup	170	189%	227%	Vegetable
RDA	75 - 90	100%	100%	

*RDA = adult male 90 mg and female 75 mg; Daily value = 60 mg.

Some cereals and other foods and beverages have been fortified with vitamin C. The product labels describe the amount of vitamin C is in the product. Cooking vitamin C-rich foods or storing them for a long period of time can decrease the content of vitamin C. This could cause deficiency of this vitamin. Microwaving and steaming vitamin C-rich foods may minimize cooking losses (Wardlaw and Smith, 2011).

SIDE EFFECTS

Serious side effects from high intake or high doses of vitamin C are very rare, because the body does not store vitamin C. However, the upper limit of vitamin C is 2,000 mg per day because high doses can lead to stomach upset and diarrhea (Wardlaw and Smith, 2011).

GROUPS AT RISK

The daily amount of vitamin C should be increased at any age by 35 mg per day above the RDA in smoking individuals or those who are around (secondhand smoke). Women, who are pregnant or breastfeeding, need higher intake of vitamin C (Wardlaw and Smith, 2011, American Dietetic Association, 2005).

VITAMIN C DEFICIENCY

Scurvy is a severe form of vitamin C deficiency and it mainly affects older, malnourished adults. No vitamin C intake for over 20 days can lead to the appearance of scurvy symptoms. Scurvy was a disease that was common among marine travelers throughout the history since they did not have access to fresh fruits and vegetables during the journey. Inadequate intake of vitamin C can lead to deficiency signs and symptoms, including: bleeding gums, decreased ability to fight infection, easy bruising, gingivitis (inflammation of the gums), nosebleeds, weakened tooth enamel, possible weight gain due to slowed metabolism, dry and splitting hair, rough-dry-scaly skin, decreased wound-healing rate, swollen and painful joints (Wardlaw and Smith, 2011).

WATER

Water is essential for life (Fig. **17**). The adequate intake of water per day is 2.7 liters for adult women and 3.7 liters for adult men. This water is used mostly to produce urine and the rest is used to compensate typical body water losses. Humans can only survive a few days without drinking water. It dissolves body compounds such as NaCl and enables chemical reactions to occur by serving as medium. Water makes up 50-70% of body weight (~ 10 gal). Lean body tissue contains 73% and the adipose tissue contains 20% water. Ion concentration and movement controls the level of water in both compartments, intra- and extra-cellular. Osmosis is used to control the movement of ions such as sodium (Na^+), potassium (K^+), chloride (Cl^-), phosphate (PO_4^-), magnesium (Mg^{++}), and calcium (Ca^{++}). The volume of intracellular water depends on the concentration of K^+ and PO_4^- while the extracellular water depends on Na^+ and Cl^- (Wardlaw and Smith, 2011, American Dietetic Association, 2005).

Water has great ability to hold heat. Molecules of water are attracted to each other so energy is needed to separate them and due to the type of bonds much energy is needed to heat water than it is needed to heat fat. Perspiration is the way the body uses to control its temperature. As perspiration evaporates through skin pores, heat energy is moved away from the skin, cooling it in the process and preventing elevation in body temperature. Dissipation of the heat from the body allows enzyme systems to function efficiently (Wardlaw and Smith, 2011).

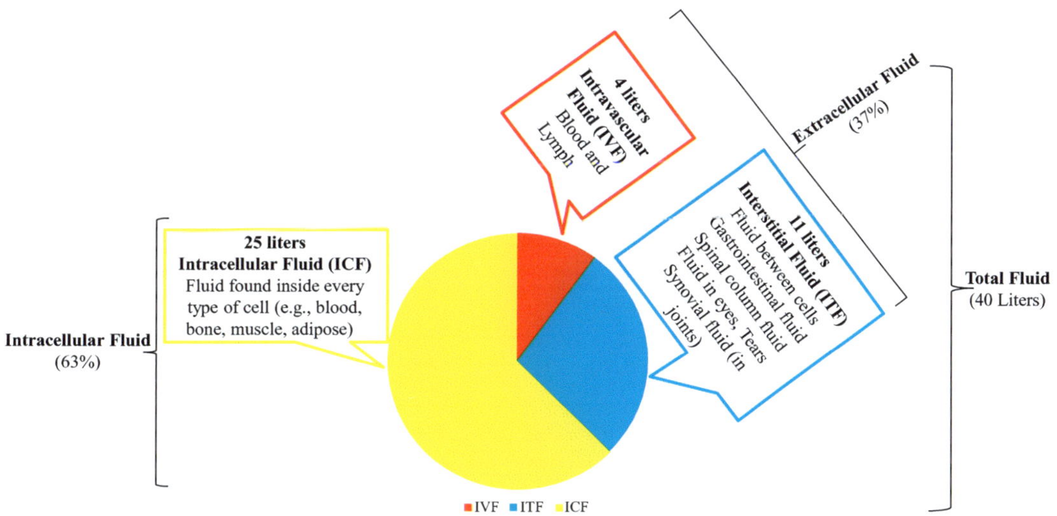

Fig. (17). Water in body composition (Wardlaw and Smith, 2011).

Lack of drinking enough water signals your brain to communicate the need to drink by the warning sign of thirst. If the signal of thirst is ignored, the body identifies the shortage and begins the process of fluid conservation through the pituitary gland by releasing antidiuretic hormone. Excessive water intake can overwhelm the kidneys, create an unbalance of blood electrolyte concentration and result in blurred vision (Wardlaw and Smith, 2011).

WATER SOURCES

Water is found in many of the food items consumed as part of the diet. Some food items contain higher % of water that others. Examples of products from seven different categories are presented in the figure below (Fig. **18**) in addition to apple (75-100%), banana (50-75%), bread (25-50%), lettuce (75-100%), potato (50-75%), steak (25-50%), ham (25-50%), and honey (1-25%) (Wardlaw and Smith, 2011).

BEVERAGE CONSUMPTION

According to the Beverage Guidance System, fluids from a healthy diet should not provide significant amount of calories (<10% of total calories consumed) or nutrients (Wardlaw and Smith, 2011).

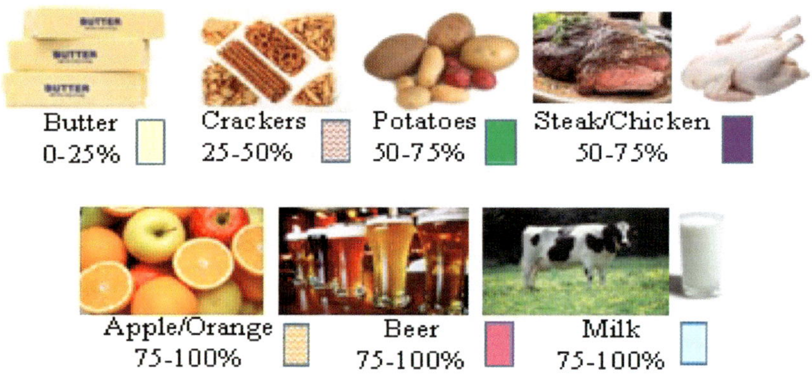

Fig. (18). Water in different categories of dietary products (Wardlaw and Smith, 2011).

WATER SUPPLY AND SAFETY

Bottled water has become the preferred source. Both bottled and tap water are regulated by the FDA and Environmental Protection Agency (EPA), respectively. Contamination of public water by *Cryptosporidium*, a parasite, could be a concern. Chlorine and ammonia are added to kill bacteria present in the water. Additionally, contamination by other substances such as lead and nitrates creates concern mainly in the preparation of infant formulas. Local municipal water departments are required to mail customers each year the results of analysis of contaminants including bacteria, various chemicals and heavy metals (Wardlaw and Smith, 2011).

MINERALS

Minerals are classified based on the amount needed per day. Recommended amount for major minerals is greater than 100 mg; trace minerals require less than that (Fig. **19**). The bioavailability of these minerals depend on factors such as natural source, presence of binding agents in the natural source that hinder absorption, *etc.* Examples of these binders include fiber, oxalic acid, phytic acid, *etc* (Wardlaw and Smith, 2011, American Dietetic Association, 2005).

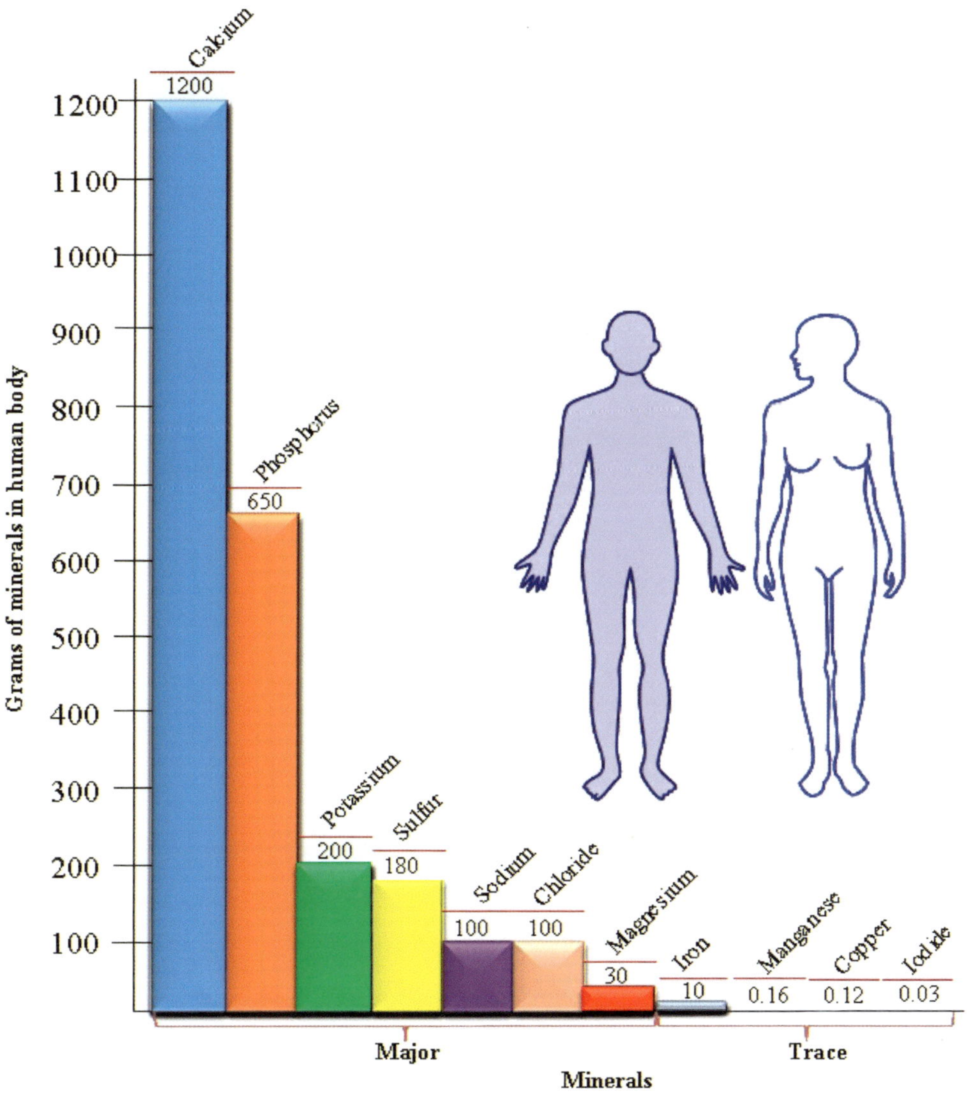

Fig. (19). Major and trace minerals in the diet (Wardlaw and Smith, 2011).

MACROMINERALS OR MAJOR MINERALS

Sodium

The main source of sodium (Na) is table salt that contains sodium chloride. Sodium chloride contains 40% sodium and 60% chloride. A teaspoon of table salt contains about 2 g of sodium. The body absorbs almost all consumed Na, which is then used to retain body water as it becomes the major positive ion in the extracellular fluid. Adequate intake of sodium is 1500 mg for adults under age 51. Older adults require between 100 and 200 mg less than that. The daily value used in food and dietary supplements labels to express Na is 2400 mg (Wardlaw and Smith, 2011).

Sources

As can be seen on Fig. **20**, most of the sodium consumed is added during food preparation. Most natural food products contain small amount of sodium, except milk that contains 120 mg per cup (Wardlaw and Smith, 2011).

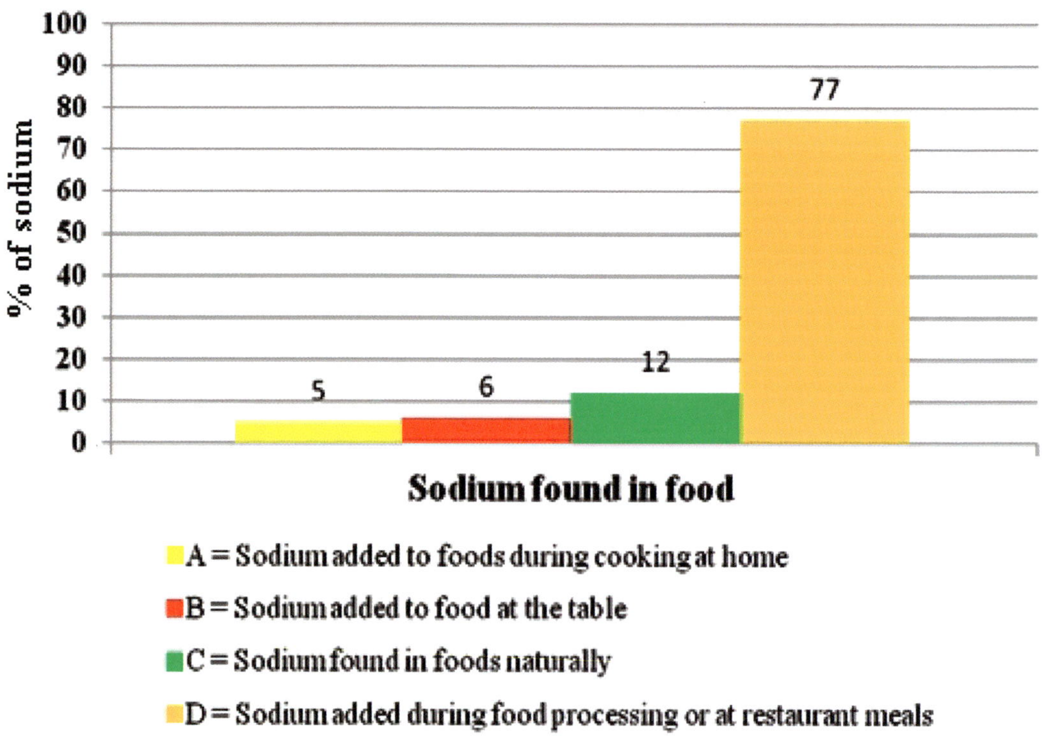

Fig. (20). Sodium found in food. (Wardlaw and Smith, 2011)

Humans can adapt to salt content in foods. To become accustomed to low levels of sodium in food the sodium taste can be substituted by herbs, lemon juice, and spices. Different sources of sodium from four different categories (Table **15** for main sources) include animal crackers (112 mcg covers to 7% AI), canned green beans (390 mcg covers to 26% AI), Cheddar cheese (176 mcg covers to 12% AI), hard pretzels (486 mcg covers to 32% AI), macaroni salad (561 mcg covers to 37% AI), non-fat milk (127 mcg covers to 8% AI), peanut butter (78 mcg covers to 5% AI), Saltine crackers (39 mcg covers to 3% AI), and seven grain bread (126 mcg covers to 8% AI) (Wardlaw and Smith, 2011).

Sodium Deficiency and Side Effects

Depletion of body sodium can lead to symptoms such as dizziness, muscle cramps, nausea vomiting, shock and coma. The upper level of sodium is 2300 mg for adults. Higher levels increase blood pressure and certain individuals are sodium sensitive (Wardlaw and Smith, 2011).

Table 15. Sodium food sources (USDA, 2016).

Product	Sodium (mg)	% AI*	Category
Pepperoni pan crust pizza, 1 slice	664	44%	Protein
Ham, honey, smoked, 1 ounce	255	17%	Protein
Chicken noodle soup, canned, 1 cup	1689	113%	Grains
V8 vegetable juice, 1 ounce	60	4%	Vegetable
Hamburger with bun, 1 each	194	13%	Protein
Grape juice, 1 ounce	3	0.2%	Fruits
AI	1500	100%	

*AI = male and female 1500 mg; Daily value = 2400 mg.

Potassium

Potassium (K) also participates in fluid balance and nerve impulse transmission as Na does. The intracellular fluids contain about 95% of the K in the body. The adequate intake for K is 4700 mg per day for adults. The daily value used in food and dietary supplements to express K is 3500 mg. Even though fruits and vegetables contain K, diets are likely low in K since K is not added to foods during preparation (Wardlaw and Smith, 2011).

Sources

The main sources of potassium include dried beans, fruits, meats, milk, vegetables, and whole grains. Different sources of potassium from four different categories (Table **16** for main sources) include artichoke (425 mg covers to 9% AI), baked potato (385 mg covers to 8% AI), banana (470 mg covers to 10% AI), buttermilk (370 mg covers to 8% AI), cantaloupe (495 mg covers to 11% AI), Lima beans (480 mg covers to 10% AI), pinto beans (400 mg covers to 9% AI), sirloin steak (115 mg covers to 2% AI), soybeans (440 mg covers to 9% AI), tomato juice (113 mg covers to 3% AI), and zucchini (450 mg covers to 10% AI) (Wardlaw and Smith, 2011).

Table 16. Potassium food sources (USDA, 2016).

Product	Potassium (mg)	% AI*	Category
Kidneys beans, 1 cup	2587	55%	Protein
Winter squash, 1 cup cubes	486	10%	Vegetables
Plain yogurt, 1 cup	380	8%	Dairy
Orange juice canned, 1 cup	458	10%	Fruits
AI	4700	100%	

*AI = male and female 4700 mg; Daily value = 3500 mg.

POTASSIUM DEFICIENCY AND SIDE EFFECTS

Over consumption of K is associated with lower blood pressure. Hence, a balanced diet rich in potassium could help people at risk of high blood pressure. People with alcoholism and people consuming food deficient in potassium can suffer severe potassium deficiency. Other individuals at risk include athletes and those with kidney problems. A balanced diet will not lead to K toxicity; hence, no upper limit has been set (Wardlaw and Smith, 2011).

Chloride

Chloride (Cl) is an important negative ion found in the extracellular fluid that plays a role in acid-base regulation. It is also part of the stomach acid and participates in immune responses when white cells fight foreign cells. Adequate intake of chloride is 2300 mg per day for adults. The daily value used in food and dietary supplement labels to express chloride is 3400 mg (Wardlaw and Smith, 2011).

Sources

Most of the chloride consumed comes from the salt added to the food. Some fruits and vegetables are good sources of chloride as well as chlorinated water. Chloride should not be confused with chlorine, which is a poisonous gas (Wardlaw and Smith, 2011).

Chloride Deficiency and Side Effects

Due to the high consumption of salt, deficiency of chloride is unlikely, except in cases of lengthy periods of vomiting as stomach acid contains much chloride. The upper level for chloride is 3600 mg per day for adults (Wardlaw and Smith, 2011).

Calcium

Calcium (Ca) is needed for growth and bone development as well as to strengthen bones and teeth. Ca participates in blood clotting and muscle contraction as well. Adequate intake of Ca is 1000-1200 mg per day for adults. The daily value used in food and dietary supplement labels to express Ca is 1000 mg (Wardlaw and Smith, 2011).

Sources

About 75% of Ca in American diet comes from dairy products. Other sources rich in Ca include canned salmon, leafy green vegetables, and sardines. To efficiently absorb Ca, an acidic pH is needed and the amount of Ca in the body depends on the level of absorption of Ca from the diet or from the dietary supplement. Additional factors that enhance Ca absorption include levels of parathyroid hormone in the blood, motility of digestive contents (chime) towards the intestine, and presence of glucose and lactose in the diet.

Different sources of Ca from five different categories (Table **17** for main sources) include buttermilk (285 mg covers to 29% RDA), Cheddar cheese (200 mg covers to 20% RDA), chocolate pudding (160 mg covers to 16% RDA), Parmesan cheese (390 mg covers to 39% RDA), Romano cheese (300 mg covers to 30% RDA), sardines (85 mg covers to 14% RDA), Swiss cheese (275 mg covers to 28% RDA), and tofu (140 mg covers to 14% RDA) (Wardlaw and Smith, 2011).

Table 17. Calcium food sources (USDA, 2016).

Product	Calcium (mg)	% RDA*	Category
Plain yogurt, 1 cup	296	30%	Dairy
Fortified orange juice, 1 cup	349	35%	Fruits
Skim milk fortified, 1 cup	504	50%	Dairy
Spinach, 1 cup	30	3%	Vegetables
Salmon (with bones), 1 ounce	71	7%	Protein
Total Raisin Bran cereal, 1 cup	1000	100%	Grains
RDA	1000	100%	

*RDA = male and female 1000 mg; Daily value = 1000 mg.

Most of the Ca present in leafy green vegetables is not absorbed because of the oxalic acid found in these sources. Other factors limiting the absorption of Ca include diarrhea, high consumption of phosphorous and magnesium in the diet, high content of phytic acid in the fiber consumed from grains, old age, presence of polyphenols in tea, and vitamin D deficiency (Wardlaw and Smith, 2011).

Calcium Deficiency and Side Effects

Tetany and failing of nerve functions can result when Ca levels fall below a critical point because muscles cannot relax and ions cannot flow in and out of nerve cells due to lack of enough Ca. Intake of Ca has been associated with different disease states including cancer, high cholesterol, hypertension, kidney stones, and obesity. The upper level of Ca is 2500 mg per day for adults based on the risk of kidney stones. Excessive intake of Ca causes headache, kidney failure, soft tissue calcification, and reduction in the absorption of other minerals (Wardlaw and Smith, 2011).

Magnesium

Magnesium (Mg) is mainly found as part of the plant pigments such as chlorophyll. It is an important mineral because it is used by enzymes and in many energy-yielding reactions inside the cells. The daily RDA for Mg is 400 mg for men and 310 mg for women. The daily value listed on food and dietary supplement labels to express Mg is 400 mg (Wardlaw and Smith, 2011, Food and Nutrition Board, 1997).

Sources

The plant kingdom is a rich source of Mg including beans, nuts, seeds, and whole grains. Additional sources include meats and milk (Wardlaw and Smith, 2011). Different sources of Mg from five different categories (Table **18** for main sources) include black-eyed peas (46 mg covers to 12% RDA male and 15% RDA female), broccoli (34 mg covers to 9% RDA male and 12% RDA female), Kidney beans (41 mg covers to 11% RDA male and 14% RDA female), oatmeal (28 mg covers to 7% RDA male and 9% RDA female), peanut butter (25 mg covers to 7% RDA male and 8% RDA female), squash (105 mg covers to 26% RDA male and 34% RDA female), Sunflower seeds (37 mg covers to 10% RDA male and 13% RDA female), watermelon (32 mg covers to 8% RDA male and 10% RDA female), wheat germ (90 mg covers to 23% RDA male and 29% RDA female), and whole-wheat bread (25 mg covers to 6% RDA male and 8% RDA female) (Wardlaw and Smith, 2011).

Table 18. Magnesium food sources (USDA, 2016).

Product	Magnesium (mg)	Adult Male % RDA*	Adult Female % RDA*	Category
Spinach, 1 cup	24	6%	8%	Vegetables
Raisin Bran cereal, 1 cup	32	8%	10%	Grains
Navy beans, 1 cup	105	26%	34%	Protein
Plain yogurt, 1 cup	29	7%	9%	Dairy
Banana, 1 medium	32	8%	10%	Fruits
1% milk, 1 cup	34	9%	11%	Dairy
RDA	400 & 310	100%	100%	

*RDA = male 400 mg and female 310 mg; Daily value = 400 mg.

Magnesium Deficiency and Side Effects

People consuming diuretics and those with long periods of vomiting and diarrhea could be at risk of Mg deficiency. People with alcoholism are also at risk of Mg deficiency due to increased urine excretion. Some of the symptoms associated with

Mg deficiency include disorientation, muscle pain, seizures, and weakness. The upper level for Mg is 350 mg per day. The main complication of excessive Mg; diarrhea, is avoided by ingesting less than the upper level amount per day. Toxicity of Mg can occur in individuals with kidney issues (Wardlaw and Smith, 2011).

Phosphorous

Phosphorus (P) is found in bones, cell membranes, DNA (genetic material), and enzymes as well as in the bloodstream and inside cells. The RDA is 700 mg per day for adult. The daily value used in food and dietary supplement labels to express P is 1000 mg (Wardlaw and Smith, 2011, Food and Nutrition Board, 1997).

Sources

Bread, cheese, meat, and milk are good sources of P in American diet. Other sources include bran, breakfast cereals, eggs, fish, and nuts. Different sources of P from three different categories (Table **19** for main sources) include Cheddar cheese (147 mg covers to 21% RDA), chicken breast (60 mg covers to 9% RDA), hard broiled eggs (100 mg covers to 15% RDA), Lean ham (55 mg covers to 8% RDA), pot roast (57 mg covers to 8% RDA), roasted turkey (60 mg covers to 9% RDA), Sunflower seeds (330 mg covers to 47% RDA), and Swiss cheese (345 mg covers to 49% RDA) (Wardlaw and Smith, 2011).

Table 19. Phosphorus food sources (USDA, 2016).

Product	Phosphorus (mg)	% RDA*	Category
Plain yogurt, 1 cup	233	33%	Dairy
Almonds, 1 cup	688	98%	Protein
1% Milk, 1 cup	245	35%	Dairy
Salmon, 1 ounce	80	11%	Protein
Raisin Bran cereal, 1 cup	100	14%	Grains
Sirloin steak, 1 ounce	53	8%	Protein
American cheese, 1 slice	135	19%	Dairy
RDA	700	100%	

*RDA = male and female 700 mg; Daily value = 1000 mg.

Phosphorus Deficiency and Side Effects

The upper level of P is 3-4 g per day. This value is reduced in those with kidney impairment. High intake of P is correlated with low absorption of Ca and can contribute with bone loss (Wardlaw and Smith, 2011).

Microminerals

Iron

Iron (Fe) is found in every cell and is mainly contained in the hemoglobin of the red blood cells. The importance of Fe in the diet has been recognized for centuries. The type of Fe present in the foods determines the level of absorption. Heme iron, from animal sources, is absorbed 2-3 times more efficiently than non-heme iron (elemental iron). When both types are consumed together, the absorption of non-heme iron is increased. This is the only mineral for which young women have a higher RDA than men. The RDA for women between 18 and 50 years of age is 18 mg. The RDA is 8 mg per day for men and for women over 50 years of age. The daily value used in food and dietary supplement labels to express Fe is 18 mg (Wardlaw and Smith, 2011, Food and Nutrition Board, 2001).

Sources

The best sources of Fe are animal sources since they contain the most bioavailable form, heme iron. Other sources include bakery products, legumes, peas, and ready-to-eat breakfast cereals (Wardlaw and Smith, 2011). Quinoa is also a rich source of iron from plant origin. Different sources of Fe from three different categories (Table **20** for main sources) include artichoke (1.7 mg covers to 21% RDA male and 9% RDA female), baked potato (1.7 mg covers to 21% RDA male and 9% RDA female), Braunschweiger sausage (2.7 mg covers to 34% RDA male and 15% RDA female), flour tortilla (2.4 mg covers to 30% RDA male and 13% RDA female), fried beef liver (3.6 mg covers to 45% RDA male and 20% RDA female), garbanzo beans (2.4 mg covers to 30% RDA male and 13% RDA female), Kidney beans (5.3 mg covers to 66% RDA male and 29% RDA female), Navy beans (2.3 mg covers to 29% RDA male and 13% RDA female), parsley (3.7 mg covers to 46% RDA male and 21% RDA female), pot roast (1 mg covers to 12% RDA male and 6% RDA female) shrimp (0.9 mg covers to 11% RDA male and 5% RDA female), and sirloin steak (1 mg covers to 12% RDA male and 4% RDA female) (Wardlaw and Smith, 2011).

Table 20. Iron food sources (USDA, 2016).

Product	Iron (mg)	Male % RDA*	Female % RDA*	Category
Oat bran cereal, 100 g	0.97	12%	5%	Grains
Raw clams, 1 ounce	0.46	6%	3%	Protein
Spinach, 1 cup	0.81	10%	5%	Vegetables
RDA	8 & 18	100%	100%	

*RDA = adult male 8 mg and adult female 18 mg; Daily value = 18 mg.

Iron Deficiency and Side Effects

The daily upper level for iron is 45 mg. Stomach irritation is more likely to occur at intakes greater than the daily value. Symptoms of iron deficiency include apathy, fatigue loss of appetite, pale skin, and poor temperature regulation. Iron deficiency is the major type of anemia worldwide. People at risk of developing iron deficiency include children depending on milk and pregnant women. Toxicity symptoms can also develop by over consumption of Fe since iron can easily build up in the body (Wardlaw and Smith, 2011).

Zinc

Zinc (Zn) absorption is influenced by the type of source. Additionally, other minerals compete with Zn or decrease its absorption such as Ca, copper and iron. Zn is necessary for many body functions including cell membrane structure and function, DNA synthesis, development of genitals and bones, growth, immune function, protein metabolism, and wound healing. The RDA for Zn is 11 mg and 8 mg for adult men and women, respectively. The daily value used in food and dietary supplement labels to express Zn is 15 mg (Wardlaw and Smith, 2011, Food and Nutrition Board, 2001).

Sources

Major sources of Zn include protein rich sources such as beef, milk, poultry as well as other sources such as bread and fortified breakfast cereals. In a similar fashion as in the case of iron, animal sources are the best because Zn is not bound to phytic acid, which interferes with absorption. Good plant sources that cannot be discounted include legumes, peanuts, and whole grains (Wardlaw and Smith, 2011). Different sources of Zn from three different categories (Table **21** for main sources) include black-eyed peas (2.2 mg covers to 20% RDA male and 28% RDA female), Cheddar cheese (0.9 mg covers to 8% RDA male and 11% RDA female), enriched white rice (1.1 mg covers to 10% RDA male and 14% RDA female), lamb chops (0.9 mg covers to 8% RDA male and 11% RDA female), lean ham (0.6 mg covers to 6% RDA male and 8% RDA female), peanuts (2.4 mg covers to 22% RDA male and 30% RDA female), pot roast (1.5 mg covers to 14% RDA male and 19% RDA female), ricotta cheese (1.7 mg covers to 15% RDA male and 21% RDA female), sirloin steak (1.9 mg covers to 17% RDA male and 23% RDA female), Sunflower seeds (1.5 mg covers to 14% RDA male and 19% RDA female), Swiss cheese (1.1 mg covers to 10% RDA male and 14% RDA female), and wheat germ (3.5 mg covers to 32% RDA male and 44% RDA female) (Wardlaw and Smith, 2011).

Table 21. Zinc food sources (USDA, 2016).

Product	Zinc (mg)	Male % RDA*	Female % RDA*	Category
Raw oysters, 6 units	33	300%	413%	Protein
Special K cereal, ½ cup	0.83	8%	10%	Grains
Plain yogurt, 1 cup	2.2	20%	28%	Dairy
RDA	11 & 8	100%	100%	

*RDA = adult male 11 mg and adult female 8 mg; Daily value = 15 mg.

Zinc Deficiency and Side Effects

The daily upper level for Zn is 40 mg. Excessive Zn intake can result in cramps, diarrhea, nausea, vomiting, suppress immune function, and interference with copper metabolism (Wardlaw and Smith, 2011).

Selenium

Selenium (Se) is part of an enzyme (glutathione peroxidase) that is involved in reducing cell membrane damage and contributes to thyroid hormone metabolism. The daily RDA for Se in adults is 55 mcg. The daily value used in food and dietary supplement labels to express Se is 70 mcg (Wardlaw and Smith, 2011, Food and Nutrition Board, 2000).

Sources

Animal sources of Se include eggs, fish, organ meats, and shellfish. Good plant sources include grains and seeds (Wardlaw and Smith, 2011). Different sources of Se from two different categories (Table **22** for main sources) include chicken breast (7 mcg covers to 12% RDA), clams (14 mcg covers to 75% RDA), cooked oatmeal (10 mcg covers to 18% RDA), egg noodles (35 mcg covers to 64% RDA), lean ham (14 mcg covers to 25% RDA), Oat bran cereal (14 mcg covers to 25% RDA), Raisin bran cereal (4 mcg covers to 7% RDA), Salmon (13 mcg covers to 24% RDA), and Special K cereal (17 mcg covers to 31% RDA) (Wardlaw and Smith, 2011).

Table 22. Selenium food sources (USDA, 2016).

Product	Selenium (mcg)	% RDA*	Category
Tuna, 3 ounces	51	93%	Protein
Sirloin steak, 100 g	30	75%	Protein
Wheat flour, 1 cup	74	135%	Grains
Barley flour, 1 cup	56	102%	Grains
RDA	55	100%	

*RDA = adult male and female 55 mcg; Daily value = 70 mg.

Selenium Deficiency and Side Effects

The daily upper level for Se in adults is 400 mcg. If this level is exceeded, hair loss is a primary sign of toxicity (Wardlaw and Smith, 2011).

Iodide

Because iodine is found in foods in the form of an ion, it is called iodide (I). The RDA for iodide in adults is 150 mcg per day. The daily value used in food and supplement labels to express iodide is the same as the RDA (Wardlaw and Smith, 2011, Food and Nutrition Board, 2001).

Sources

Iodide is found in various forms in dairy, grains, iodized salt, saltwater fish, and seafood. Many countries require iodide fortification of the salt (Wardlaw and Smith, 2011). Different sources of I from four different categories (Table **23** for main sources) include buttermilk (60 mcg covers to 40% RDA), 1% cottage cheese (28 mcg covers to 19% RDA), Luna bar (38 mcg covers to 25% RDA), 1% Milk (59 mcg covers to 39% RDA), soy protein bar (38 mcg covers to 25% RDA), and Mozzarella cheese (10 mcg covers to 7% RDA) (Wardlaw and Smith, 2011).

Iodide Deficiency and Side Effects

The daily upper level for iodide in adults is 1.1 mg per day. Excessive consumption of iodide inhibits thyroid hormone synthesis as in deficiency. Enlarged thyroid gland (goiter) is observed with iodide deficiency (Wardlaw and Smith, 2011).

Table 23. Iodide food sources (NIH, 2016).

Product	Iodide (mcg)	% RDA*	Category
Iodized table salt, ¼ tsp	71	47%	---
Plain yogurt, 1 cup	75	50%	Dairy
Shrimp, 3 ounces	35	23%	Grains
Egg, 1 unit	24	16%	Protein
RDA	150	100%	

*RDA = adult male and female 150 mcg; Daily value = 150 mcg.

Copper

Copper (Cu) is an important mineral as it participates in the metabolism of Fe. Cu is needed by many enzymes including the one involved in the release of Fe from storage. Absorption of Cu can be reduced by fiber, Fe, phytates, and Zn. The RDA for Cu in adults is 900 mcg per day. The daily value used in food and supplement labels to express Cu is 2 mg (Wardlaw and Smith, 2011, Food and Nutrition Board, 2001).

Sources

The main sources of Cu are cereals, cocoa, legumes, liver, nuts, seafood, seeds, and whole grain breads (Wardlaw and Smith, 2011).

Copper Deficiency and Side Effects

Deficiency of Cu can develop anemia, bone loss, low white blood cell count, poor growth, and even cardio vascular diseases. People at risk of developing Cu deficiencies include infants and those recovering from intestinal surgery. The daily upper level for Cu in adults is 10 mg per day based on potential risk of toxicity symptoms such as vomiting (Wardlaw and Smith, 2011).

Fluoride

Fluoride (F) is found in foods in the form of an ion. Fluoride is an important mineral as it has been shown that it reduces the rate of dental caries. F aids the synthesis of acid resistant tooth enamel, making teeth strong and resistant to dental caries. The adequate intake for F in adults is 3.1-3.8 mg per day (Wardlaw and Smith, 2011, Food and Nutrition Board, 1997).

Sources

The main sources of F include seafood, seaweed, some water sources, and tea. Fluoride should not be confused with fluorine, which is a poisonous gas (Wardlaw and Smith, 2011).

Fluoride Deficiency and Side Effects

Lack of F in drinking water increases chances of caries. The daily upper level for F in children under 9 years of age is 1.3-2.2 mg and 10 mg for anyone over 9 years of age based on potential skeletal and tooth damage. High consumption of F can cause small spots on the teeth (called mottling) (Wardlaw and Smith, 2011).

Chromium

Chromium (Cr) has been shown to participate in the maintenance of glucose uptake into cells. Marginal consumption of Cr can increase the risk of developing Type 2 diabetes. The adequate intake for Cr in adults is 25-35 mcg per day. The daily value used in food and dietary supplement labels to express Cr is 120 mcg (Wardlaw and Smith, 2011, Food and Nutrition Board, 2001).

Sources

The main sources of Cr include beer, egg yolks, mushrooms, nuts, organ meats and whole grains (Wardlaw and Smith, 2011).

Chromium Deficiency and Side Effects

Cr deficiency has been associated with impaired blood glucose control and higher levels of blood cholesterol and triglycerides. People on total parental nutrition have shown Cr deficiency. Few toxicity symptoms have been reported, but no upper limit has been set (Wardlaw and Smith, 2011).

Manganese

Manganese (Mn) is sometimes confused with magnesium (Mg) in both name and in its use as part of the metabolic process. It is an important mineral in bone formation. Mn is also needed by different enzymes including those participating in CHO and free-radical metabolism (superoxide dismutase). The adequate intake for Mn in adults is 1.8-2.3 mg per day. The daily value used in food and dietary supplement labels to express Mn is 2 mg (Wardlaw and Smith, 2011, Food and Nutrition Board, 2001).

Sources

The main sources of Mn include beans, leafy vegetables, nuts, rice, oats, and whole grains (Wardlaw and Smith, 2011).

Manganese Deficiency and Side Effects

Mn deficiency has not been associated with any disease symptom. The daily upper level for Mn in adults is 11 mg per day based on the potential risk of developing nerve damage (Wardlaw and Smith, 2011).

Molybdenum

Molybdenum (Mo) is used by several human enzymes. The RDA for Mo in adults is 45 mcg per day. The daily value used in food and dietary supplement labels to express Mo is 75 mcg (Wardlaw and Smith, 2011, Food and Nutrition Board, 2001).

Sources

The main sources of Mo include beans, dairy products, nuts, and whole grains (Wardlaw and Smith, 2011).

Molybdenum Deficiency and Side Effects

Mo deficiency has not been associated with any disease symptom. The daily upper level for Mo in adults is 2 mg per day based on toxicity observed in laboratory animals such as weight loss and decreased growth (Wardlaw and Smith, 2011).

Dietary Supplements

Dietary supplements are products with the major purpose of supplementing the diet. A supplement contains one or more of the following components: amino acid, herb or other botanical, mineral, vitamin, or a dietary substance to supplement the diet which could be an extent or a combination of the 1st four ingredients on the list. Individuals take dietary supplements to decrease susceptibility to health problems (*e.g.* colds), prevent heart disease or cancer, reduce stress and improve or increase 'energy'. A possible reason for consuming supplements is the lack of interest or ability to change food habits to include recommended servings of fruits, vegetables and whole grains (Wardlaw and Smith, 2011, Ulbricht and Seamon, 2010, ODS, 2015).

Food experts and United States government agency recommendations are to use a savvy approach to your use of dietary supplements with a primary focus on ingesting a healthy diet rich in vitamins and minerals prior to considering a supplement. However, 15% of American households are unable to secure adequate food to meet their needs. Others ingest less than optimal quantities of certain nutrients even though they have adequate resources for a healthy diet, but lack of knowledge regarding RDA and corresponding natural sources of the macro and micronutrients. It is emphasized that **'nutrient needs should be met primarily through consuming foods'** (Wardlaw and Smith, 2011). However, there are those where supplement use is often needed or recommended (see Table **24** below).

Table 24. People Most Likely to Need Supplements.

Individual	Supplement
Women of childbearing age	Folic acid
Women with excessive bleeding	Iron
Women: pregnant or breast feeding	Iron, Folic acid, Calcium
Low caloric intakes (<1200 Cal per day)	Range of vitamins and minerals
Strict Vegans	Calcium, iron, zinc, Vitamin B-12 and K
Newborns	Vitamin K
Older infants	Fluoride supplements
Limited milk intake and sunlight exposure	Vitamin D
Lactose maldigestion or lactose intolerance, allergies to dairy	Calcium

products	
Age > 50	Vitamin B-12
Low Fat diets or diets low in plant oils and nuts	Vitamin E
Consume a large part of their diet as refined foods rather than as fruits, vegetables, or whole grains	Vitamins and minerals

Multivitamin and mineral supplements have been described as a 'cure-all' approach promoted by the supplement industry, health-food stores, pharmacies and supermarkets ($28-29 billion in annual sales) (ODS, 2015).

An example of a label is presented below. This label contains some of the micronutrients discussed in this chapter (Fig. **21**).

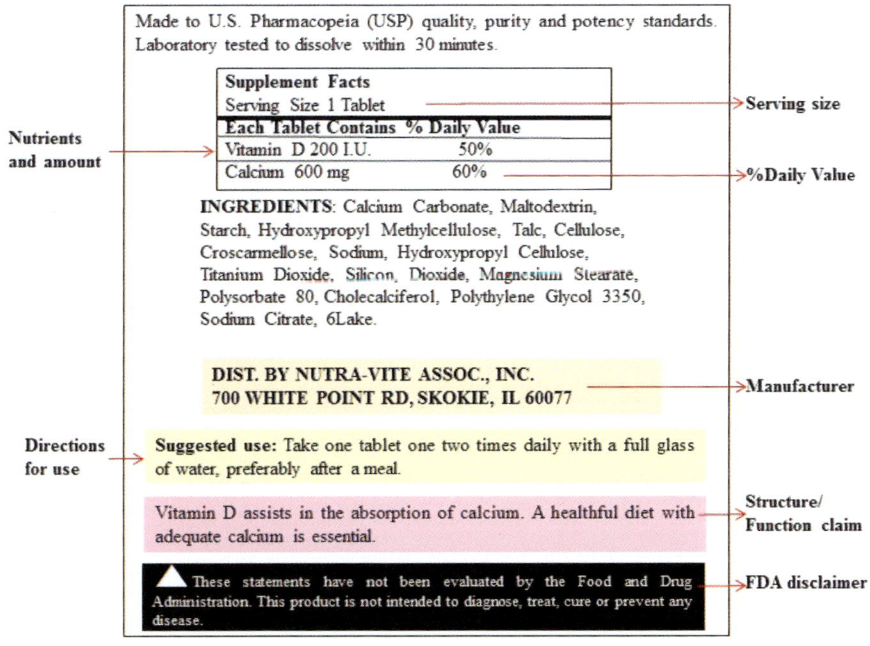

Fig. (21). Example of a dietary supplement label. Information in this figure is not accurate; it is only used for providing an example.

Some labels are more complex than others, but all should contain the basic information required by the FDA, based on Dietary Supplement Health and Education Act (DSHEA) of 1994 (Wardlaw and Smith, 2011, Ulbricht and Seamon, 2010, ODS, 2015). According to the FDA, the information required on the labels of dietary supplements includes:

- Declaration of identity

- Net measure of contents
- 'Structure-function claim and the statement "This statement has not been evaluated by the Food and Drug Administration. This product is not intended to diagnose, treat, cure, or prevent any disease".'
- Instructions for use
- Supplement-Facts section (lists active ingredient, amount, and dose)
- Other ingredients in descending order of amount and by common name or proprietary blend
- Name and place of business or manufacturer, packer or distributor.

In addition to the micronutrients discussed in this chapter, there are other nutrients that are also classified as dietary supplements that will discussed in the next chapter (s).

Are Dietary Supplements Safe?

The Food and Drug Administration does not regulate dietary supplements as drugs. Dietary supplements may be sold without proof that they are safe and effective. The FDA will regulate dietary supplements when they are: found to be inherently dangerous or marketed with an illegal claim (see Chapter 2 for more details) (ODS, 2015).

Quality of Dietary Supplements

The United States Pharmacopeia (USP) (Fig. **22**) verifies the active and inactive ingredients used in the production of these products, including: amino acids, botanical extracts, fine chemicals, non-botanicals, minerals, and vitamins. Participation in the quality control program is voluntary and open to companies that market products for use in the dietary supplement industry worldwide. The USP Verified Ingredient Mark is issued for the products that meet its highly demanding program requirements.

The Certificate of Analysis that accompanies the USP Verified Mark displayed on dietary ingredients assures the following as stated by USP:

- The ingredients are reliable in quality from batch to batch.

- The ingredients meet label or certificate of analysis entitlements for identity, strength, purity and quality.

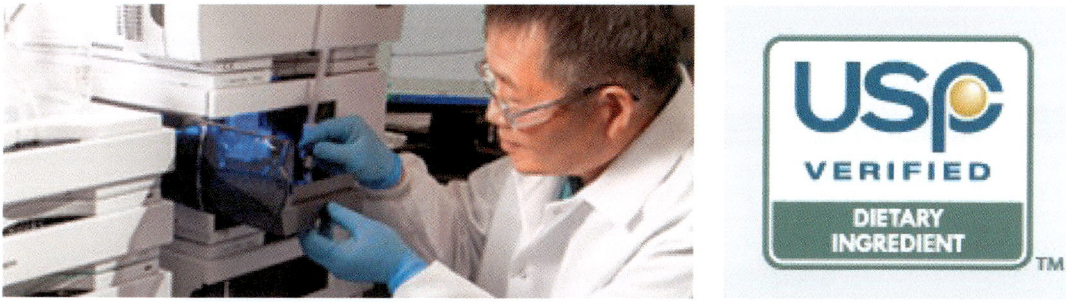

Fig. (22). Example of a USP ingredient label. Taken from the United States Pharmacopoeia Website (United States Pharmacopeia, 2015a).

- The ingredients are prepared in agreement with approved manufacturing practices.

- The ingredients meet requirements for satisfactory levels of contamination.

The USP Dietary Supplement Verification Program (Fig. **23**) is a voluntary testing and auditing platform that helps dietary supplement manufacturers guarantee the production of quality products for consumers. Manufacturers that meet the stringent USP criteria are endowed the USP Verified Mark for use on labels, packaging, and promotional materials.

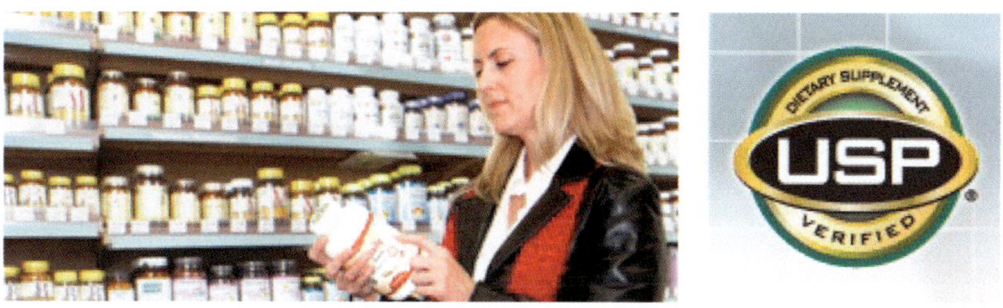

Fig. (23). Example of a USP dietary supplement label. Taken from the United States Pharmacopoeia Website (United States Pharmacopeia, 2015b).

Seeing the USP Verified Mark on a label specifies that the dietary supplement product inside:

- Contains the components listed on the label, in the stated potency and amounts.

- Does not contain unsafe levels of specified contaminants.
- Will break down and release into the body within a defined amount of time.
- Has been made according to FDA present Good Manufacturing Practices using sanitary and well-controlled techniques.

CONCLUDING REMARKS

The human body requires different micronutrients in different amounts in order to have a balanced nutrition and to function properly. This chapter have discussed the major classes of micronutrients that the body needs as part of a balanced diet, including vitamins, minerals, and water. The chapter also discussed the sources of these nutrients and how these nutrients can be absorbed and used in the metabolic process by the human body. Additionally, this chapter has given a brief overview of dietary supplements as some of these micronutrients are consumed in the form of dietary supplements. In summary, this chapter presented elements that are essential in understanding the importance of micronutrients in a balanced diet to have an adequate nutrition for the proper function of a healthy human body.

CONFLICT OF INTEREST

The authors confirm that this ebook contents have no conflict of interest.

ACKNOWLEDGMENTS

None declared.

REFERENCES

American Dietetic Association. (2005). ADA Reports: Position of the American Dietetic Association: fortification and nutritional supplements. *Journal of American Dietetic Association,* 105: 1300-1311.

Andrès, E., Affengerger, S., Vinzio, S., Kurtz, J. E., Noel, E., Kaltenbach, G., Maloisel, F., Schlienger, J. L. & Blicklé, J. F. (2005). Food-cobalamin malabsorption in elderly patients: clinical manifestations and treatment. *American Journal of Medicine,* 118: 1154-9.

American Dietetic Association. (2005). Position of the American Dietetic Association: fortification and nutritional supplements. *Journal of American Dietetic Association,* 105: 1300-1311.

De Wals, P., Tairou, F., Van Allen, M. I., Uh, S. H., Lowry, R. B., Sibbald, B., Evans, J. A., Van Den Hof, M. C., Zimmer, P., Crowley, M., Fernandez, B., Lee, N. S. & Niyonsenga, T. (2007). Reduction in neural-tube defects after folic acid fortification in Canada. *The New England Journal of Medicine,* 357: 135-42.

Edible Science. (2015). *Vitamin D3 1000IU soft-gels.* Sarasota, FL: Edible Science. Available at: http://www.ediblescience.com/store/p/55-Vitamin-D3-1000IU-soft-gels.aspx (Accessed: 2.26.2015).

Food and Nutrition Board, I. O. M. (1997). *Dietary Reference Intakes for Calcium, Phosphorus, Magnesium, Vitamin D, and Fluoride.* Washington, DC: National Academies Press.

Food and Nutrition Board, I. O. M. (1998). *Dietary Reference Intakes for Thiamin, Riboflavin, Niacin, Vitamin, B-6, Folate, Vitamin B-12, Pantothenic acid, Biotin, and choline.* Washington, DC: National Academies Press.

Food and Nutrition Board, I. O. M. (2000). *Dietary Reference Intakes for Vitamin C, Vitamin E, Selenium, and Carotenoids.* Washington, DC: National Academies Press.

Food and Nutrition Board, I. O. M. 2001. *Dietary reference Intakes for Vitamin A, Vitamin K, Arsenic, Boron, Chromium, Copper, Iodine, Iron, Manganese, Molybdenum, Nickel, Silicon, Vanadium, and Zinc.* Washington, DC: National Academies Press.

Garland, C. F., Gorham, E. D., Mohr, S. B., Grant, W. B., Giovannucci, E. L., Lipkin, M., Newmark, H., Holick, M. F. & Garland, F. C. (2007). Vitamin D and prevention of breast cancer: pooled analysis. *Journal of Steroid Biochemistry and Molecular Biology,* 103: 708-711.

Graham Solomons, T. W., Fryhle, C. B. & Snyder, S. A. (2013). *Organic Chemistry.* 11th ed. Hoboken, NJ: John Wiley and Sons, Inc.

Holick, M. F. (2004). "Sunlight and vitamin D for bone health and prevention of autoimmune diseases, cancers, and cardiovascular disease". *American Journal Clinical Nutrition*, 80:1678S-1688S.

Holick, M. F. (2007). Vitamin D deficiency. *The New England Journal of Medicine,* 357: 266-281.

Lemke, T. L. & Williams, D. A. (2008). *Foye's Principles of Medicinal Chemistry.* Baltimore, MD: Lippincott Williams & Wilkins.

Lichtenstein, A. H. & Russell, R. M. (2005). Essential nutrients: food or supplements? Where should the emphasis be? *JAMA,* 294: 351-358.

Medline Plus. (2015). *Vitamin C.* Bethesda, MD: U.S. National Library of Medicine. Available at: http://www.nlm.nih.gov/medlineplus/ency/article/002404.htm (Accessed 2.18.2015).

Nield, L. S., Mahajan, P., Joshi, A. & Kamat, D. (2006). Rickets: not a disease of the past. *American Family Physician,* 74: 619-626.

NIH (2016). Iodine. Facts Sheet for Health Professionals. National Institute of Health. Office of Dietary Supplements. Available at: https://ods.od.nih.gov/factsheets/Iodine-HealthProfessional/ (accessed 02.19.2016). (Updated 06.24.2011)

ODS. (2015). *About the Office of Dietary Supplements at the National Institutes of Health.* Bethesda, MD: National Institutes of Health. Available at: http://ods.od.nih.gov/About/ODS_Overview.aspx (Accessed 2.18.2015).

Ross, A. C., Taylor, C. L., Yaktine, A. L. & Del Valle, H. B. (2011). *Dietary Reference Intakes for Calcium and Vitamin D.* Washington, DC: National Academies Press.

Staggs, C. G., Sealey, W. M., McCabe, B. J., Teague, A. M. & Mock, D.M. (2004). Determination of the biotin content of select foods using accurate and sensitive HPLC/avidin binding. Journal Food Composition Analysis, 17(6): 767–776.

Massachusetts General Hospital. (2009). *Vitamin D Deficiency May Increase Risk Of Colds, Flu.* Rockville, MD: Science Daily. Available at: http://www.sciencedaily.com/releases/2009/02/090223221242.htm (Accessed 2.25.2015).

Ulbricht, C. & Seamon, E. (2010). Natural Standard Herbal Pharmacotherapy: An Evidence-Based Approach. *Ulster Medical Journal*. St. Louis, MO: Mosby, Elsevier, Inc.

United States Pharmacopeia. (2015a). *USP Verified Dietary Ingredients*. Rockville, MD: US Pharmacopeial Convention. Available at: http://www.usp.org/usp-verification-services/usp-verified-dietary-ingredients (Accessed 2.25.2015).

United States Pharmacopeia. (2015b). *USP Verified Dietary Supplement*. Rockville, MD: US Pharmacopeial Convention. Available at: http://www.usp.org/usp-verification-services/usp-verified-dietary-supplements (Accessed 2.25.2015).

USDA (2016). National Nutrient Database for Standard Reference. Available at: http://ndb.nal.usda.gov/ndb/foods/show/3491?fgcd=&manu=&lfacet=&format=&count=&max=35&offset=&sort=&qlookup=Sweet+potato, 11876, 09176, 01151, 04073 (accessed 02.02.2016).

USDA (2016). National Nutrient Database for Standard Reference. Available at: http://ndb.nal.usda.gov/ndb/foods/show/4714?man=&lfacet=&count=&max=&qlookup=&offset=&sort=&format=Abridged&reportfmt=other&rptfrm=&ndbno=&nutrient1=&nutrient2=&nutrient3=&subset=&totCount=&measureby=&_action_show=Apply+Changes&Qv=1&Q8892=1&Q8893=0.5, 15236, 42290, 01253, 08247 (accessed 02.22.2016).

USDA (2016). National Nutrient Database for Standard Reference. Available at: http://ndb.nal.usda.gov/ndb/foods/show/679?manu=&fgcd=, 04506, 12037, 18385, 09038, 11233, 04044, 07026, 20078, 11482, 14163, 09326, 08200, 17204, 01116, 11260, 15117, 11260, 08261, 08089, 11992, 01294, 25017 (accessed 02.15.2016).

USDA (2016). National Nutrient Database for Standard Reference. Available at: http://ndb.nal.usda.gov/ndb/foods/show/2824?manu=&fgcd=, 11011, 16070, 42297, 09206, 15076, 11363, 09040, 08067, 15157, 01116, 08020 (accessed 02.16.2016).

USDA (2016). National Nutrient Database for Standard Reference. Available at: http://ndb.nal.usda.gov/ndb/foods/show/2287?manu=&fgcd=, 09203, 11363, 11099, 11540, 21275, 07938, 06019, 31005, 28394, 14202, 01123, 01085, 08084 (accessed 02.17.2016).

USDA (2016). National Nutrient Database for Standard Reference. Available at: http://ndb.nal.usda.gov/ndb/foods/show/4766?manu=&fgcd=, 16027, 11482, 01116, 09207, 01116, 09210, 42290, 11457, 15180, 08247, 11457, 08247, 11046, 01116, 09040, 01083, 01116, 12061, 01083, 15079, 08247, 13929, 01253, 08236, 15157, 11457, 15185, 23051, 20080, 20130, 15167, 08587, 01117 (accessed 02.19.2016).

Voutilainen, S., Nurmi, T., Mursu, J. & Rissanen, T. H. (2006). Carotenoids and cardiovascular health. *American Journal of Clinical Nutrition,* 83: 1265-1271.

Wardlaw, G. M. & Smith, A. M. (2011). *Contemporary Nutrition.* 8th ed. New York, NY: McGraw Hill Education, Inc.

CHAPTER 6

Micronutrients: Nutritional Requirement Applications

Nicole Eggers, Preston Manwill, Jay Mirtallo* and Esperanza J. Carcache de Blanco*

College of Pharmacy, The Ohio State University, Columbus, Ohio, USA

Abstract: Micronutrients are required in minor quantities by the human body, but are important components of human diet. The most important groups of micronutrients include vitamins, minerals, and water. Adequate intake of these micronutrients has been associated with a good diet and good health. Analysis of the use of these micronutrients as part of the diet and the application of the concepts learned in chapter five will be presented and discussed in this chapter.

Keywords: Biotin, calcium, copper, cyanocobalamin, folate, hydrosoluble vitamins, iodide, iron, liposoluble vitamins, macrominerals, magnesium, manganese, molybdenum, niacin, pantothenic acid, potassium, riboflavin, sodium, thiamine, trace minerals, vitamin A, vitamin C, vitamin D, vitamin E, vitamin K, water, water, zinc.

INTRODUCTION

The aim of this chapter is to apply concepts learned in Chapter 5 regarding micronutrients such as vitamins, minerals, and water. For the purpose of performing calculations, RDA, RAE, and AI values will be used per dietary guidelines.

MICRONUTRIENT APPLICATIONS

The aim of this chapter is to apply concepts learned in Chapter 5 regarding micronutrients: lipo- and hydro-soluble vitamins, major minerals, and trace minerals. Every one of these micronutrients has an established daily requirement. Table **1** below outlines the daily requirements for micronutrients necessary for a healthy diet:

***Corresponding authors Esperanza J. Carcache de Blanco and Jay Mirtallo:** College of Pharmacy, The Ohio State University, Columbus, OH 43210, USA; E-mails: carcache-de-blan.1@osu.edu; mirtallo.1@osu.edu

Esperanza J. Carcache de Blanco and Jay Mirtallo (Eds)

Table 1. Daily Requirements for Water-Soluble Vitamins and Minerals.

Vitamin/Mineral	RDA		Daily Value
	Male	Female	
Vitamins			
Thiamine, mg	1.2	1.1	1.5
Riboflavin, mg	1.3	1.1	1.7
Niacin, mg (NE*)	16	14	20
Pantothenic acid, mg	5		10
Biotin, mcg	30		30
Vitamin B-6, mg	1.7	1.3	2
Folate (Folic Acid), mcg	400		400
Vitamin B-12, mcg	2.4		6
Vitamin C, mg	90	75	60
Smokers	+35		
Choline, mg	550	425	
Minerals			
Electrolytes			
Sodium, mg	1500		2400
Potassium, mg	4700		3500
Chloride, mg	2300		
Calcium, mg	1300		1000
Phosphorus, mg	700		1000
Magnesium	400-700	310-320	400
Sulfur	None		
Trace elements			
Iron, mg	8	18	18
Zinc, mg	11	8	
Selenium, mcg	55		70
Iodide, mcg	150		
Copper, mcg	900		
Fluoride, mg	3.8	3.1	
Chromium, mcg	25-35		
Manganese, mg	1.8-2.3		
Molybdenum, mcg	45		

*NE = niacin equivalents.

6.1. VITAMINS: LIPOSOLUBLE VITAMINS OVERVIEW

6.1.1. Vitamin A (Wardlaw and Smith, 2011, American Dietetic Association, 2005, Institute of Medicine, 2000, Institute of Medicine, 2001)

- The RDA for vitamin A is 700 to 900 micrograms of retinol activity equivalents (RAEs).
- The Daily Value used on food and supplement labels is 1000 micrograms (5000 IU).
- Upper limit intake is 3 mg RAE (10,000 IU)/ day.
- Women in childbearing age should limit intake to 100% of daily value (5000 IU), especially in early months of pregnancy to avoid malformations.
- Above upper limits, there is increased risk in birth defects, liver toxicity, hip fracture, and poor pregnancy outcome.

6.1.2. Vitamin D (Institute of Medicine, 1997, Nield *et al.*, 2006, Wardlaw and Smith, 2011, American Dietetic Association, 2005)

- Dietary needs are correlated to age and skin color: age under 51 the need is 5 μg/day (200 IU/day) and increases 2-3 times for older adults.
- Daily value used in food and supplements is 10 mcg (400 IU).
- Recommendations suggest adults 70 and over with limited sun exposure receive 25 μg (1000 IU) from fortified food and supplements.
- Upper limit intake for vitamin D is 50 μg (2,000 IU)/ day.
- Too much Vitamin D results in over absorption of calcium with deposits in kidneys and other organs.
- Vitamin D toxicity can also result from tanning even though the body regulates the amount made in the skin.

6.1.3. Vitamin E (Wardlaw and Smith, 2011, Institute of Medicine, 2000)

- RDA for adults is 15 mg/day of alpha-tocopherol, the most active form of vitamin E.

- A Daily Value of 30 IU expresses the vitamin E content on food and supplement labels.
- The maximum dose the body can retain on a daily basis is 200 mg and represent 300 IU of *d* -isomer (200/0.67 = 300) to 450 IU of dl isomer (200/0.45 = 450).
- The Upper Level of Vitamin E is 1000 mg/day of supplemental alpha-tocopherol.
- Higher intake of vitamin E can interfere with vitamin K's role in the clotting mechanism, leading to hemorrhage.

6.1.4. Vitamin K (Institute of Medicine, 2001, Wardlaw and Smith, 2011)

- Adequate Intake for vitamin K is 90 - 120 µg/day for adult women and men.
- A Daily Value of 80 µg is used to express vitamin K content on food and supplement labels.
- Older adults may be at risk of a deficiency because of low consumption of green vegetables.
- Oral vitamin K generally poses no risk of toxicity; hence, no Upper Level has been set.
- Megadoses reduce effectiveness of oral medications used to reduce blood clotting (*e.g.*, Coumadin).

6.2. VITAMINS: HYDROSOLUBLE VITAMINS OVERVIEW

6.2.1. Vitamin C (Institute of Medicine, 2000, Wardlaw and Smith, 2011)

- Adult RDA of Vitamin C is 75-90 mg/day.
- Daily value of 60 mg/day is used to express content on food and supplement labels.
- Upper limit for Vitamin C is 2 g/day.
- Smokers need 35 mg/day extra due to great stress on their lungs from oxygen and toxic by-products.

- Deficiency of Vitamin C is mostly observed in alcoholic people and the elderly.
- Kidneys rapidly excrete excess Vitamin C starting from 100 mg/day.
- Over upper limit may cause stomach inflammation and diarrhea.

6.2.2. Carnitine, inositol, lipoic acid, taurine (Wardlaw and Smith, 2011)

- Carnitine is needed to transport fatty acids into the mitochondria.
- Inositol is found as part of cell membranes.
- Lipoic acid participates in CHOs metabolism and acts as an antioxidant.
- Taurine is found as part of bile acids.

6.2.3. Choline (Wardlaw and Smith, 2011, Institute of Medicine, 1998)

- Adequate intake of Choline for adult is 425-550 mg/day.
- Americans consume ample choline from food between 700 and 1000 mg/day.
- Deficiency is mostly observed in alcoholic people and the elderly.
- Upper level for adults is 3.5 g/day (based on fishy body odor and low blood pressure).

6.2.4. Thiamin (B_1) (Wardlaw and Smith, 2011, Institute of Medicine, 1998)

- Adult RDA of thiamine is 1.1-1.2 mg/day.
- Daily value of 1.5 mg is used to express thiamin content on food and supplement labels.
- No upper level has been set because excess thiamin is rapidly lost in the urine.
- Consumption of highly processed and unenriched foods, sugar, fat, and alcohol creates potential for deficiency.

- Population at risk includes low-income and older people.

6.2.5. Riboflavin (B_2) (Wardlaw and Smith, 2011, Institute of Medicine, 1998)

- Adult RDA of riboflavin is 1.1-1.3 mg/day.
- Daily value of 1.7 mg is used to express riboflavin content on food and supplement labels.
- No upper level has been set since excess riboflavin is rapidly lost in the urine and no specific symptoms indicate that megadoses are toxic.
- Population at risk includes people with alcoholism because of nutrient poor diets.

6.2.6. Niacin (B_3)(Institute of Medicine, 1998, Wardlaw and Smith, 2011)

- Adult RDA for niacin is 14-16 mg/day expressed as Niacin Equivalents (NE) to account for niacin from diet and tryptophan as well.
- Daily value of 20 mg is used to express Niacin content on food and supplement labels.
- Population at risk includes people with alcoholism and those with rare disorders of tryptophan metabolism.
- Upper level for niacin is 35 mg/day of the nicotinic acid form.
- Body can synthesize niacin from tryptophan, up to 50% of the RDA.

6.2.7. Pantothenic acid (B_5)(Institute of Medicine, 1998, Wardlaw and Smith, 2011)

- Adequate intake of pantothenic acid for adults is 5 mg/day.
- Daily value of 10 mg is used to express pantothenic acid content on food and supplement labels.
- Population at risk includes people with alcoholism having a nutrient deficient diet.
- No upper level has been set and no toxicity is known.

6.2.8. Pyridoxine (B_6)(Institute of Medicine, 1998, Wardlaw and Smith, 2011, ADA, 2005)

- Adult RDA for pyridoxine is 1.3-1.7 mg/day.
- Daily value of 2 mg is used to express vitamin B6 content on food and supplement labels.
- Upper limit is set to 100 mg/day, based on risk of developing nerve damage.
- Intakes of 2-6 g/day for $\geq$ 2 months lead to irreversible nerve damage.
- Cirrhosis and hepatitis disable liver tissue from metabolizing vitamin B_6.
- Pregnancy supplementation of 30-75 mg/day is used to reduce nausea.

6.2.9. Biotin (B_7 or Vitamin H) (Wardlaw and Smith, 2011, Institute of Medicine, 1998)

- Adequate intake for biotin is 30 μg/day.
- On average, the daily intake is about 40-60 mcg/day.
- Daily value of 30 mcg is used to express biotin content on food and supplement labels.
- Population at risk includes people missing a large part of the small intestine or take antibiotics for many months.
- No upper level has been set and no toxicity is known.

6.2.10. Folate (B_9) (Institute of Medicine, 1998, Wardlaw and Smith, 2011)

- Adult RDA for folate is 400 μg/day.
- On average, daily intake is 520 mcg for men and 420 mcg for women.
- Daily value of 400 mcg is used to express folate content on food and supplement labels.

- Population at risk include: a) pregnant women, need extra folate (600 mcg DFE) to prevent birth defects: b) older people with inadequate folate intake and decreased absorption: c) alcoholism with inadequate folate intake and decreased absorption.

6.2.11. Cobalamin (B_{12}) (Institute of Medicine, 1998, Wardlaw and Smith, 2011)

- Adult RDA for cobalamin is 2.4 μg/day.
- On average, the daily intake is two times the RDA in the US.
- Daily value of 6 mg is used to express vitamin B_{12} content on food and supplement labels.
- Levels above RDA intake are non-toxic; hence, no Upper Level has been set.
- Vegans and people over age 50 are risk of developing pernicious anemia.

6.3. MAJOR MINERALS OVERVIEW

Citations for the summary: (Wardlaw and Smith, 2011, Institute of Medicine, 1997)

- Na, K, and Ca aid in the transfer of nerve impulses.
- Ca and P participate in growth and development.
- Na, K, Ca, and P are required for water balance.
- Major minerals require at least 100 mg/day.
- Na - Adequate Intake for adults under age 51 is 1500 mg. In older adults, it is reduced by 100-200 mg. Body proper function needs only 200 mg/day. Daily value for Na is 2400 mg/day. Na Upper Level for adults is 2300 mg/day. Individuals with hypertension, middle-age and older people recommended no more than 1500 mg/day.
- K - Adequate Intake for adults is 4700 mg/day. Daily Value used is 3500 mg. Average consumption in North America is 2000-3000 mg/day.

- Cl - Adequate Intake for adults is 2300 mg/day based on ratio of NaCl (40:60) (1500 mg Na: 2300 mg Cl). Daily Value used is 3400 mg/day. Upper Limit of Cl is 3600 mg/day.

- Ca - Daily Value used is 1000 mg. Adequate Intake for adults is 1000-1200 mg/day. Consumption in the US is for men 1000 mg and women 800 mg. Upper Level is 2500 mg/day.

- P - RDA for adults (>18 y/o) is 700 mg/day. Daily Value is 1000 mg. Upper Level of P is 3-4 g/day.

- Mg - RDA of magnesium in men is 400mg/day and women 310 mg/day. Daily value is 400 mg. Consumption in the US is for men 320 mg/day and women 200 mg/day. Upper level is 350 mg/day based on the risk of developing diarrhea.

- S – It is found in amino acids (methionine) and vitamins (biotin and B_1). S helps in the balance of acids and bases in the body. It is an important part of the liver drug detoxifying enzymes.

6.4. TRACE MINERALS OVERVIEW

Citations for the summary: (Institute of Medicine, 1997, Institute of Medicine, 2001, Institute of Medicine, 2000, Wardlaw and Smith, 2011)

- Trace mineral require less than 100 mg/day.

- Copper and selenium work as cofactors and enable proteins and enzymes to function.

- Fe - Iron is a component of red blood cells. The RDA for > 50 y/o is 8 mg. RDA between 19 and 50 y/o is 18 mg. Daily value is 18 mg. Average daily intake is for women 13 mg and men 18 mg. Upper level is 45 mg/day

- Se - RDA for adults is 55 µg/day. The Daily Value is 70 µg. Average consumption is 105 µg /day. Upper Level is 400 mcg/day based on signs of selenium toxicity (hair loss).

- Other trace minerals include I, Cu, F, Cr, Mn, Mo, and Zn.

6.5. TEST YOUR KNOWLEDGE

Match Puzzle 1: Macronutrients and Vitamins

Each term must be matched to one number and one letter from below (select the best option).

Nutrient	Number	Letter
Vitamin A	__________	__________
Vitamin D	__________	__________
Vitamin E	__________	__________
Vitamin K	__________	__________
Vitamin C	__________	__________
9 kcal/g	__________	__________
Complex CHO	__________	__________
Simple CHO	__________	__________
Carbohydrates	__________	__________
Lipids	__________	__________
Proteins		

1	Composed mostly of C, H, O, and 15-25% N.	**A**	Hydrosoluble vitamin (not B).
2	Metabolized in the liver and stored as glycogen or fat, depending on amount consumed.	**B**	Smoking destroys this nutrient in the lungs.
3	Deficiency causes scurvy, treated by eating citrus fruit.	**C**	Monosaccharides, disaccharides, and polysaccharides.
4	Most important source of this vitamin is from UVB rays.	**D**	The average Caloric density that predominates in the non-protein portion of mackerel.
5	Natural form exists in d-isomer while synthetic form is the dl-isomer.	**E**	Beta carotene is a precursor.
6	Causes a spike in blood sugar, followed by a crash.	**F**	Eliminate this by drinking diet soda instead of regular.
7	More branched chains, slower to digest, typically lower in fat content.	**G**	70% of this macronutrient in the American diet comes from animal sources.
8	*Trans* unsaturation makes your metabolism work harder to burn this form of energy.	**H**	Eat your green vegetables every day to get enough of this, as the nutrient is retained in your body for only one day.
9	RDA for this nutrient is measured in retinol activity equivalents (RAE).	**I**	Pyridoxine
10	Important for the synthesis of coagulation and anticoagulation proteins.	**J**	Considered a hormone and has 5 forms.
11	The macronutrient made of a carbon chain with a carboxylic acid on one end has this Caloric density.	**K**	Starches.

Match Puzzle 2: Macronutrients and Vitamins

Each term must be matched to one number and one letter from below (select the best option).

Nutrient	Number	Letter
Vitamin A	______	______
Vitamin D	______	______
Vitamin E	______	______
Vitamin K	______	______
Vitamin C	______	______
4 kcal/g	______	______
Complex CHO	______	______
Simple CHO	______	______
Carbohydrates	______	______
Lipids	______	______
Proteins	______	______

1	Average Caloric density of carbohydrates.	**A**	Increasing the intake of this nutrient can be beneficial for those with low iron stores.
2	This nutrient is resistant to being cooked out of food sources.	**B**	One sugar molecule or two sugar molecules that have joined together.
3	Consumption of this nutrient prevents your body from resorting to ketogenesis for energy.	**C**	Deficiency can cause rickets.
4	Helps regulate calcium and bone metabolism.	**D**	Soy is a complete source of this macronutrient while many others introduce cholesterol & fat.
5	L-Ascorbic Acid, antioxidant.	**E**	Triglycerides, phospholipids, and sterols
6	75-80% of the Calories in avocado, bacon, and peanut butter can be classified as what?	**F**	Megadoses of this nutrient reduce the effectiveness of orally administered pharmaceuticals such as Coumadin.
7	Chain of amino acids joined by peptide bonds.	**G**	Average Caloric density of protein.
8	Natural form is also called tocopherol.	**H**	Important sources of this macronutrient include grains, rice, breads, and potatoes.
9	Whole grain bread	**I**	Plant oils are the best source of this nutrient.
10	In the American diet, 65% of this vitamin comes from preformed sources whereas developing countries rely on the provitamin sources.	**J**	Polysaccharide with large fiber content.
11	High fructose corn syrup	**K**	Plays an important role in vision.

Match Puzzle 3: Vitamins

Each term must be matched to one number and one letter from below (select the best option).

Nutrient	Number	Letter
Vitamin B (general)	__________	__________
Vitamin C	__________	__________
Vitamin B1	__________	__________
Vitamin B2	__________	__________
Vitamin B3	__________	__________
Vitamin B5	__________	__________
Vitamin B6	__________	__________
Vitamin B7	__________	__________
Vitamin B9	__________	__________
Vitamin B12	__________	__________
Vitamin-like	__________	__________
Vitamin-like	__________	__________

1	Increasing intake is beneficial for those with low iron stores	**A**	Choline: part of a neurotransmitter & part of a phospholipid
2	Thiamin	**B**	Riboflavin
3	Inositol: part of cell membrane. Taurine: part of bile acids	**C**	Synthesized by intestinal bacteria; only those on antibiotics long-term at risk of deficiency
4	Biotin	**D**	Carnitine: needed to transport fatty acids to mitochondria
5	Lipoic Acid: participates in carbohydrate metabolism & acts as antioxidant	**E**	Required to synthesize coenzyme A
6	Plays role in synthesis of hemoglobin, white blood cells, and neurotransmitters	**F**	Milling grains leads to loss of this vitamin:
7	Major source: grains	**G**	Can synthesize up to 50% of this requirement from tryptophan
8	Family of compounds containing cobalt, synthesized by bacteria and fungi	**H**	Maintains myelin sheaths; 20yrs of deficiency can result in nerve damage
9	Pantothenic Acid	**I**	Pyridoxine
10	Folate	**J**	Glutamic acids must be cleaved from natural form before absorption (1.7x conversion)
11	Name comes from Latin word for yellow because of yellow color	**K**	Important in collagen protein synthesis
12	Niacin; in body as nicotinic acid and nicotinamide	**L**	Deficiency of this vitamin causes a disease called beriberi

Match Puzzle 4: Major Minerals

Each term must be matched to one number and one letter from below (select the best option).

Nutrient	Number	Letter
Sodium		
Potassium		
Chloride		
Calcium		
Phosphorus		
Magnesium		
Sulfur		

1	Diuretics deplete the body of this mineral:	**A**	Table salt is 40% composed of this major mineral:
2	Important cofactor in many enzymatic reactions	**B**	Efficient absorption of this mineral requires an acidic pH in the GI tract and active Vitamin D hormone
3	Body absorbs the same amount of this mineral that is eaten, and deficiency is rare while overconsumption is common in US.	**C**	Most Americans consume this mineral in excess; most is excreted by the kidneys while some is lost through perspiration
4	About 85% of this mineral in the body is found in bone (hint: not calcium!)	**D**	This mineral is not considered an essential nutrient because proteins provide the S we need
5	This mineral represents 40% (by weight) of all minerals in the body	**E**	No upper limit has been set for this mineral, but if your kidneys function poorly, the buildup can be fatal.
6	Found in amino acids and vitamins: methionine, biotin, and B1	**F**	Most people have deficiency of this mineral, especially those who perspire heavily, have diarrhea, vomiting, or alcoholism
7	Component of stomach acid	**G**	20-30% of this mineral in our diet comes from baked goods, cheeses, processed meats, and many soft drinks

Match Puzzle 5: Trace Minerals

Each term must be matched to one number and one letter from below (select the best option).

Nutrient	Number	Letter
Chromium		
Copper		
Fluoride		
Iodide		
Iron		
Manganese		
Molybdenum		
Selenium		
Zinc		

1	Good source: fish, meat, eggs, shellfish. This mineral works together with vitamin E as an antioxidant.	**A**	Toxicity symptoms have only been seen in laboratory animals, which exhibit poor growth. This mineral is found in beans, grains, and nuts.
2	Deficiency & toxicity are rare. Deficiency may occur in those hospitalized on a liquid diet for long periods. Toxicity is from industrial contamination, such as on cooking pans.	**B**	Countries with soil deficient of this mineral may use a fertilizer containing this in order to prevent dietary deficiencies associated with poor growth and development.
3	Young women have a greater RDA than men for this trace mineral; vitamin C can increase absorption of the non-animal source.	**C**	The cation of this mineral works with superoxide dismutase (SOD) as the principal antioxidant in mitochondria.
4	Aids in iron metabolism, and a symptom of deficiency is therefore anemia, along with low white blood cell counts.	**D**	Important for a well-functioning thyroid gland.
5	This mineral aids in the action of some enzymes. Deficiency has not been observed in healthy humans; only in those being fed intravenously for extended periods of time.	**E**	Deficiency of this mineral is the most common deficiency worldwide.
6	Populations at greatest risk of deficiency are those who live inland with no access to saltwater fish.	**F**	Toothpaste often contains this mineral as it prevents dental caries.
7	Required for the proper functioning of nearly 200 enzymes.	**G**	Consumption of this mineral helps to have normal blood glucose after eating.
8	Drinking well water as opposed to city tap water may increase your risk of deficiency of this trace mineral.	**H**	Upper level: 400µg/day. This is based upon signs of toxicity such as hair loss.
9	Cofactor of enzymes involved in metabolism of carbohydrates, amino acids, and cholesterol. Hint: starts with an M.	**I**	Toxicity causes nervous disorders resulting in tingling of extremities, loss of coordination, and reduced peripheral vision.

6.6. CALCULATIONS

- Dietary Intake of 10 g of salt translate into

    a. How many g of Na?

    - ____________g of Na

    b. If an adult consumes 9 g salt a day, how much chloride would they have ingested?

    - ____________mg of Cl

6.7. PRACTICE SESSION I: ASSESSMENT OF MICRONUTRIENT DAILY INTAKE FROM A DIET HISTORY

A friend is concerned whether they are eating properly and whether they should be taking a dietary supplement. They have a diary of their dietary intake from yesterday and ask that you evaluate the content for vitamins and minerals

The person is a female and weighs 60 kg and is 5'4" tall.

Nutritional Intake

Breakfast: Protein Crunchy Granola with 2 ounces of 2% milk, 2 slices of whole-wheat toast including 2 teaspoon of margarine enriched with calcium and vitamin D, Coffee with 2% milk, 8 ounces

Lunch: 1 cup of Chicken-noodle soup, 6 saline crackers, ½ ham and cheese sandwich with 1 tablespoon of mayonnaise, a small bag of potato chips, and Coca-Cola® with 2 refills.

Dinner: Garden-Fresh Salad with dressing, Spaghetti with Marinara Sauce, 2 Breadsticks with garlic butter spread, 1 serving of and Coca-Cola® with 2 refills.

1. Using Table **2** below (provides the micronutrient content for each item ingested with the meals), calculate the amount of micronutrient ingested at each meal and as well as the total for the day

Table 2. Itemized nutritional content of meals.

Micronutrient Content						
Breakfast	Vit C, mg	B-1, mg	Folate, mcg	Na, mg	K, mg	Ca, mg
Cereal	0	0	0	165	125	390
Toast	0	0.2	32	380	25	208
Coffee	0	0	0	15	0	180
Meal Total						
Lunch						
Soup with crackers	0	0	0	715	445	260
Ham and cheese Sandwich	18	0.2	32	1110	0	208
Potato Chips	9	0	0	140	340	0
Coca-Cola x3	0	0	0	15	0	0
Meal Total						
Dinner						
Salad	27	0	30	470	0	60
Spaghetti with Marinara	3.6	0.36	110	480	0	260
Breadsticks	0	0	0	642	122	260
Coca-cola x 3	0	0	0	15	0	0
Meal Total						
Total per Day						

2. Assess the daily nutritional intake as compared with that recommended for a healthy diet for this person's age and weight as it relates to vitamin C, thiamine and folic acid as well as sodium, potassium and calcium. Circle the value (<, Nl, >) that best represents the relationship between intake and the healthy recommendation

	Water-Soluble Vitamin Content			**Mineral Content**		
	C, mg	**B-1, mg**	**Folate, mcg**	**Na, mg**	**K, mg**	**Ca, mg**
Healthy Diet*	90	1.2	400	1500	4700	1300
Assessment	<, Nl, >	<, Nl, >	<, Nl, >	<, Nl, >	<, Nl, >	<, Nl, >

* Based on 2000 Calorie Diet.

< = less than the RDA, > = greater than the RDA.

Nl = adequate intake (allow for a variance of 10% to answer this question).

a. What adjustments in this individual's diet should be made to improve their nutritional health?

b. Should this individual begin taking a calcium supplement?

6.8. DIETARY SUPPLEMENTS

Dietary Supplements Overview

Most vitamins and minerals are available in the form of dietary supplements. Some of these micronutrients have required amount to be contained in a product in order to be sold as a dietary supplement. Individuals usually take dietary supplements to prevent diseases such as heart disease or cancer, reduce stress, and improve or increase 'energy'. Sometimes, dietary supplements are taken to reduce susceptibility to diseases such as colds. Dietary Supplement Label is similar in some ways to a nutrition label but different: the label must list: ingredient(s), amount(s) per serving, suggested use, % daily value. A sample label is provided below in Fig. **1**:

Supplement Facts

Serving Size 1 Tablet

	Amount Per Serving	% Daily Value
Vitamin A (as retinyl acetate and 50% as beta-carotene)	5000 IU	100%
Vitamin C (as ascorbic acid)	60 mg	100%
Vitamin D (as cholecalciferol)	400 IU	100%
Vitamin E (as dl-alpha tocopheryl acetate)	30 IU	100%
Thiamin (as thiamin mononitrate)	1.5 mg	100%
Riboflavin	1.7 mg	100%
Niacin (as niacinamide)	20 mg	100%
Vitamin B_6 (as pyridoxine hydrochloride)	2.0 mg	100%
Folate (as folic acid)	400 mcg	100%
Vitamin B_{12} (as cyanocobalamin)	6 mcg	100%
Biotin	30 mcg	10%
Pantothenic Acid (as calcium pantothenate)	10 mg	100%

Other ingredients: Gelatin, lactose, magnesium stearate, microcrystalline cellulose, FD&C Yellow No. 6, propylene glycol, propylparaben, and sodium benzoate.

Fig. (1). Sample Dietary Supplement Label: Multivitamin with Minerals.

Practice Session II: Assessment of Dietary Supplement Content

Use Table **3** below along with recommended daily values from Table **1** to answer the following questions:

1. Of those water soluble vitamins with more than 1000% of the daily value what are the potential toxic effects possible with long term daily ingestion of Ultra Mega® and Ultra Mega Gold®?

2. Which minerals are in amounts <50% of the Daily Value?
3. Which trace mineral content is in excess of its Daily value? What are toxic symptoms of this trace element?

Table 3. Dietary Supplement Examples: Multivitamins with Minerals

Ingredient	Amount per Serving	% Daily Value
	Vitamins	
Fat-Soluble		
A, IU	5000	100
D, IU	400	100
E, IU	30	100
Water-Soluble		
C, mg	180	333
Thiamine, mg	80	5000
Riboflavin, mg	80	4412
Niacin, mg	80	375
Pyridoxine, mg	80	3750
Folic acid, mcg	600	150
Vitamin B-12, mcg	80	1250
Biotin, mg	80	25
Pantothenic Acid, mg	80	750
	Minerals	
Calcium, mg	200	12
Magnesium, mg	60	15
Potassium, mg	4	<1
	Trace Minerals	
Iron, mg	20	100
Iodine, mcg	150	100
Zinc, mg	20	100
Selenium, mcg	220	300
Copper, mg	3	100
Manganese, mg	3	100
Chromium, mcg	140	100
Molybdenum, mcg	80	100

Practice Session III. SuperTracker Assessment of Personal Diet

Using information from the SuperTracker exercise in Chapter 4 answer the following questions:

1. Using your 24 hour Nutrients Report, look at your intake of sodium. Compared to the recommended intake, please circle or underline what corresponds to your particular case:

   * Less than Daily Value Equal to Daily Value Greater than Daily Value.

2. Look at your Food Details Report. Calculate the percent of the RDA you achieved for each of those nutrients below, and include those values (these should be percent less than 100%).

   a. If you ate three types of micronutrients (other than sodium) in amounts <70% of the RDA, give the name of these micronutrients and the food source. Please make sure you use the micronutrients included in your report.

MICRONUTRIENT (<70% RDA) FOOD SOURCE

   b. If you consumed three micronutrients over 70% of the RDA, give the name of these micronutrients and the food source. Please make sure you use the micronutrients included in your report.

MICRONUTRIENT (>70% RDA) FOOD SOURCE

   c. Explain what you could do to compensate for the micronutrients you listed in Question 2a with <70% of the RDA requirements as well as for those in Question 2b with over 70% of the RDA. For instance, list which product sources you could remove or reduce from your diet and which one you could add to your diet to balance (a food that you could have eaten that would be a relatively good source).

MICRONUTRIENT RDA (70%) FOOD SOURCE______ADD/REMOVE_

Explanation:

3. Next, look at your fiber intake. Was your fiber intake above, below or about equal as the recommended amount? List the two main food sources of your fiber intake. Which other two sources could have you used?

Data Analysis and Dietary Counseling

Look at all of your reports. Pretend these reports are client data. How would you, as a nutritionist, instruct your client to alter his or her diet? You can critique Caloric intake, type of nutrients consumed, and Caloric expenditure. Limit your answer to 200 words, but keep in mind that content, rather than length, is the most important factor of the essay.

CONCLUDING REMARKS

This chapter has presented and applied concepts related to micronutrient intake as part of a balanced diet. After completing the exercises above, the reader should have understood importance of micronutrients as part of a balanced diet and applied concepts to be able to design a healthy diet.

CONFLICT OF INTEREST

The authors confirm that this ebook contents have no conflict of interest.

ACKNOWLEDGEMENTS

Declared none.

REFERENCES

American Dietetic Association. (2005). ADA Reports: Position of the American Dietetic Association: fortification and nutritional supplements. Journal of American Dietetic Association, 105: 1300-1311.

Institute of Medicine, 1997, Dietary Reference Intakes for Calcium, Phosphorus, Magnesium, Vitamin D, and Fluoride: Washington DC, National Academies Press.

Institute of Medicine, 1998, Dietary Reference Intakes for Thiamin, Riboflavin, Niacin, Vitamin, B-6, Folate, Vitamin B-12, Pantothenic acid, Biotin, and choline: Washington DC, National Academies Press.

Institute of Medicine, 2000, Dietary Reference Intakes for Vitamin C, Vitamin E, Selenium, and Carotenoids: Washington DC, National Academies Press.

Institute of Medicine, 2001, Dietary reference Intakes for Vitamin A, Vitamin K, Arsenic, Boron, Chromium, Copper, Iodine, Iron, Manganese, Molybdenum, Nickel, Silicon, Vanadium, and Zinc, Washington DC, National Academies Press.

Nield, L. S., Mahajan, P., Joshi, A. & Kamat, D. (2006). Rickets: not a disease of the past. American Family Physician, 74: 619-626.

Wardlaw, G. M. & Smith, A. M. (2011). Contemporary Nutrition. 8th ed. New York, N. Y., McGraw Hill, Inc. Learning Solutions.

CHAPTER 7

Phytochemicals in Nutrition and Health

Nicole A. Eggers and Esperanza J. Carcache de Blanco*

College of Pharmacy, The Ohio State University, Columbus, Ohio, USA

Abstract: Some phytochemicals, or chemical compounds produced by or present in plants, may be nutritious for human consumption. Phytochemicals are not essential nutrients for humans, but they may contribute to preventing or treating diseases such as cancer, diabetes, diseases of the eye, and cardiovascular disease. In this chapter, some of the most important phytochemicals for human health and nutrition are detailed, along with their mechanisms of action, chemical structures, and specific health benefits. These health-promoting phytochemicals are present in familiar plant sources of fruits, vegetables, and legumes. The carotenoids in tomatoes, for example, are studied for anticancer effects and reduced risk of cardiovascular diseases. The proanthocyanidins in cranberries can prevent or treat urinary tract infections. The isoflavonoids in soybeans mimic hormones, which contribute to the possible effectiveness in some breast cancers. The sulfur-containing phytochemicals in broccoli and Brussels sprouts have potential anticancer effects. A few sulfur-containing compounds in garlic are very good antibacterial agents. The study of chemical compounds present in common edible plants, allows students to correlate nutrition to disease prevention or treatment by functional foods; perhaps this chapter even facilitates thinking about foods as drugs.

Keywords: Aglycones, antioxidants, cancer, cardiovascular disease, carotenoids, chemical structures, chemopreventative agents, diabetes, eye diseases, flavonoids, glycosides, inflammation, natural colorants, obesity, organosulfur compounds, phytochemical index, phytochemicals, phytoestrogens, steroids, terpenoids.

7.1. INTRODUCTION TO PHYTOCHEMICALS

Phytochemicals, where *phtyo* is from the Greek for plant, are chemical compounds that naturally occur in plant organisms. Phytochemicals are not essential nutrients for the plant or for humans, but which may have protective or disease preventative properties. The plant produces such phytochemicals to protect itself from predators, poor conditions, or disease; but recent research demonstrates that they can also protect humans against disease and even serve as functional foods. For example, glucosinolates are sulfur-containing

***Corresponding author Esperanza J. Carcache de Blanco:** College of Pharmacy, The Ohio State University, Columbus, OH 43210, USA; E-mail: Carcache-de-blan.1@osu.edu

Esperanza J. Carcache de Blanco and Jay Mirtallo (Eds)

phytochemicals found in broccoli, cabbage, horseradish, and garlic. The pungent taste of glucosinolates deter pests such as the cotton bollworm from feeding on the leaves of these types of plants, but glucosinolate metabolites have also been studied for their potential cancer chemopreventative effects in humans (Shroff *et al.,* 2008; Hecht, 1995).

Phytochemicals that play a role in human nutrition and disease prevention are naturally present in plant-based foods such as fruits and vegetables. Manufacturers may alternatively formulate phytochemicals into nutraceuticals or functional foods. Some food advertising companies even run campaigns that food products have a certain disease-preventative property; the label or claim may or may not advertise the phytochemical responsible for the effect. Many different phytochemicals are studied for their use in weight loss, general well-being, and disease prevention. Some farmers and scientists make an effort to elevate the amount of phytochemicals in crops, such as tomatoes or peppers, so that consumers can achieve optimal intake of these substances regularly. In addition, increasing the amount of phytochemicals in products enables those who do not eat many plant-based foods to achieve higher levels of phytochemicals when they do. To elevate levels of these phytochemicals, farmers and scientists selectively breed the most potent members of various fruit or vegetable families in specific climates and environmental conditions. For example, chile peppers are often bred to be bigger, spicier, or sweeter; and tomatoes are sometimes selectively bred to have more red, round, or sweet characteristics.

Consuming more phytochemicals can promote maintenance of a healthier weight by lowering blood sugar and affecting insulin production, affecting the life cycle of adipose cells, reducing the levels of inflammatory markers, and acting as probiotics:

- Blood Sugar – Consuming phytochemicals tends to lower blood glucose and the corresponding over-production of insulin. Specifically, phytochemicals may help moderate our post-meal blood sugar response. Stable blood glucose levels are important for metabolism, maintaining healthy body weight, preventing abdominal obesity, and limiting cardiovascular health risks.

- Effects on Adipose Cells – Certain phytochemicals including genistein, quercetin, and ajoene, which will all be discussed throughout this chapter, directly impact the life cycle of fat cells. These phytochemicals and others may increase the breakdown of adipose tissue in two ways:

by inducing apoptosis, or by inhibiting adipogenesis (generation of new fat cells) (Rayalam *et al.,* 2008; Nelson-Dooley *et al.,* 2005).

- Inflammation – Several phytochemicals can aid in the management of chronic inflammation, particularly in cancer, neurological, cardiovascular, and metabolic disorders. In such conditions, patients exhibit higher levels of inflammatory markers. Inflammation is thought to contribute to weight gain and associated diseases. However, a diet rich in phytochemicals and low-glycemic produce lower expression of inflammatory markers in the body, so a phytochemical-rich diet may relieve some inflammation and related symptoms of diseases linked to chronic inflammation (Chun *et al.,* 2008; Tosetti *et al.,* 2009; Holt *et al.,* 2009; Woo *et al.,* 2007).

- Probiotics – Recent studies demonstrate that the inclusion of probiotics, tannins, proanthocyanidins, and/or antioxidants in the human diet reduces inflammation and supports the growth of beneficial bacteria in the digestive system. Having too small a proportion of beneficial bacteria in the intestines may contribute to obesity by promoting inflammation and insulin resistance. This may explain why post-surgery probiotic supplementation helped gastric bypass patients lose more weight than those who did not receive the post-operative probiotic intervention (Cani *et al.,* 2007; Burcelin *et al.,* 2009; Woodard *et al.,* 2009; Osman *et al.,* 2007; Bialonska *et al.,* 2009; DiBaise *et al.,* 2008).

In 2010, a study published in the *Journal of Human Nutrition and Dietetics* drew a correlation between plant food consumption and weight management. Study participants (n = 54) categorized into normal weight and overweight groups kept a food diary for three days. The food logs were evaluated for total caloric intake (energy), food groups, and a new assessment value called the phytochemical index (PI). The PI was defined in the study design as the ratio of energy from high-nutrient, phytochemical-rich foods, to the overall daily energy consumed. A lower intake of phytochemicals, and therefore a lower PI, was observed for those individuals who were overweight and obese. A poor PI was correlated with a higher BMI, larger waist circumference, higher waist-to-hip ratios, and more oxidative stress. This study afforded the conclusion that, "The PI is inversely related to adiposity and oxidative stress in healthy young adults, and the PI is responsive to body weight changes" (Vincent *et al.,* 2010).

Overall, substances that produce many of the beneficial effects associated with a diet include fruits, vegetables, beans, and grains. There are more than one thousand known phytochemicals, and they belong to different classes of chemical compounds including carotenoids, flavonoids, polyphenols, proanthocyanidins, phytoestrogens, terpenes, isothiocyanates, *etc*. Some of the most well-studied phytochemicals are included in Table **1**.

Table 1. Common and well-studied phytochemicals.

Alkaloids	**Hydroxycinnamic Acids**	**Terpenoids**
Caffeine	Chicoric acid	Isoprene
Cocaine	Coumarin	Geraniol
Ephedrine	Ferulic acid	Menthol
Morphine	Caffeic acid	Geranylgeraniol
Nicotine	Curcumin	Taxadiene
Quinine	Cinnamic acid	Squalene
Theobromine	**Lignans**	Lupeol
Carotenoids	Podophyllotoxin	Phytoene
Astaxanthin	Silymarin	Limonene
Beta-carotene	**Organosulfurs**	***Saponins***
Beta-cryptoxanthin	Allicin	Ginsenosides
Canthaxanthin	Allyl sulfides	Diosgenin
Lutein	Glucosinolates	Sarsasapogenin
Lycopene	Indole-3-carbinol	***Phytosterols***
Zeaxanthin	Isothiocyanates	Beta-sitosterol
Flavonoids	Sulforaphane	Stigmasterol
Daidzein	Ajoenes	Fucosterol
Epicatechin	Vinyl dithiins	Ergosterol
Genistein	**Phenolic Acids**	**Others**
Hesperidin	Capsaicin	Eugenol
Myricetin	Ellagic acid	Thymol
Naringin	Gallic acid	Carvacrol
Quercetin	Rosmarinic acid	Anethole
Anthocyanidins	Tannic acid	1,8-cineole
Cyanidin	**Stilbenes**	Limonene
Delphinidin	Pterostilbene	Linalool
Malvidin	Resveratrol	Digoxin
Proanthocyanidins	Combretastatin A-4	Phytic acid

7.2. COMMON MECHANISMS OF PHYTOCHEMICALS

How do phytochemicals work? There are many types of phytochemicals and each works differently. Some possible actions include:

- Antioxidant – Many phytochemicals act as antioxidants to prevent cellular damage by free radicals and oxidative stress, thereby reducing the risk of developing cancer. Phytochemicals with potent antioxidant activity include carotenoids found in red to yellow produce, flavonoids in a vast array of fruits and vegetables, and sulfur-containing compounds from garlic.

- Anti-microbial properties – Several sulfur-containing phytochemicals from garlic, such as the compound allicin, have antibacterial properties. Many common food-flavoring spices including cloves, cinnamon, and rosemary also possess antimicrobial activity.

- Enzyme action – Indoles found in cruciferous vegetables, most notably indole-3-carbinol, stimulate enzymes involved in food and drug metabolism. Phytochemicals in grapefruit juice interfere with cytochrome P450 enzyme action, and protease inhibitors found in soybeans can inhibit the breakdown of proteins in the body if consumed in too high quantities.

- Hormonal action – Isoflavones, a sub-type of flavonoid often found in soybeans and other legumes, are similar in structure to human estrogen and have the ability to mimic the hormone. Phytochemicals that exhibit hormonal action can sometimes serve as therapeutic agents for hormone-related diseases and conditions such as in menopause, osteoporosis, or some breast cancers.

- Interference with DNA replication – Saponins interfere with DNA replication and are sometimes explored as antiviral agents due to their ability to disrupt replication of the viral DNA. Phytochemicals with numerous conjugated double bonds such as some fatty acids, polyketides, and sterols may also interfere with cellular DNA replication.

- Physical action – Some phytochemicals physically wrap around pathogens or coat surfaces for a therapeutic effect. Large phytochemicals in cranberries, called proanthocyanidins, wrap around bacterial cells to prevent bacteria from adhering to human cell walls and causing infections. Phytochemicals in licorice, upon consumption, will coat the throat to soothe minor pharyngitis. Anthraquinones may coat the inside of some digestive organs, smoothing the organ surface and acting as a laxative for easier bowel movement.

7.3. MAJOR GROUPS OF PHYTOCHEMICALS

7.3.1. Carotenoids

Carotenoids are chemical compounds found in fruits and vegetables which are often responsible for the red, orange, and yellow pigments. Dark green vegetables and fruits like kiwi also contain carotenoids, but green chlorophyll masks the red, orange, and yellow colors. In addition, some algae produce carotenoids or carotenoid precursors, and when crustaceans, shrimp, or flamingos feed on the algae, they absorb the pigment, developing pinkish color (Fox, 1955; Fox, 1976). Carotenoids are divided into two main structural groups: the carotenes (hydrocarbon carotenoids) and the xanthophylls (oxygenated carotenoids) (Fig. **1**) (Mordi, 1993). In addition to serving as natural colorants, several carotenoids including lutein, zeaxanthin, lycopene, and beta-carotene (Fig. **1**) have been indicated in eye and heart health. Carotenoids may also help prevent cardiovascular diseases, cancers, and degenerative brain diseases (Voutilainen *et al.,* 2006). Structures of common carotenoids, their classification, and common foods containing these carotenoids are included in Fig. **1**.

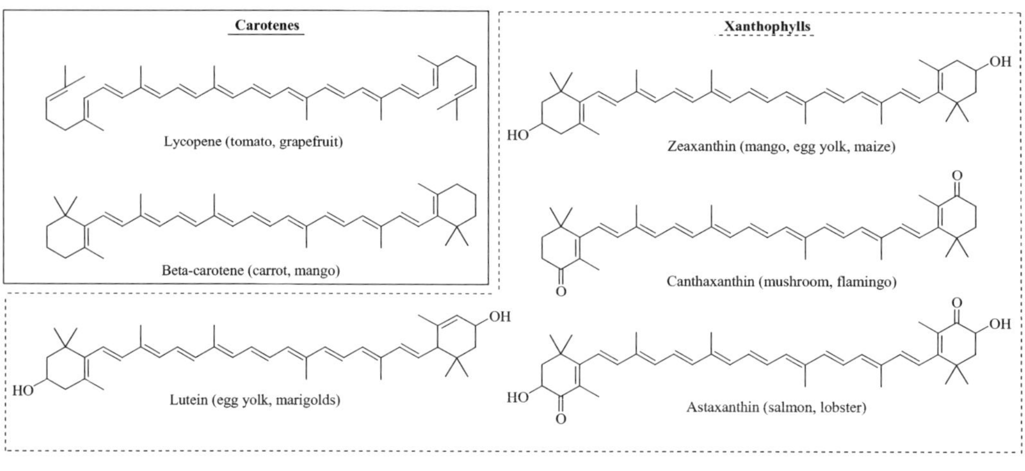

Fig. (1). Examples of carotenoids (examples of sources) and structural classification of each example (adapted from Mordi, 1993).

7.3.1.1. Beta-Carotene

Beta-carotene (Fig. **1**), along with two other carotenoids not shown (alpha-carotene and beta-cryptoxanthin), are precursors to vitamin A. The human body is capable of converting all three of these phytochemicals into vitamin A (also called retinol), but the body is most efficient at converting beta-carotene. As such, these phytochemicals contribute significantly to meeting daily nutritional requirements.

Beta-carotene has been incorporated into golden rice, a functional food or genetically modified organism, to prevent vitamin A deficiency. It consists of rice that has been genetically modified to produce beta-carotene in the edible part of the grain. In this way, people who rely heavily on rice (and consume very few fruits and vegetables) for daily sustenance, may consume enough of the vitamin A precursor to prevent vitamin A deficiency. The beta-carotene in the grain turns the rice a golden yellow color, hence the name. Golden rice is surrounded by controversy concerning genetically modified organisms, but as with other carotenoids, beta-carotene (and golden rice) must be consumed with other lipids for the greatest absorption of the phytochemical. Unfortunately, populations suffering from vitamin A deficiency tend to have very low-fat diets and thus may not absorb an adequate amount of beta-carotene to prevent vitamin A deficiency. In the United States, beta-carotene is commercially available as a dietary supplement.

Beta-carotene was included in the Carotene and Retinol Efficacy Trial (CARET) and Alpha-Tocopherol Beta-Carotene (ATBC) clinical studies. The *in vitro* and animal *in vivo* studies of beta-carotene suggested that the phytochemical may prevent cellular damage caused by free radicals, which is one of the common contributing factors in the progression phase of cancer development. Both trials were designed to investigate cancer prevention in patients at high risk of developing lung cancer, *i.e.* smokers and those exposed to asbestos. Unfortunately, both trials reported an increase in lung cancer incidence and mortality in the beta-carotene intervention group *versus* the placebo group. The most widely accepted hypothesis to explain the unexpected results is that in the presence of an overload of free radicals produced by cigarette smoke or asbestos exposure, beta-carotene instead undergoes oxidation, resulting in a pro-oxidant (rather than antioxidant) effect (Duffield-Lillico and Begg, 2004). The undesired effects in the CARET and ATBC trials may also have been due to the mega doses of supplemental beta-carotene instead of increasing the dietary intake of fruits and vegetables that contain beta-carotene as well as other health-promoting phytochemicals. Despite the unfortunate outcome of the clinical studies, it has been suggested that non-smokers, former smokers, and patients with micronutrient deficiencies may still benefit from increased beta-carotene consumption.

7.3.1.2. Lutein

Lutein (Fig. **1**) is a yellow-to-orange carotenoid found in carrots, egg yolks, kale, marigold flowers, spinach, squash, and other dark green, orange, and yellow fruits and vegetables. Lutein is also found commercially as a dietary supplement. It works as an antioxidant in the body to reduce the damage done by free radicals. Lutein is a necessary component of normal vision, and like most carotenoids, it is a fat-soluble compound.

Lutein is not produced in the human body and must be consumed in the diet. Once it is in the body, lutein (as well as zeaxanthin) is deposited as a pigment in the macula of the eye. There, the pigment selectively absorbs high-energy and eye-damaging blue light, preventing photoreceptor damage. The incorporation of lutein into the diet has been shown to reduce the risk of developing age-related macular degeneration (AMD). Researchers studied various vitamins, minerals, and phytochemicals as part of the supplement formula used in the Age Related Eye Disease Study (AREDS). The first formulation in 2001 included vitamin C, vitamin E, beta-carotene, zinc, and copper. To improve the formulation in 2006 (AREDS-2), the same group tried vitamin C, vitamin E, zinc, copper, omega-3 fatty acids, lutein, and zeaxanthin. The study indicated that while lutein and zeaxanthin were safe alternatives for beta-carotene (which was associated with increased risk of lung cancer in smokers), the omega-3 fatty acids had no effect (National Eye Institute 2013b; National Eye Institute 2013a). The researchers found, overall, that the second formulation may help slow the progression of macular degeneration. Unfortunately, lutein does not appear effective in preventing or treating cataracts.

Consumption of lutein may slow the progression of macular degeneration, but it may also decrease the risk of cardiovascular disease according to one correlation study. Epidemiological data revealed that of 573 healthy adults, those who had higher plasma levels of lutein, zeaxanthin, and two other carotenoids also had healthier blood vessels (Dwyer *et al.,* 2004). Keep in mind, however, that lutein was not the only antioxidant present, and there was not a specific baseline or constant diet among the participants. There may be several lifestyle factors that also contributed to the evidence that lutein is inversely associated with atherosclerosis.

One of the most bioavailable food sources of lutein is the egg yolk because of its fat content, which enables better absorption of the fat-soluble compound; however, eating a diet with a sufficient amount of colorful fruits and vegetables with a little fat would provide ample amounts of lutein. Egg producers often feed chickens marigold-supplemented feed in order to produce yolks with more orange color (due to the high level of lutein found in the marigold-supplemented feed), and marigolds are farmed in several Central and South American countries for this reason.

7.3.1.3. Zeaxanthin

Zeaxanthin is another important phytochemical, and it is present in orange bell peppers, leafy green vegetables, and egg yolks. Zeaxanthin is also present in paprika, spirulina (a dietary supplement made from blue-green algae), and marigolds. It is difficult to separate lutein and zeaxanthin in the laboratory, so many foods and supplements report combined levels of lutein and zeaxanthin on their labels.

As is the case for lutein, zeaxanthin is deposited in the macula and protects the photoreceptors and the retina from damaging light. Zeaxanthin and the macular pigment are thus essential in preventing AMD, the most common cause of vision impairment in the elderly. It is estimated that more than 733 million people worldwide suffer from symptoms of AMD. Irreversible vision loss due to AMD can be devastating to the point of inability to read or even distinguish different facial expressions of friends.

Goji berries are often referred to as superfruits and were traditionally used for eye health in Traditional Chinese Medicine. Many AMD patients still try and see some efficacy in consuming goji berries, usually as a tea or dried fruit. They are in fact very high in zeaxanthin, as well as lutein and three other carotenoids, and several vitamins, minerals, and amino acids.

7.3.1.4. Lycopene

Lycopene gives fruits and vegetables the red or pink pigment that is most recognized in tomato products. Other rich sources of lycopene include watermelon, guava, papaya, red bell peppers, and pink grapefruit. Eating a diet rich in lycopene has been associated with a lower risk of cardiovascular disease and pancreatic cancer (Giovannucci *et al.,* 1995; Stahl and Sies, 1996).

Lycopene is located inside the chromoplasts of tomatoes, in a crystalline conformation. Cooking or pulverizing tomatoes disrupts the chromoplasts, melts the crystals, and expels more lycopene into the dish or meal. Lycopene is a fat-soluble compound like vitamin A and the other carotenoids, so the human body absorbs more lycopene when it is consumed with a little fat. Lycopene is more readily absorbed by the human body from tomato sauce than from fresh tomatoes because chemical modifications occurred during the preparation, in addition to the presence of lipids; more specifically, the tomato sauce has undergone thermal processing, pulverization, and also includes a little fat. In most cases, fresh fruits and vegetables contain more phytochemicals than their cooked counterparts; however, tomatoes are an exception in terms of lycopene. Although, if interested in consuming tomato products for their vitamin C content, the more the tomato products are cooked, the more vitamin C they will lose. Availability of phytochemicals and/or nutrients therefore depends on the chemical structure as well as storage compartment of the compound.

The structure of lycopene in Fig. **1** is drawn as all-*trans*-lycopene. However, there are several other forms of lycopene including 5-*cis*-lycopene, 9-*cis*-lycopene, 13-*cis*-lycopene, and finally tetra-*cis* or 7,9,9',7'-*cis*-lycopene. Most tomato products contain a majority of all-*trans*-lycopene, but the lycopene present in the blood or tissues of those who have consumed products containing lycopene, are more commonly the *cis*-isomers. In fact, products such as the tangerine tomato, which contain more *cis*-lycopene, are more readily absorbed forms of the phytochemical. In addition, the cooking or thermal processing of products containing all-*trans*-lycopene in oil may convert them to a *cis*-isomer, enhancing the benefits of heating tomatoes to achieve greater amounts of available lycopene in general.

7.3.2. Flavonoids

Flavonoids are another class of phytochemicals; they are often found in grains, fruits, and vegetables, especially in the colorful skins. The flavonoid family includes many sub-classifications of compounds, such as flavanones, flavanols, isoflavonoids, and proanthocyanidins (Fig. **2**) (Dewick, 2009). Flavonoids as a whole, are generally classified as having a C6-C3-C6 organization around the A, B, and C rings, respectively (Fig. **2**). However, they vary in having a ketone at C4, a double bond between C2 and C3, the ring B connection through C2 or C3, the number of hydroxyl groups attached at different positions on each of the rings, the presence and location of linked sugars, and even the opening or closure of the C ring.

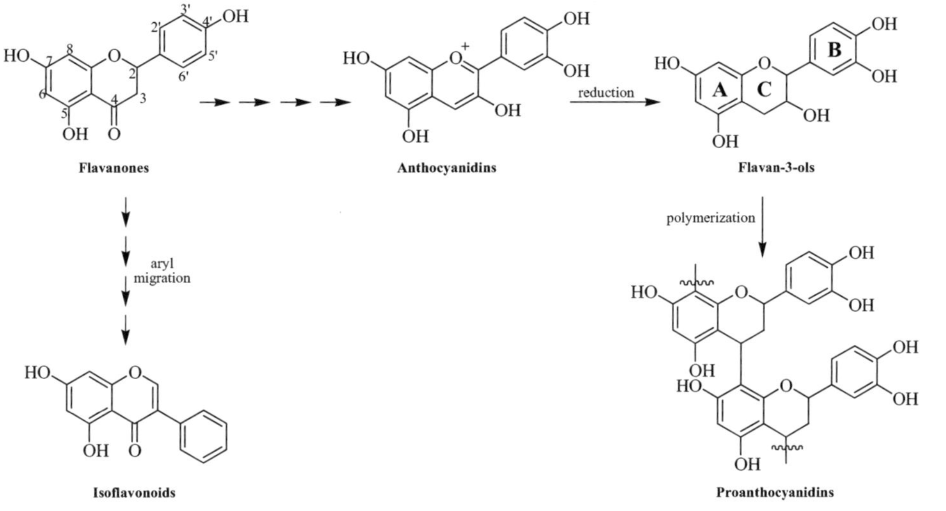

Fig. (2). Flavonoids and the relationship among several sub-classifications of flavonoids (Dewick, 2009).

An example of a very important flavonoid is quercetin (Fig. **3**). Quercetin is one of the most ubiquitous flavonoids, and as an antioxidant, it has a broad range of health benefits. Quercetin is commonly found in produce, tea, and wine; it is also available as a dietary supplement. Sources with the greatest amount of quercetin include apples, red bell peppers, and onions.

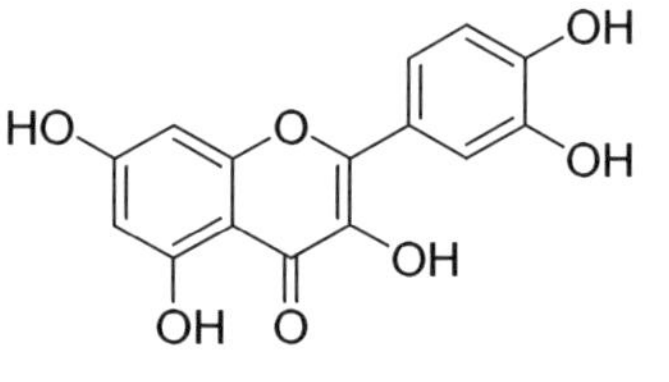

Fig. (3). Quercetin, a nutritionally important flavonone.

Other common flavonoids include naringenin, hesperidin, and kaempferol found in citrus fruits, and epicatechin found in green tea and numerous other plant sources.

Flavonoids in general are beneficial for human health, because they may work as antioxidants in the body, protecting cells from damage caused by free radicals. Free radicals are unstable and react easily with essential molecules of the body, including DNA, lipids, and proteins. Free radicals are formed endogenously as part of natural metabolism, but also exogenously by environmental factors including cigarette smoke, pesticides, pollution, and radiation.

Free radicals are one electron away from being stable, so they try to steal or donate electrons to other molecules. Once the free radical is electronically stabilized, the molecule that accepted or donated the extra electron becomes a free radical itself. This chain reaction goes on to damage the cell, sometimes leading to uncontrolled cellular growth or even tumors.

Antioxidants have the ability to neutralize free radicals without contributing to the chain reaction. When antioxidants accept or donate an electron to the free radical, they do not become radicals themselves because antioxidants are stable in both electronic states. Hence, antioxidants truncate the chain reaction and prevent further damage. However, when an antioxidant neutralizes a free radical, the antioxidant becomes inactive and cannot perform the task again. Therefore, the human body must be continuously supplied with antioxidants from the diet. The damage caused by free radicals could increase the risk of developing cancer and heart problems, and could accelerate aging. Well-known examples of antioxidants are the vitamins A, C, E (and/or vitamin A precursor, beta-carotene). These vitamins are often added to the so-called ACE drinks, but there are numerous other comparatively unknown antioxidants such as lycopene, lutein, and several other carotenoids as well as flavonoids such as quercetin.

Antioxidants are found in berries, broccoli, carrots, celery, citrus fruits, fish oil, kale, liver, mangos, nuts, red peppers, soybeans, spinach, sweet potatoes, tea, and tomatoes. Intensely colored fruits and vegetables tend to contain more antioxidants as the carotenoids are excellent antioxidants, as well as natural colorants. A study in 2006 by Dr. Henry Thompson and the Cancer Prevention Laboratory at Colorado State University, demonstrated that consuming a small quantity but very diverse variety of antioxidants and phytochemicals from produce may be more beneficial than consuming a few phytochemicals in large amounts (Thompson *et al.,* 2006).

7.3.2.1. Isoflavonoids

One subdivision of flavonoids, the isoflavonoids, contains phytochemicals that are particularly important in the diet of individuals with diseases, conditions, or who are on treatments that are affected by hormones. Some plant isoflavonoids, especially isoflavones, have chemical structures that behave in a similar fashion to estrogens (Fig. **4**) and are called phytoestrogens due to their ability to mimic estrogenic activity. Daidzein and genistein (Fig. **4**), for example, act as hormone-like compounds in many fruits and vegetables. Phytoestrogens are mostly limited to the plant family of Leguminosae, which includes soybeans, chickpeas, and licorice; and they are typically present in small amounts within these foods. Although most phytoestrogens have very weak estrogen-like activity, they can compete with estrogens, or replace estrogens in their absence, to interact with the estrogen receptors in the body. In this way, phytoestrogens may help work against some types of cancer that rely on estrogens for tumor growth, or replace estrogens after menopause or a hysterectomy. Researchers are therefore studying flavonoids to evaluate their ability to reduce the risk of certain types of cancers and heart diseases, and to treat some women's health conditions.

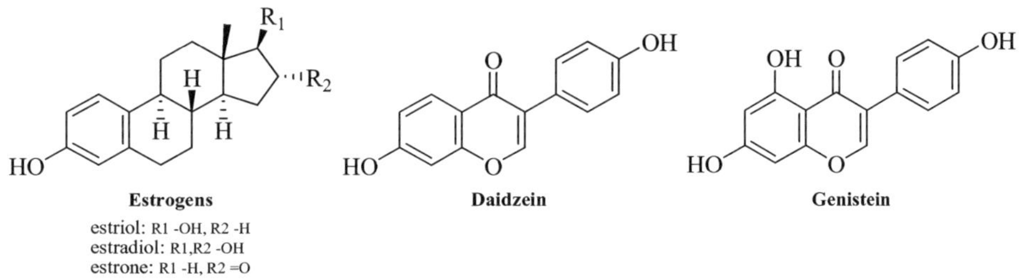

Fig. (4). Chemical structures of estrogens and two isoflavone phytoestrogens.

Isoflavones have received a great deal of attention in research, especially for possible cancer and heart disease preventative properties. However, most of the research has been done *in vitro* or in animal studies rather than clinical trials. There are many types of phytoestrogen isoflavones, but not all of them are in edible plants. The edible plant with the most concentrated amount of phytoestrogens, is the legume, soybean (Fig. **5**). Exact chemical analysis was done on a wide variety of soy foods, and there was considerable variability in the amounts of the isoflavones, as well as their chemical forms in each of the different soy foods.

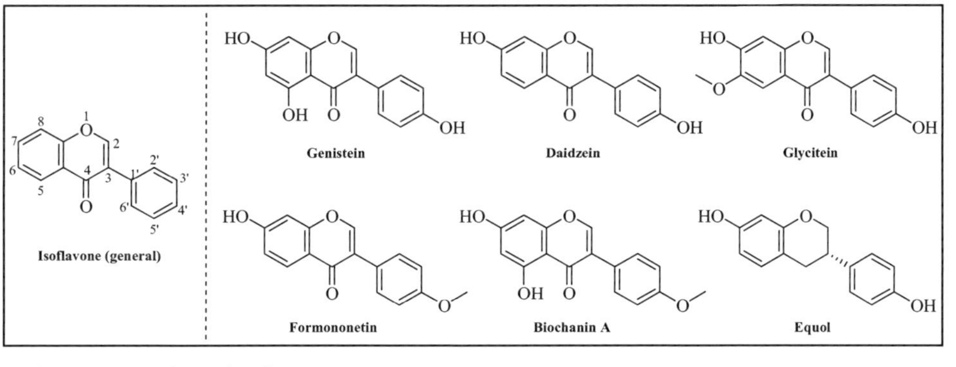

Fig. (5). Structures of soy isoflavones.

The predominant isoflavones in soy are genistein and daidzein, and their sugar-containing analogs, genistin and daidzin. During digestion, intestinal bacteria cleave the sugar molecules, resulting in more genistein and daidzein. Soy isoflavones act in at least four distinct ways: as estrogen mimics, antioxidants, enzyme regulators, and immune system boosters.

With chemical structures so similar to the endogenous estrogens produced in women, isoflavones are sometimes considered nonsteroidal estrogens. In a comparative absence of estrogen, isoflavones tend to have an estrogen-like effect. Christine Conrad and co-workers reported that soy isoflavones and other phytoestrogens are effective hormone replacements post-hysterectomy (Laux and Conrad, 1997). There have also been several Japanese and US patents since 1996 for the formulation of isoflavone-containing products that are estrogenic enough to promote bone formation or to prevent osteoporosis and fracture. In addition, the European drug ipriflavone, used to prevent and treat osteoporosis, is a synthetic isoflavone; it is often synthesized from daidzein, and daidzein is one of its human drug metabolites (Bassleer *et al.,* 1996). Isoflavones also act as antiestrogens by competing for estrogen receptors with endogenous estrogens, interfering with tumor growth in estrogen-dependent cancers. The use of isoflavones as antiestrogens will be discussed further in the cancer section of chapter 10.

Isoflavones, as part of the flavonoid family, are powerful antioxidants. Genistein, followed by daidzein, are among the most potent isoflavonoid antioxidants (Ruiz-Larrea *et al.,* 1997). In addition to quenching free radicals, genistein may also increase production of superoxide dismutase (SOD) in the body (Cai and Wei, 1996). SOD is a powerful endogenous enzyme that quenches superoxide radicals to prevent cellular damage. In a combination of *in vitro* and mice *in vivo* studies, daidzein was demonstrated to act as an immune stimulator (Wang *et al.,* 1997; Zhang *et al.,* 1997).

7.3.2.2. Anthocyanidins

Anthocyanidins are a subdivision of flavonoids with an electric charge on the heteroatom of the C ring (Figs. **2**, **6**). Anthocyanidins are often responsible for the red, purple, and blue colors in fruits such as berries, grapes, and currants, and in flowers such as peonies and petunias. Anthocyanidins with sugar molecules bonded in one to three locations, are called anthocyanins (Fig. **6**). The anthocyanins from grapes are responsible for the different aromas, tastes, and colors of wine.

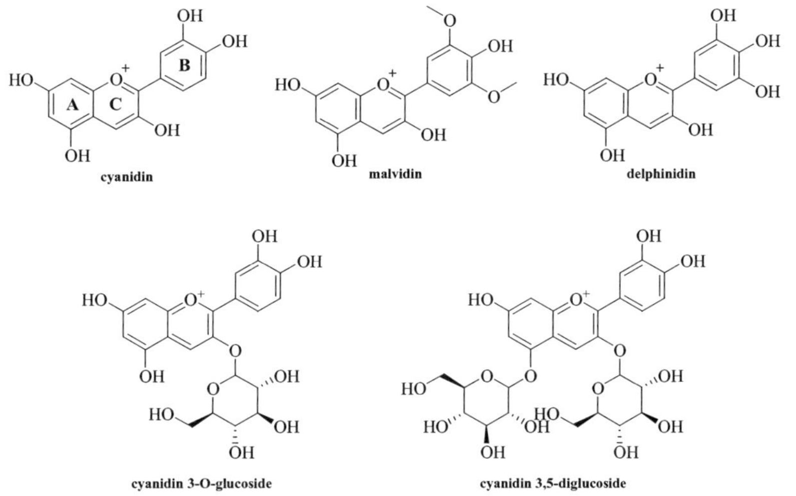

Fig. (6). Examples of anthocyanidins (top) and anthocyanins (bottom).

Blueberries and the related bilberries (common to Europe), with their deep blue color, contain anthocyanins. In a study with a rat model of cataracts and macular degeneration, 25mg/kg of bilberry extract (containing just 4.5mg/kg of anthocyanins) prevented both vision impairments (Fursova *et al.,* 2005).

Anthocyanidins, rather than the sugar-containing anthocyanins, are typically responsible for the therapeutic value of these types of phytochemicals. In fact, when producers standardize a dietary supplement that will contain anthocyanins, the sugar portions are often removed in the processing. However, incorporation of the sugar moiety onto the anthocyanidin core drastically improves its water solubility, allowing for a higher quantity of anthocyanidins in juices and wines. In fact, if making blueberry muffins with canned blueberries, anthocyanins often leach out of the berries and into the canning syrup; draining the syrup before adding the blueberries to the muffin mix rinses away many of the anthocyanins (Brownmiller *et al.,* 2008). In addition, the improved solubility of anthocyanins may allow greater absorption into the bloodstream. The two most common anthocyanidins in the human diet are cyanidin and malvidin; both are well absorbed when administered in anthocyanin forms.

Several anthocyanins have been shown to have antioxidant effects, antiviral properties, anti-inflammatory activity, and even anti-tumor properties. The suggestion to drink one glass of red wine per day to reduce the risk of cardiovascular disease may also be related to the anthocyanin content of wine.

7.3.2.3. Proanthocyanidins

When many anthocyanidins or flavan-3-ols (Fig. **6**) are linked, the resulting polymer is called a proanthocyanidin. The most prominent dietary sources of proanthocyanidins include cocoa nibs, apples, cranberries, deep red to purple grapes, and red wines (Hammerstone *et al.,* 2000).

Cranberry extract is available as a dietary supplement or over the counter therapy for preventing urinary tract infections. The active phytochemical ingredient in the cranberry extracts are proanthocyanidins, which act by preventing infection-causing bacteria from adhering to the cell walls in the urinary tract. Proanthocyanidins wrap around the bacteria, interfering with peripheral adhesion proteins on the bacterial cell. Bacteria that cannot adhere to the walls of the bladder or urethra are excreted in the urine before an infection can occur (Howell, 2007). The use of preventing or even the possibility of treating urinary tract infections with cranberry is an excellent alternative to using prescription antibacterial drugs as bacteria are rapidly gaining drug resistance.

Some pine tree bark extracts that contain numerous phenolic compounds (*e.g.*, proanthocyanidins and flavonoids) have been proposed to treat cardiovascular diseases, hypertension, and blood circulation and clotting disorders. An eight-week clinical trial in coronary artery disease patients indicated that treatment with 200mg/day of the pine tree bark extract (Pycnogenol) significantly reduced oxidative stress and improved endothelial cell function (Enseleit *et al.,* 2012). Although the evidence for Pycnogenol or other proanthocyanidin formulations for effectively treating cardiovascular diseases is not advanced enough for FDA drug approval, Pycnogenol and similar pine tree bark extracts are sold as dietary supplements for treating a number of conditions.

7.3.3. Terpenoids and Steroids

Terpenoids make up the largest group of natural products, and terpenoids and steroids are made through a common biosynthetic pathway, which will not be discussed in detail. Terpenoids vary in size, typically from molecules with five to 40 carbon atoms; however, they almost always contain a number of carbons that is a factor of five. This is due to the head-to-tail arrangement of the 5-carbon isoprene units (Table **2**). Monoterpenes have two isoprene units (10 carbons), diterpenes have four isoprene units (20 carbons), triterpenes have six (30 carbons), and tetraterpenes include eight (40 carbons) (Table **2**). Some terpenoids are straight-chained, and many of the larger terpenoids are cyclized. From the cyclized triterpenes, two important classes of phytochemicals are derived: the sapogenins (Fig. 7) and the phytosterols (Fig. 9). Both groups have structures similar to plant and animal steroids, with their core structures consisting of three linked six-membered rings and one five-membered ring. Sapogenins and phytosterols differ in their substitution of the five-membered ring (D ring).

Table 2. Terpenoid classifications with colored indicators of individual isoprene units in examples of each terpenoid class (hemi-, sesqui-, and sester-terpenoids not shown) (Dewick, 2009).

Terpenoid Type (# of Carbons)	Isoprene Units	Examples of Corresponding Terpenoids
Isoprene Unit (C_5)	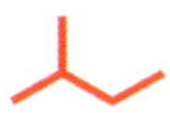	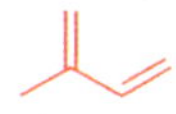 isoprene
Monoterpenes (C_{10})	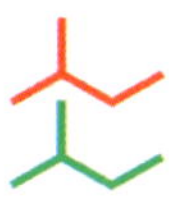	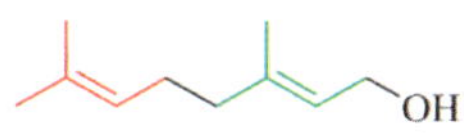 geraniol 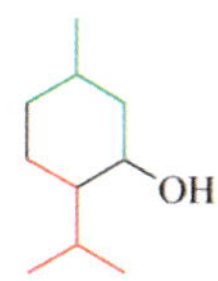 menthol
Diterpenes (C_{20})	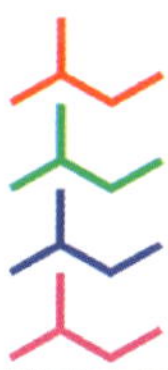	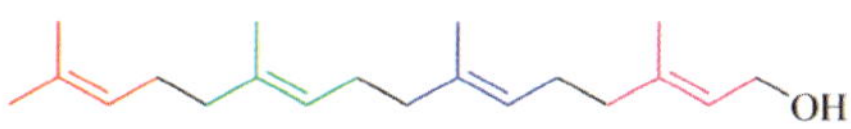 geranylgeraniol 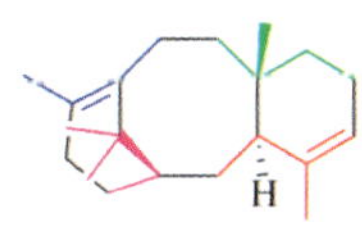 taxadiene
Triterpenes (C_{30})	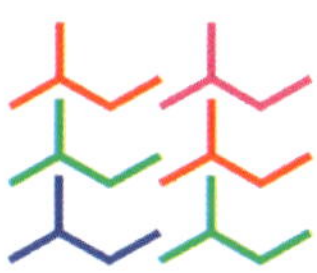	lupeol 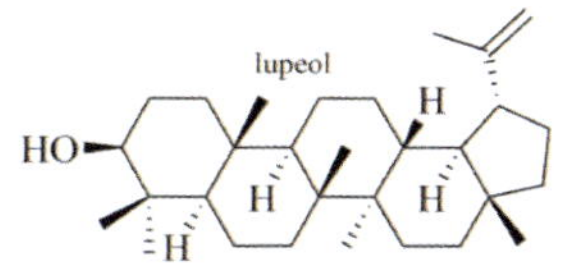 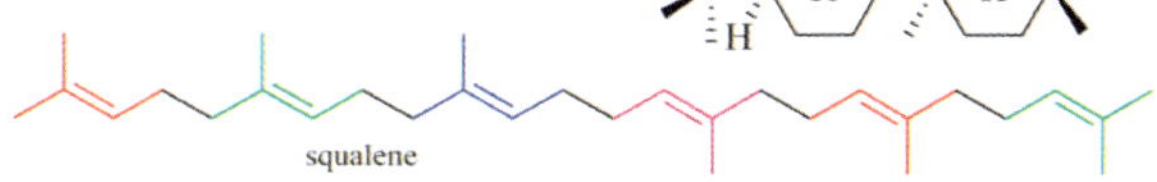 squalene
Tetraterpenes (C_{40})	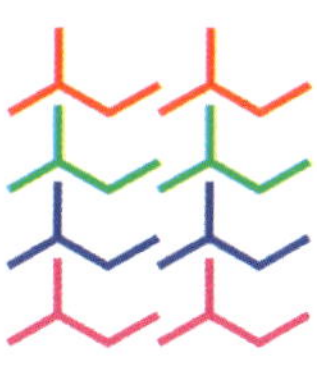	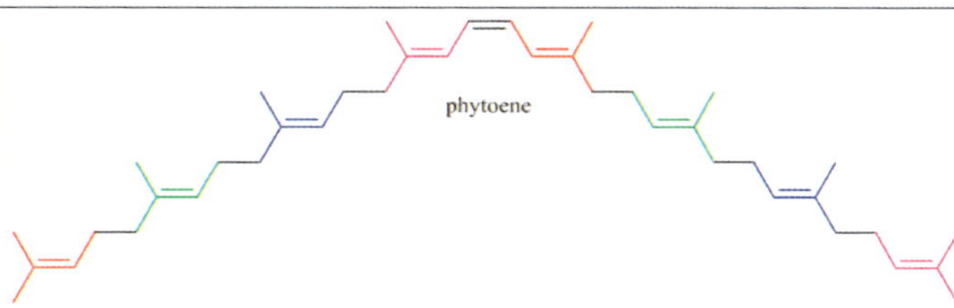 phytoene

7.3.3.1. Sapogenins

Sapogenins with sugars attached are called saponins. *Sapon*, which means soap, refers to the tendency of saponins to foam or become sudsy when agitated in water. Notice that some package directions for cooking quinoa grains, depending on how the product was processed, call for the grains to be rinsed before cooking. This is to rid the quinoa grains of extra sapogenins, which impart a bitter taste. Just as with anthocyanidins and anthocyanins, the molecule with sugars attached (saponins or anthocyanins) are more water-soluble than their non-sugar counterparts (sapogenins and anthocyanidins). Therefore, saponins may be more easily extracted into beverages or more bioavailable for a pharmacological effect, than are sapogenins (although neither forms appear to be very bioavailable as saponins have only been detected in the intestine or feces, and have not been found in blood or urine) (Kang *et al.,* 2010; Tsukamoto and Yoshiki, 2005; Gestetner *et al.,* 1968). Saponins and sapogenins have been studied for therapeutic potential as antioxidant, antiviral, antihepatotoxic, immunostimulatory, antihyperlipidemic, anti-diabetes, hormone stimulatory, and anticarcinogenic agents (Leela and Shafeekh, 2008; Basu and Srichamroen, 2010; Park *et al.,* 2005; Shibata, 2001; Tantry and Khan, 2013).

The most important and most abundant sapogenin is called diosgenin (Fig. 7). In the pharmaceutical industry, diosgenin is often extracted from plant material to serve as starting material for the semi-synthesis of androgenic, anti-inflammatory, contraceptive, and estrogenic steroidal drugs (Sautour *et al.,* 2007; Leela and Shafeekh, 2008). Diosgenin is also known to act through NFκB to increase apoptosis, an indicator of a potential cancer chemopreventative or chemotherapeutic agent (Leela and Shafeekh, 2008). The most common sources of saponins and sapogenins from food or dietary supplements are fenugreek, ginseng, soybeans, and wild yams.

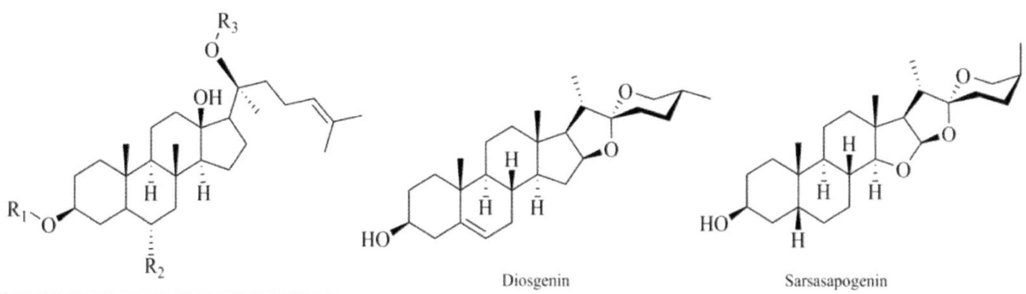

	R_1	R_2	R_3
Ginsenoside Rb1	$Glc^{2}\text{-}^{1}Glc$	H	$Glc^{6}\text{-}^{1}Glc$
Ginsenoside Rg1	H	O-Glc	Glc

Fig. (7). Saponin aglycones, also called sapogenins, from ginseng, yam and fenugreek, and sarsaparilla (from left to right).

Fenugreek (*Trigonella foenum-graecum*) is commonly incorporated into foods and spices in India, and in the United States, it is the primary flavoring agent used in the production of imitation maple syrup (Basu and Srichamroen, 2010). The leaves of fenugreek are also sometimes consumed as vegetables. In addition to these dietary uses, fenugreek is often used in traditional medicine for treating burns, swelling, baldness, or for use during pregnancy and lactation. The saponins from fenugreek have been studied as antihyperlipidemic agents and in treatment of several diabetes-associated symptoms (frequent urination, insatiable thirst, and weight loss) (Basu and Srichamroen, 2010). Diosgenin makes up about five percent of the fenugreek seed; the three most abundant sapogenins in fenugreek are diosgenin, tigogenin, and gitogenin (from most abundant to least) (Leela and Shafeekh, 2008). The antihyperlipidemic effect of fenugreek is thought to occur by interacting with bile acids and increasing cholesterol degradation (Basu and Srichamroen, 2010; Sidhu and Oakenfull, 2007; Bhaumick *et al.,* 2008). In both diabetic and normal rats, fenugreek saponins decreased cholesterol levels in the plasma (Petit *et al.,* 1995; Leela and Shafeekh, 2008).

Ginseng (*Panax ginseng* and other closely related *Panax* species) contains numerous saponins, typically referred to as ginsenosides. Ginseng is used in traditional medicine for innumerable ailments and conditions, but the ginsenosides have been primarily identified with the pharmacological activities listed in Table **3** In addition to those, a ginseng berry extract with the major component ginsenoside Re had anti-hyperglycemic and anti-obesity properties. In a 1985 study, diabetic rats treated with ginsenoside Rb2 experienced a significant decrease in blood glucose concentration (Yokozawa *et al.,* 1985).

Table 3. Pharmacological activity of saponins from ginseng (adapted from Shibata, 2001).

Possible Pharmacological Activity (includes *in vitro* and *in vivo* data/results)	Ginsenosides									
	R0	Rb1	Rb2	Rc	Rd	Re	Rg1	Rg2	Rg3	Rh2
Anti-platelet aggregation	■						■	■		
Vasodilating action		■			■		■			
Cholesterol decreasing and HDL increasing		■	■	■						
Hormone stimulation		■	■	■		■				
Stimulation of RNA or protein synthesis		■		■			■			
Anticancer activity (any mechanism/phase)			■					■	■	■

Soybeans are the primary dietary source of saponins and sapogenins. The saponins from soybeans foam or bubble in the process of making tofu. Some methods for the production of tofu skim the bubbles (and saponins) off, while other techniques leave the saponin components in the product (Tsukamoto and Yoshiki, 2005). Soy saponins affect cholesterol metabolism through interaction with bile acids as discussed for fenugreek, but soy saponins also form insoluble complexes with cholesterol, which inhibits cholesterol from being absorbed in the intestines (Kang *et al.,* 2010). The medicinal value of soybean phytochemicals is often thought to be due only to the isoflavone components. In fact, saponins in soy have long been regarded as anti-nutrients because of their undesirable effects on the absorption and utilization of protein (Kang *et al.,* 2010). Alfalfa (*Medicago sativa*) too, is a high-protein food rich in saponins, and many farmers refuse to feed livestock the grain because the saponins act as anti-nutrients and affect protein utilization and digestion in the animals (Sen *et al.,* 1998). However, more recent research suggests that soy saponins may be responsible for some of the other therapeutic effects of soybean that were not traceable to soy isoflavones. Among these possible therapeutic effects from soy saponins are cholesterol-lowering and some anticarcinogenic activities (Cabrera-Orozco *et al.,* 2013).

Wild yams (*Dioscorea villosa* and other closely related *Dioscorea* species) are a significant source of saponins and sapogenins. It should also be noted, however, that most "yams" that are consumed in the United States are actually sweet potatoes (*Ipomoea* species), which are taxonomically unrelated to *Dioscorea* species. Wild yams, often bitter from their high saponin content, are more typically used for traditional medicine than for food. As a traditional medicine, there are several formulations containing wild yam, for the relief of menopausal symptoms. It was previously thought that the saponins in wild yam were converted into sapogenins, and in turn into progesterone, in the body. However, a small, 3-month clinical trial in menopausal women compared a commercial topical cream that included wild yam extract in the formulation, to a placebo topical cream, with no statistical difference between the two groups (Komesaroff *et al.,* 2001). Moreover, the wild yam group did not experience a change in hormone levels, and the menopausal symptoms did not subside (Komesaroff *et al.,* 2001). Several other herbal treatments have shown more clinical efficacy in relieving menopausal symptoms than the sapogenins from wild yam, and the ability of those sapogenins to be converted into hormones *in vivo* is highly disputed. Interestingly, due to the abundance of diosgenin in the *Dioscorea* species, yams are the most common source of diosgenin for the semi-synthesis of steroidal drugs in the pharmaceutical industry (Sautour *et al.,* 2007).

Sarsaparilla (*Smilax officinalis* and other closely related *Smilax* species) is also a source of sapogenins, though not one common to the North American diet. Sarsaparilla is used in traditional medicine to treat gout, arthritis, inflammation and many inflammation-associated conditions (Bernardo *et al.,* 1996; Sashida *et al.,* 1992; Challinor *et al.,* 2012). Sarsaparilla was also once used as a flavoring agent for root beer, but artificial flavoring has since replaced it. Saponins that may be isolated from sarsaparilla include sarsasapogenins (Fig. **7**), furostanol, and spirostanol glycosides (Challinor *et al.,* 2012).

The Maasai, an ethnic group from parts of Kenya and Tanzania, have long been known for their paradoxically high dietary intake of fatty foods (milk, animal blood, and meat) yet almost nonexistent incidence of cardiovascular disease. While many factors such as low overall caloric intake, more frequent exercise, or their genetics may explain the paradox, Timothy Johns and colleagues point to the inclusion of roots and barks that the Maasai add to milk-based soups (Johns *et al.,* 1999). In consulting retrospective phytochemical studies of several of the root and bark additives, a high level of saponins, polyphenols, dietary fibers, and phytosterols may be correlated to the Maasai diet conundrum. All four of these substituents, with emphasis on saponins and phytosterols within this chapter, have been individually reported for their antihyperlipidemic or cholesterol-lowering abilities. Although a comparative dietary study between a Western population and the Maasai population remains to be performed, the phytochemicals ingested in the Maasai diet offers a perceivable hypothesis for explaining the high fat consumption, yet low cardiovascular disease rate of the Maasai population. Also of interest is that the root and bark additives are cooked in a high-fat liquid, allowing for a higher yielding extraction of lipophilic compounds such as sapogenins and phytosterols into the soup broth for easier absorption.

7.3.3.2. Phytosterols

Phytosterols are plant steroid alcohols that very closely resemble the chemical structure of the animal steroid alcohol, cholesterol (Fig. **8**). Despite its negative connotation, cholesterol is essential for life and is a critical component of cellular membranes and the central nervous system.

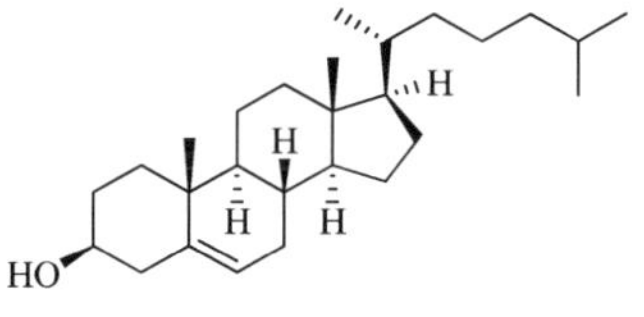

Fig. (8). Cholesterol.

Just as cholesterol is the human precursor to all steroidal hormones (*e.g.*, cortisol, estrogen, progesterone, and testosterone), beta-sitosterol (Fig. **9**) is the plant sterol precursor to growth and reproductive hormones. In fact, some phytosterols are so similar to medicinal steroids, that stigmasterol and sitosterol (Fig. **9**) from soybeans are often semi-synthetically modified to produce therapeutic steroidal hormones including androgens, progestogens, and corticosteroids (Dewick, 2009; Wang *et al.*, 2011; Schmidt *et al.*, 2008).

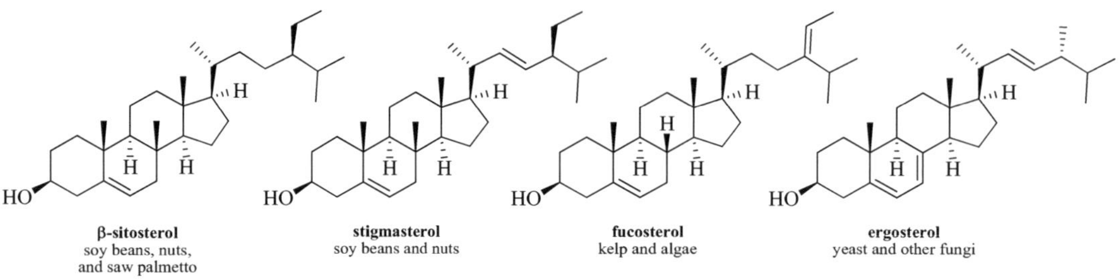

Fig. (9). Natural sterols, including phytosterols, and their sources.

Phytosterols, to an even greater extent than sapogenins, have cholesterol-lowering abilities (Kang *et al.*, 2010; Lerman *et al.*, 2008; Jenkins *et al.*, 2005). Phytosterols also have some anticancer and immunomodulatory effects, though the mechanisms for those effects have not yet been fully elucidated. The most common natural dietary sources of phytosterols are legumes, nuts, whole grains, vegetables, and oils and margarines (Lagarda *et al.*, 2006).

A recent study demonstrated the astounding antihypercholesterolemic effect of phytosterols, in accompaniment with other known antihyperlipidemic phytochemicals (Jenkins *et al.*, 2005; Denke, 2005). Hyperlipidemic patients (n = 34) followed three different 1-month diet programs in random order. The three programs consisted of a low saturated fat diet; a low saturated fat diet with 20mg lovastatin; and a diet high in phytosterols, soy protein, almonds, and fiber from grains and vegetables. The latter two diets were nearly equally effective at lowering LDL-cholesterol levels (33.3 and 29.6%, respectively) (Jenkins *et al.*, 2005). Another human study, which compared the Mediterranean diet (famous for being heart-healthy) to a modified Mediterranean diet (supplemented with phytosterols, proanthocyanidins, a hops extract, and soy protein), demonstrated that the modified diet decreased the cardiovascular disease risk score of the test subjects more than those on the standard Mediterranean diet (Lerman *et al.*, 2008).

The cholesterol-lowering abilities of phytosterols are effective and well-known enough that the US National Cholesterol Education Program recommends adding 2.0 g of phytosterols daily to the adult diet in order to decrease low density lipoprotein-cholesterol and to reduce the risk of cardiovascular disease (Executive Summary, 2001). In order to meet that 2.0 g recommendation, manufacturers are producing phytosterol-enriched functional foods; enriched margarines are the most common, but phytosterol-enriched yogurt, milk, bread, and cereal products are also appearing in grocery stores.

The antihyperlipidemic effect of phytosterols is to compete with cholesterol for absorption in the intestinal lumen (Kang *et al.,* 2010). However, the extra methyl or ethyl groups on phytosterols increase their hydrophobicity in comparison to cholesterol, so cholesterol absorption occurs preferentially. That being said, phytosterols are still absorbed, and the more phytosterols in the diet, the less cholesterol can be absorbed (to a certain extent) (Kang *et al.,* 2010; Clifton *et al.,* 2004). In fact, that very point is raising fear of phytosterol overconsumption with the increased accessibility to enriched functional foods; although hyperlipidemia is the current concern in the US, having too little cholesterol is also harmful to the body. In addition to the concern of low cholesterol levels due to overconsumption of phytosterols, it has also been demonstrated that high levels of phytosterols decrease the absorptivity of vitamin A precursors, lutein, lycopene, and vitamin E, begging the question if the same is true for numerous fat-soluble vitamins and phytochemicals (Table **4**) (Clifton *et al.,* 2004).

Table 4: Importance of cholesterol and phytosterol balance in the diet (adapted from Clifton *et al.,* 2004

	Phytosterols (g)
Human on an average Western diet consumes:	**0.15-0.4**
National Cholesterol Education Program recommends consuming:	**2**
Cholesterol-lowering effect continues in a dose-response pattern until consumption of:	**> 3.2**
No additional cholesterol-lowering effect, but decreased absorption of liposoluble vitamins and phytochemicals begin to occur after consumption of:	**> 6.6**

In addition to phytosterols produced by plants, algae and fungi also biosynthesize sterols. For example, red yeast rice, a rice dish served in Asia that is also used medicinally, produces ergosterol (Fig. **9**) and other sterols. In fact, monacolin K, also known by the pharmaceutical industry as lovastatin, is naturally produced in red yeast rice. Thus, the food has been formulated as a dietary supplement and marketed for lowering cholesterol. However, as with any dietary supplement, consumers should be cautious when selecting a particular product because companies and batches often vary in the amount of monacolin K and other sterols (and thus effectiveness) in the product. Edible fungi (*e.g.*, kelp, mushrooms, and spirulina) are known to produce fucosterol, ergosterol (Fig. **9**), and other sterols, which may have cholesterol-lowering effects similar to phytosterols.

Another important activity of phytosterols is their protective and therapeutic actions against diseases of the prostate. Saw palmetto (*Serenoa repens*), a dietary supplement, contains a high level of fatty acids and a moderate amount of phytosterols; it is thought that the combination of the fatty acids and the phytosterols in saw palmetto are effective against benign prostate hyperplasia (BPH), lower urinary tract infections, nonbacterial prostitis, and perhaps even prostate cancer (Scholtysek *et al.,* 2009). Saw palmetto is sold over the counter, but like the BPH prescription drug finasteride, the dietary supplement inhibits 5α-reductase. An *in vitro* study by Scholtysek and colleagues demonstrated that a saw palmetto berry extract (a combination of phytosterols and fatty acids) was effective against prostate cancer cells to a greater extent than individual dosages of beta-sitosterol, stigmasterol, or cholesterol (Scholtysek *et al.,* 2009). This study also reported that cholesterol actually increased the cancer cell growth; therefore, phytosterol inhibition of cholesterol absorption may also play a role in the contribution of saw palmetto to prostate health (Scholtysek *et al.,* 2009). Coleman and coworkers conducted a clinical study, in which the patients experienced improved urological symptoms and urine flow with treatment of saw palmetto in comparison to placebo (Coleman *et al.,* 2002). The beneficial effects from saw palmetto were similar to the effectiveness of finasteride in the same study. The researchers concluded "phytosterols are generally well tolerated and potentially effective in treating symptoms of BPH and in improving quality of life" (Coleman *et al.,* 2002).

As mentioned, phytosterols are commonly found in vegetables and vegetable oils. In fact, in the production of soybean oil, there is a step that is the main source of phytosterols which supply pharmaceutical companies and phytosterol functional food manufacturers (Wang *et al.,* 2011). The deodorization process in refining soybean oil produces a distillate, which contains the primary commercial source of phytosterols. Pharmaceutical companies use phytosterols, especially stigmasterol and sitosterol, in microbial cultures so the microbes metabolize the starting material into steroidal drugs (Wang *et al.,* 2011).

7.3.4. Organosulfur Phytochemicals

Some organosulfur phytochemicals, or sulfur-containing phytochemicals, have been indicated in enhancing the immune system and even in cancer chemoprevention. Common sources of these organosulfur phytochemicals in the human diet include glucosinolates and their metabolites found in cruciferous vegetables, as well as sulfides found in garlic and onions.

7.3.4.1. Cruciferous Vegetables

Cruciferous vegetables (members of the cabbage family that include bok choy, collards, broccoli, Brussels sprouts, watercress, mustard greens, kohlrabi, kale, turnip greens, and cauliflower) contain glucosinolates (Fig. **10**), and glucosinolates are metabolized by enzymatic reactions to yield isothiocyanates (and several other reaction products).

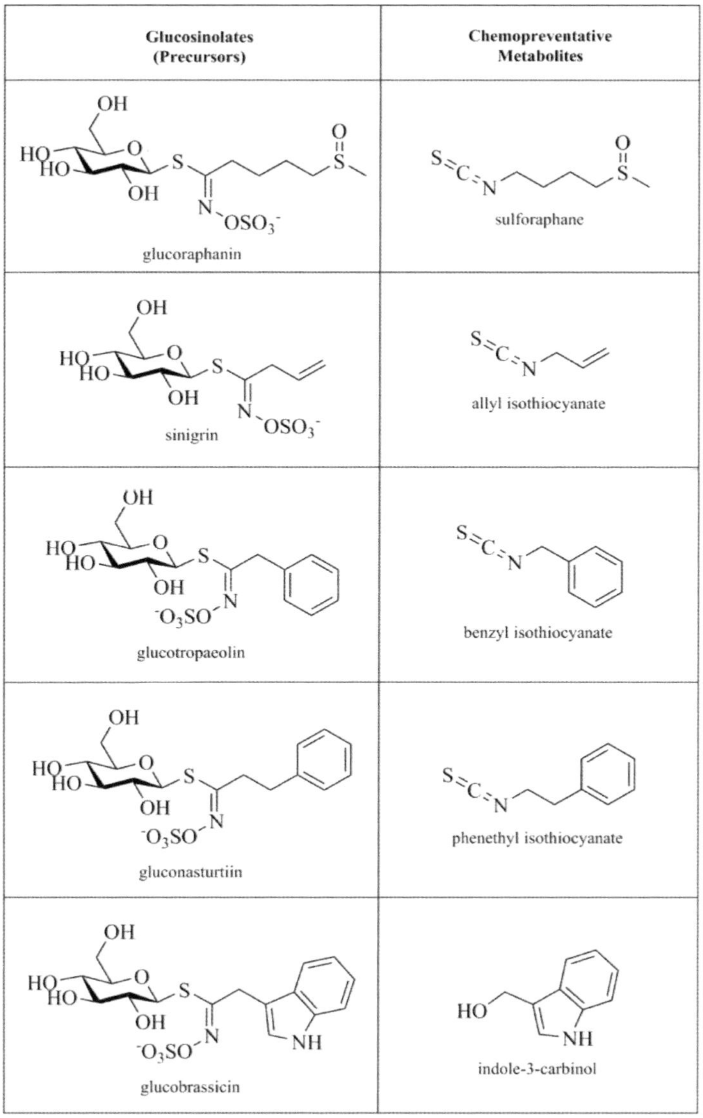

Fig. (10). Glucosinolates found in cruciferous vegetables, and their cancer chemopreventative metabolites (isothiocyanates and indoles) (Higdon *et al.,* 2007).

The isothiocyanates are responsible for the bitter or pungent tastes and smells that are most notable from boiling cabbage or broccoli, but which also flavor mustard and horseradish. In addition, these isothiocyanates (*i.e.* sulforaphane), along with another glucosinolate metabolite called indole-3-carbinol, have been investigated for their use as cancer chemopreventative agents (Fig. **10**). Although the active metabolite indole-3-carbinol does not contain a sulfur atom, its natural precursor, which is found in cruciferous vegetables, does.

The possible cancer chemopreventative activity of isothiocyanates and indoles from cruciferous vegetables (most notably sulforaphane and indole-3-carbinol from broccoli and Brussels sprouts) are in part due to their prevention of carcinogenesis by inhibiting cytochrome P450 (or more generally, phase I) enzymes from producing toxic metabolites, and by activating phase II enzymes to prevent ROS- or DNA-damage.

The enzyme myrosinase, which converts glucosinolates to their isothiocyanate or indole metabolites, is stored in separate cellular compartments away from the glucosinolates in cruciferous vegetables (Higdon *et al.,* 2007). When vegetables are chewed, the enzyme is released, coming in contact with the glucosinolates, and the active metabolites become available for absorption by the consumer.

However, extensive cooking, especially in water, will limit the availability of these compounds. Glucosinolates are water-soluble compounds, and if they are boiled, the glucosinolates and metabolites may leach out of the vegetable that will be consumed, into the cooking water to be thrown out. In addition, myrosinase may be denatured and/or deactivated by heating and cooking processes; without active myrosinase, the glucosinolates cannot be converted to their active metabolites for human absorption and a cancer chemopreventative effect. However, there is some evidence that intestinal bacteria in the human gut can metabolize glucosinolates to the cancer chemopreventative compounds, but not at as high of a rate (Higdon *et al.,* 2007).

7.3.4.2. Allium Species

Garlic, onion, and other members of the *Allium* genus also produce sulfur-containing phytochemicals, many of which are volatile compounds and give garlic or onion their smell and health-related properties. Alliin is a stable sulfoxide, and alliinase is a stable enzyme, found in different cellular storage compartments in garlic.

However, when garlic is crushed, chopped, or chewed, alliin and alliinase come into contact in the presence of water or moisture (such as in the mouth, on the countertop, or water from the disrupted cells), they are destabilized and undergo an enzymatic reaction to produce allicin (Fig. **11**).

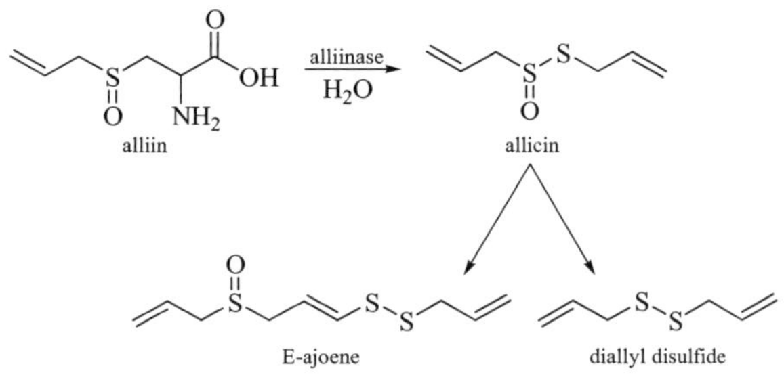

Fig. (11). Enzymatic reaction to form an active component of garlic (allicin) and two of its degradation products.

Allicin is a volatile and odiferous thiosulfinate that gives the smell most associated with the pungency of garlic. Allicin has several metabolites or degradation products, including diallyl [mono-, di-, and tri-] sulfides and Z- and E-ajoenes (Fig. **11**), which are also volatile and smelly. In most cases, the compounds responsible for the health-promoting activities are allicin or its degradation products.

Many of these organosulfur *Allium* compounds, and garlic as a whole, have been studied for their ability to treat or prevent microbial infections, carcinogenesis, or cardiovascular disease. In particular, many of the sulfur-containing compounds from the *Allium* genus have been shown to have antimicrobial activity, the allyl sulfides (*e.g.*, diallyl mono-, di-, and trisulfides) have been extensively studied for anti-cancer effects, and the ajoenes have exhibited significant antithrombotic effects. For simplicity, the vinyl dithiins from garlic are not shown; however, they are known to have some antimicrobial activity and may aid in lowering cholesterol levels (Rahman, 2007; Ohta, 1999). The degree of usefulness of these organosulfur compounds as chemopreventative or therapeutic agents is disputed within the scientific literature, due to the wide variety of preparations used in *in vitro, in vivo*, and human studies. Since many of the sulfur-containing compounds are volatile, they are lost in drying or cooking methods, so the different preparations vary in concentrations of each of the components. Any cooking methods that use high heat may also denature or inactivate the alliinase enzyme, preventing the formation of the active components allicin and degradation products.

For antibacterial activity, 1 mg of allicin has been equated to 10 μg penicillin (Kamel and Saleh, 2000). In fact, when the Russian army ran out of penicillin in World War II, they resorted to using garlic, just as was done before the discovery of penicillin in 1928. Allicin works as an antibacterial agent by reacting with bacterial enzymes that contain SH-groups, inhibiting the enzymes (Kamel and Saleh, 2000). However, most studies of allicin as an antimicrobial agent have been *in vitro*, and allicin degrades too rapidly to be detected in human blood, urine, or breath (Lawson *et al.,* 1992; Taucher *et al.,* 1996; Kamel and Saleh, 2000). It is also thought that the disulfide bond is essential for the antibacterial activity, which may explain why the ajoenes and several other *Allium* disulfide compounds have antibacterial or antimicrobial properties (Naganawa *et al.,* 1996). Some of the disulfide compounds from garlic are even mildly active against gastric ulcer- and cancer-causing bacteria (*Helicobacter pylori*) (Table **5**) (Ohta, 1999). And three disulfide compounds from *Allium stipitatum* (Persian shallot) are very active against multi-drug resistant bacteria such as MRSA (methicillin-resistant *Staphylococcus aureus*) and other *S. aureus* strains resistant to the antibacterial drugs norfloxacin, oxacillin, and/or tetracyclines (Table **6**) (O'Donnell *et al.,* 2009).

Table 5. *In vitro* antibacterial activity of three sulfur-containing compounds from garlic (adapted from Ohta, 1999).

Test Agent	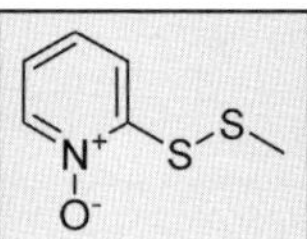	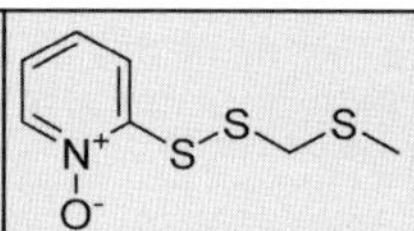	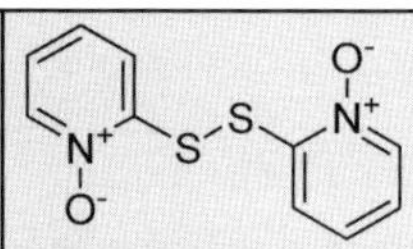	Norfloxacin	Oxacillin
Drug Resistant Bacterial Strains	*In vitro* Minimum Inhibitory Concentration (MIC) in (μg/mL)				
S. auerus (SA-1199B)	2	1	1	32	0.25
S. aureus (XU212)	1	1	1	16	128
S. aureus (EMRSA-15)	0.5	0.5	0.5	0.5	32

Consuming garlic or onion to treat a bacterial infection may be more beneficial than taking a prescription antibacterial since multi-component products or treatment agents such as functional foods (which may contain thousands of different phytochemicals) make it difficult to develop drug-resistance. In addition, physicians are cautious to prescribe antibacterial agents because they not only treat the infection, but also eliminate the good bacteria in the human digestive tract. Consuming a food product may not be as aggressive toward intestinal bacteria because many of the antibacterial compounds from edible products will have been at least partially metabolized before reaching the intestine, and may be found in smaller quantities in those products.

Table 6. Antibacterial activity of three disulfides isolated from *Allium stipitatum*, against multidrug resistant bacteria (adapted from O'Donnell *et al.*, 2009).

In vitro Minimum Inhibitory Concentration (MIC) in (µg/mL)				
Gastric Bacterial Strains	Allicin	E-ajoene	Z-ajoene	Amoxicillin
H. pylori (ATCC 43504)	20	25	20	0.025
H. pylori (ATCC 43579)	30	25	20	0.025
H. pylori (ATCC43629)	30	25	15	0.025

7.3.5. Phytochemicals in Spices

Many spices that are used to flavor foods contain hundreds of phytochemicals. Some of the phytochemicals in certain spices have been identified, while others are still unknown or have not yet been sufficiently investigated. Spices are concentrated and semi-purified in comparison to whole plants, so the disease preventative or treatment agents in spices are administered at a higher concentration than if the whole plant or fruit were consumed. Since there are so many spices, and many of them have not yet been well studied, the focus of the phytochemicals in the spices section is on those which have antimicrobial activity.

It is important to note that antimicrobial agents can be of two types: inhibitory or germicidal. Inhibitory agents inhibit the growth of the microorganism, but once removed, the microorganism may continue to grow. Germicidal antimicrobial agents act by a mechanism which kills the microorganism, and even upon removal of the agent, the organism cannot re-grow (Zaika, 1988). Fungal organisms are typically more sensitive to growth inhibition by spices than are bacteria, and gram-positive bacteria are typically more susceptible to the spices than gram-negative bacteria (Zaika, 1988).

Depending on the manufacturing process, some spices may contain microbial contaminants, and some spices even encourage growth of those microbes. However, the amount of spices that is added to foods is usually so minor that the microorganisms from the spices will not lead to food spoilage. Other spices may synergistically add to the effect of preservatives to help prevent spices or spiced foods from spoiling (Zaika, 1988). Several of the spices most used in daily cooking are listed in Table **7** and are categorized into strong, medium, and weak antimicrobial agents.

Table 7. Degree of antimicrobial activity of common spices (adapted from Zaika, 1988).

Inhibitory Effect
Strong: Cinnamon, clove, garlic, mustard
Medium: Allspice, bay leaf, caraway, coriander, cumin, oregano, rosemary, sage, thyme
Weak: Black pepper, ginger, red pepper

Although there is wide agreement among scientists that these spices have antimicrobial activity, it is difficult to indubitably rate which spice is more active than others. This is due to a number of factors including how the spice was prepared, the purity of the spice, the concentration of active components, the microbe being tested, and even the laboratory or scientist performing the experiment. Thus very few publications report results for a comprehensive list of spices that can be compared; one such report was published in 1984 with the essential oils of six common spices tested in an antimicrobial assay (Table **8**) (Shelef, 1984). In addition to the whole-spice antimicrobial activity, some scientists go on to identify the active antimicrobial components in the spices. This is time-consuming work, but several of the most common antimicrobial compounds are included in Table **8** Other important antimicrobial compounds isolated from spices but not included in the 1984 experiments are anethole, 1,8-cineole, limonene, and linalool (Fig. **12**).

anethole (star anise, fennel) | 1,8-cineole (sage, rosemary, laurel, cardemom) | limonene (celery seed, caraway, dill) | linalool (coriander, sage, rosemary, basil)

Fig. (12). Other antimicrobial compounds found in common cooking spices (Hitokoto *et al.,* 1980, Zaika, 1988, and Kellner and Kober, 1955).

7.4. INCORPORATING ADEQUATE PHYTOCHEMICALS INTO THE DIET

There is no one single miracle phytochemical; it is important to eat a balanced diet, incorporating a wide variety of fruits, vegetables, whole grains, nuts, beans, spices, and herbs. In doing so, consumers will achieve a vast array of phytochemicals that can contribute toward human health and nutrition in a

Table 8. Antimicrobial activity of essential oils of spices and active components (Shelef, 1984).

Spice/Herb (Essential Oil)	Proximate Essentail Oil Content (%)	Antimicrobial Component(s)
Garlic	0.3 - 0.5	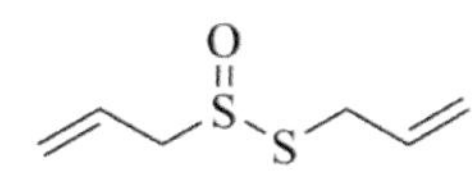 allicin
Mustard	0.5 - 1.0	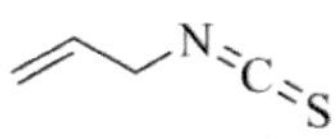 allyl isothiocyanate
Cinnamon	0.5 - 2.0	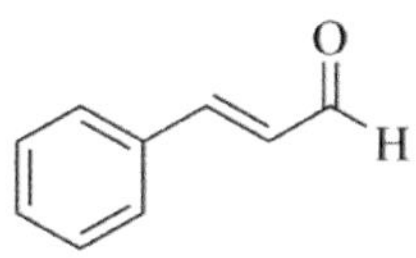 cinnamaldehyde 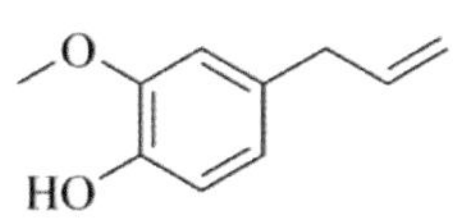 eugenol
Cloves	16 - 18	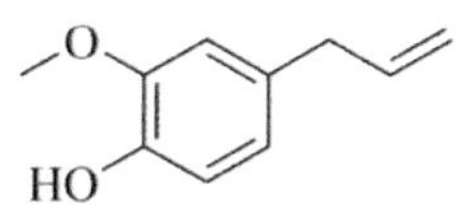 eugenol
Sage	0.7 - 2.0	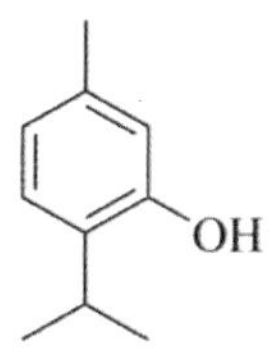 thymol 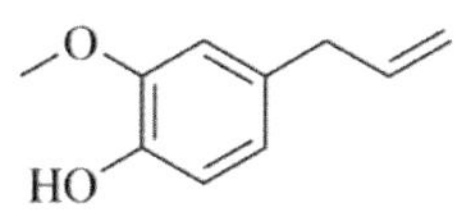 eugenol
Oregano	0.8 - 0.9	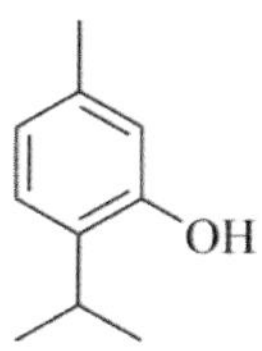 thymol 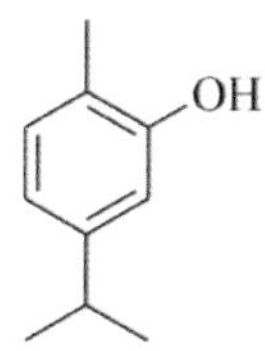 carvacrol

number of different ways. In order to get more phytochemicals in general, replace foods with refined sugars and alcohols with fresh produce. In addition to being a rich source of phytochemicals, produce is also rich in vitamins, minerals, and dietary fiber, and low in saturated fat. Aside from consuming foods rich in phytochemicals, it is also important to consume small amounts of healthy fats in order to increase absorption of liposoluble phytochemicals.

Although supermarkets are becoming more and more stocked with fresh fruits, vegetables, and herbs, the need to ship those products from far away has had a negative effect on the level of phytochemicals present in those products. In order for the produce to look fresh and ripe when it arrives in the store, many food harvesting and processing companies must harvest the produce before it is fully ripe. The un-ripened products then go through a forced chemical or physical change in order to make it appear ripe; this is most commonly achieved through application of ethylene gas (a natural, gaseous plant hormone that causes ripening), which causes flowers to open, produce to soften, and the skin on fruits and vegetables to change to their vibrant, ripeness-denoting colors. Different phytochemicals are present in the same plant throughout different phases of the growing season. Some of those phytochemicals do not develop until, or are in very low concentrations until the product is fully ripe. Many phytochemicals and even vitamins are not at their highest concentrations in the fruit or vegetable until the last few days of ripening. For example, un-ripened, hard, green tomatoes are often exposed to ethylene gas in ripening rooms of processing plants to force them to take on a red color and to soften the flesh, actions that would otherwise occur late-stage on the vine. In a study comparing tomatoes grown on the vine and off the vine, in the same environment, the former group contained 33% more lycopene, 33% more beta-carotene, and an equal amount of vitamin C than the latter (Arias *et al.,* 2000). In terms of optimal phytochemical content, it may therefore be advisable to grow tomatoes in a home garden or to purchase them from a farmer's market where the shortened shipping distance does not force an early harvest. For this same reason, it is preferred to consume fruits and vegetables that are locally grown and in-season.

In the future, it may become easier to attain adequate levels of phytochemicals in the diet, due to bioengineering and the development of new functional foods. This may be accomplished through selective breeding of edible plants, genetic modifications of the plants, or enrichment of phytochemicals into every day foods. There may even come a time when the National Academy of Science determines adequate intake or recommended daily allowance levels for phytochemicals, just as with vitamins and minerals. Further research into the health-promoting and disease-preventing and -treating properties of phytochemicals will aid such recommendations.

7.5 CONCLUDING REMARKS

While this chapter demonstrated the promising potential displayed by phytochemicals towards preventing or treating disease, it is important to remember that exploration of their role in human health, disease prevention, and treatment is still in its infancy. There is still a great deal of research that must be done before phytochemicals can be classified as preventative or therapeutic agents for human diseases. However, the traditional uses and preliminary research of phytochemicals presented in this chapter suggests that phytochemicals do play a significant role in human nutrition and health. The health benefits associated with phytochemicals are derived through several different mechanisms of action that have been detailed above, including macular pigmentation (*e.g.*, lutein and zeaxanthin), inhibition of bacterial adhesion (*e.g.*, cranberry proanthocyanidins), estrogen mimicry (*e.g.*, soy isoflavones), inhibition of cholesterol absorption (*e.g.*, phytosterols), cancer chemoprevention (*e.g.*, glucosinolate metabolites from cruciferous vegetables), and antimicrobial activity (*e.g.*, some spices and *Allium* organosulfur compounds), among others. The conscious incorporation of phytochemicals into the diet, and further study of their mechanisms, will compel increased thinking of phytochemicals as health-promoting agents or even pharmaceutical-like foods.

Test your knowledge: List the types of phytochemicals you might find in each of the following natural food products.

Products		Phytochemicals
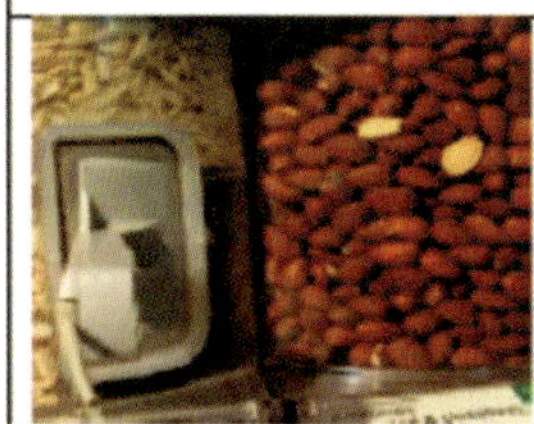	Almonds	
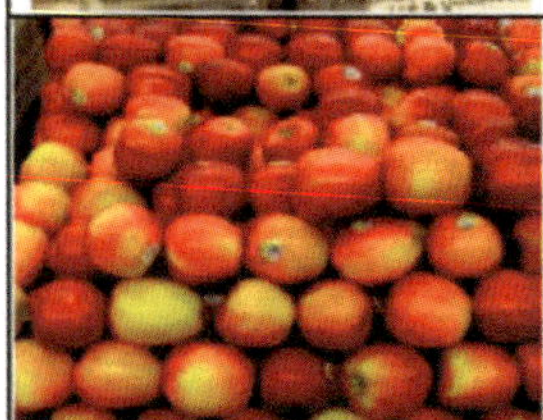	Apples	
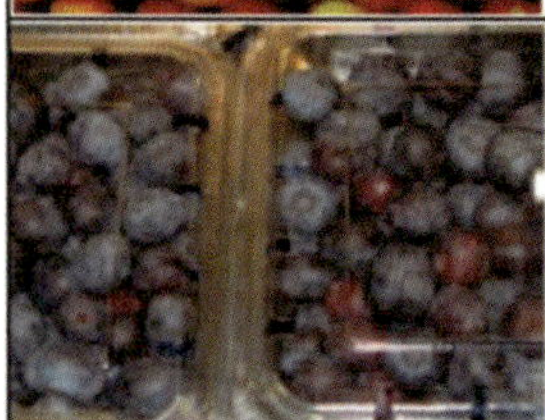	Blueberries	
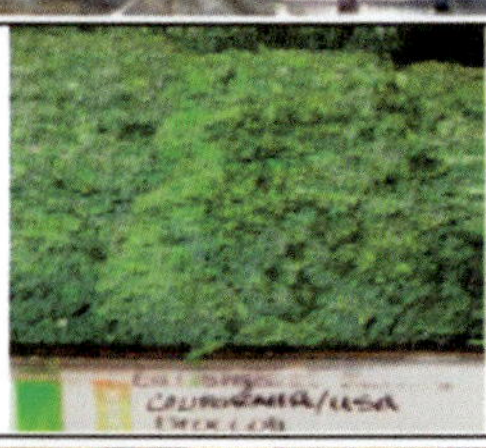	Broccoli	
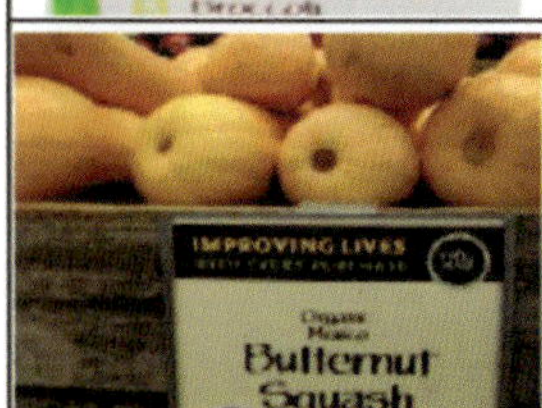	Butternut Squash	
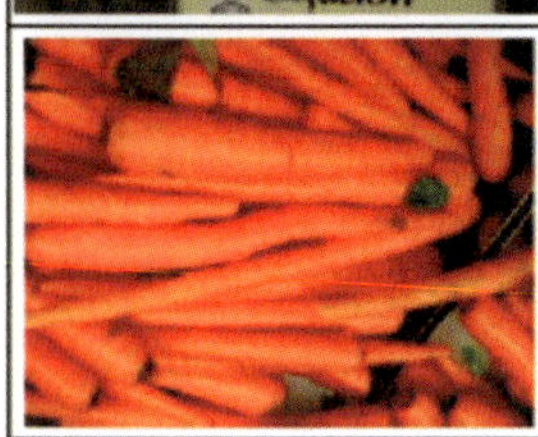	Carrots	

Test your knowledge: List the types of phytochemicals you might find in each of the following natural food products.

Products		**Phytochemicals**
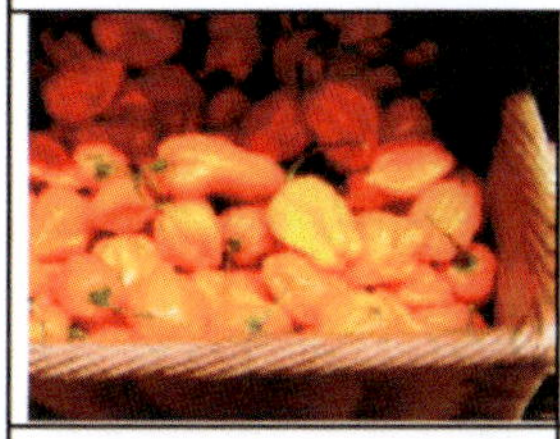	Habanero Peppers	
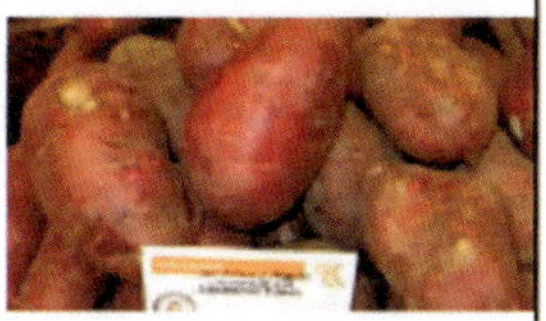	Japanese Yams	
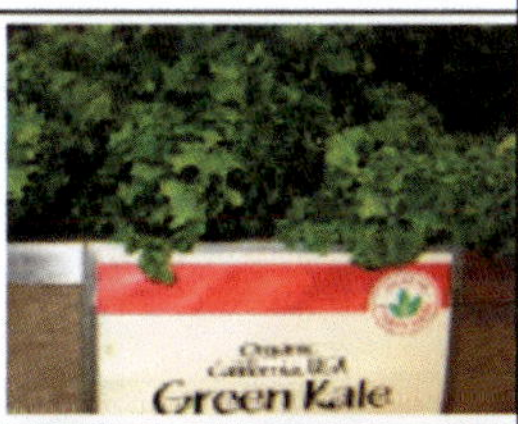	Kale	
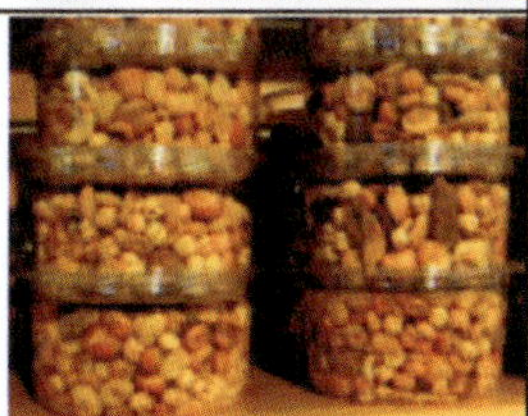	Mixed Nuts	
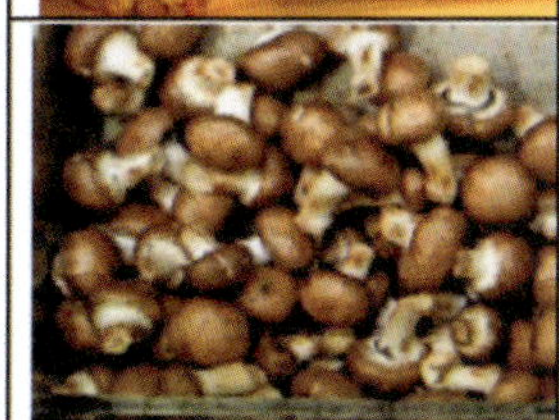	Mushrooms	
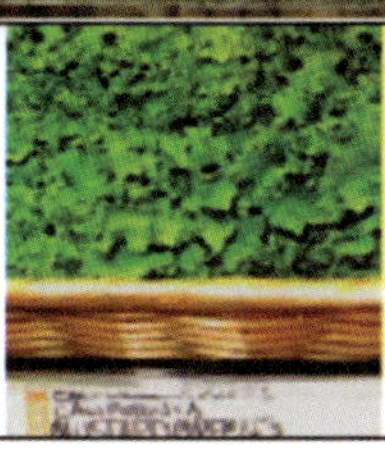	Mustard Greens	

Test your knowledge: List the types of phytochemicals you might find in each of the following natural food products.

Products		Phytochemicals
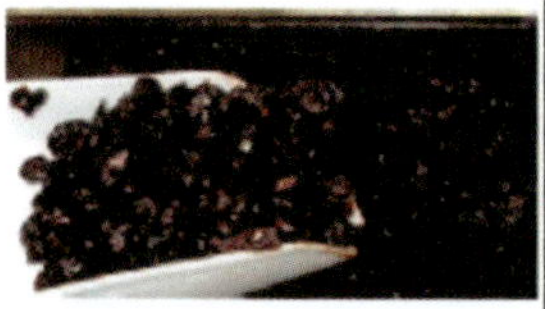	Cranberries	
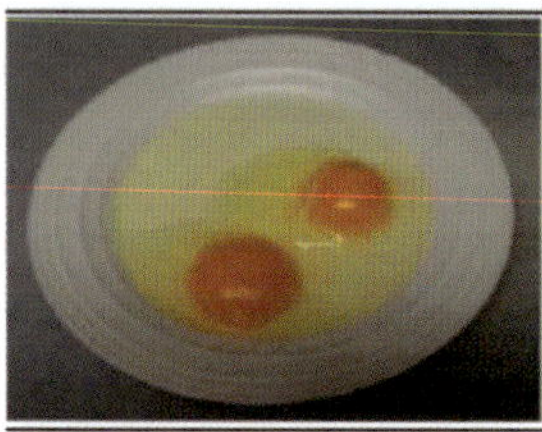	Eggs	
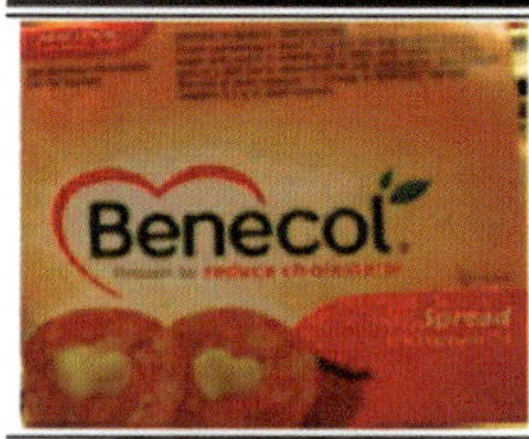	Enriched Margarine (reduces cholesterol)	
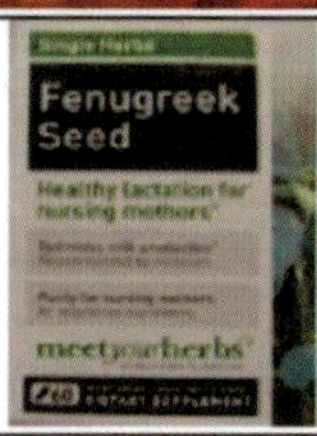	Fenugreek	
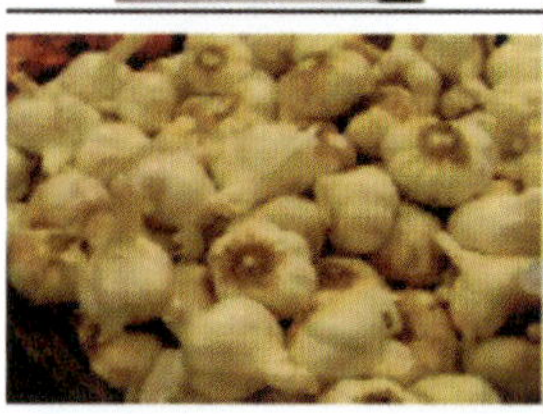	Garlic	
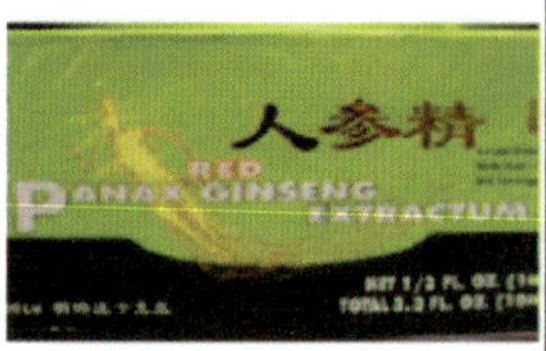	Ginseng	

Test your knowledge: List the types of phytochemicals you might find in each of the following natural food products.

Products		Phytochemicals
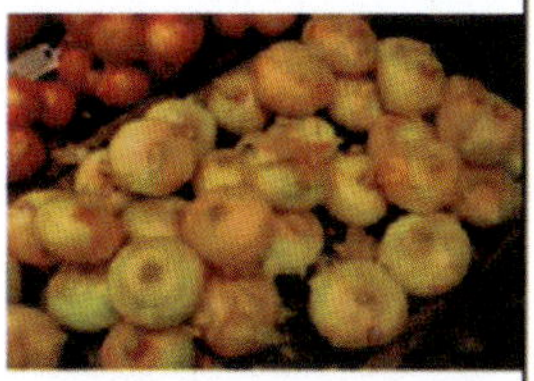	Onions	
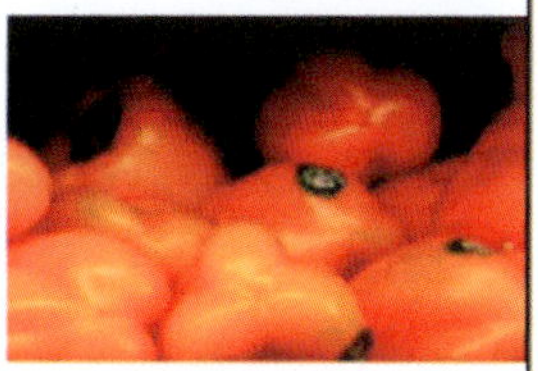	Orange Bell Peppers	
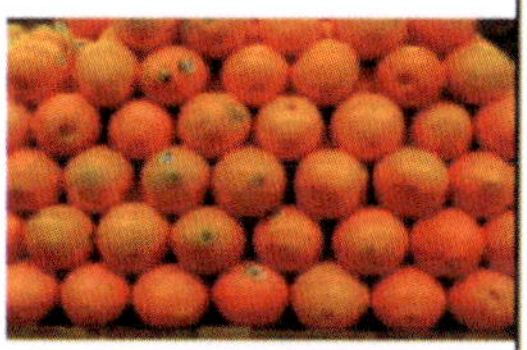	Oranges	
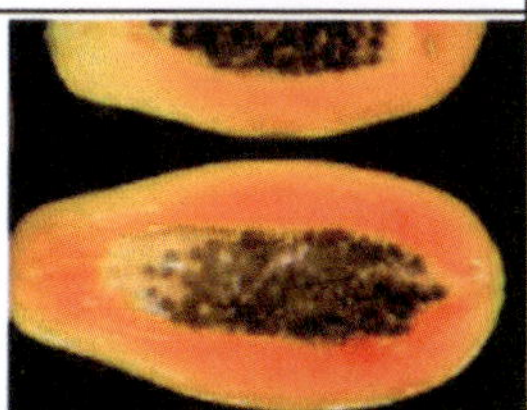	Papaya	
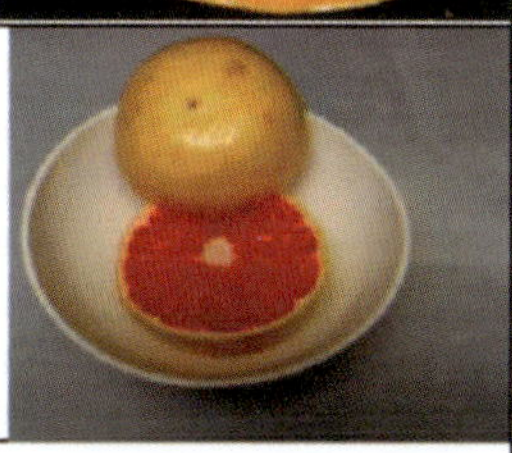	Pink Grapefruit	
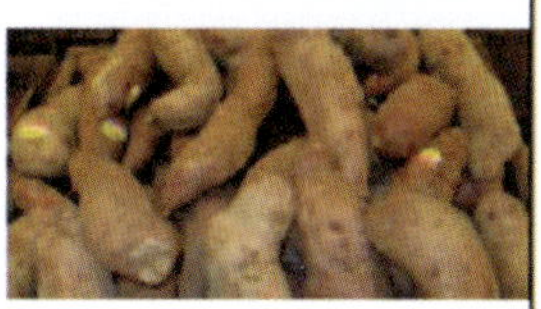	Purple Sweet Potatoes	

Test your knowledge: List the types of phytochemicals you might find in each of the following natural food products.

Products		Phytochemicals
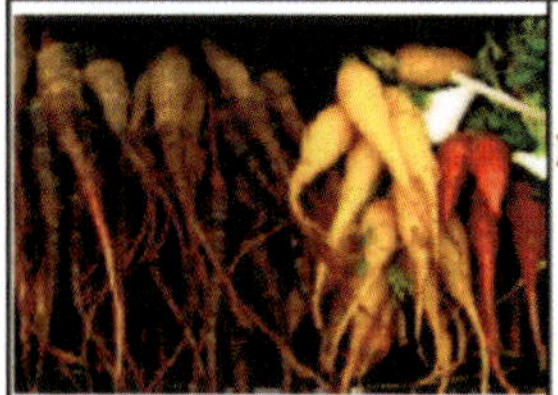	Rainbow Carrots, especially purple carrots	
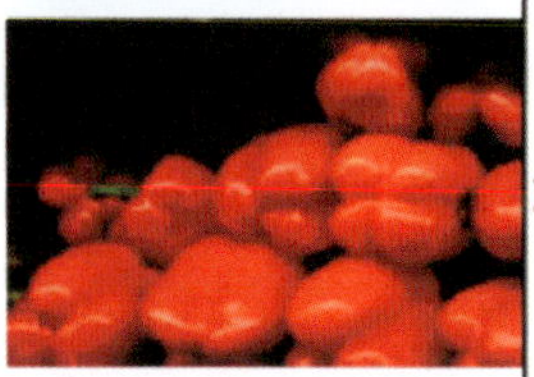	Red Bell Peppers	
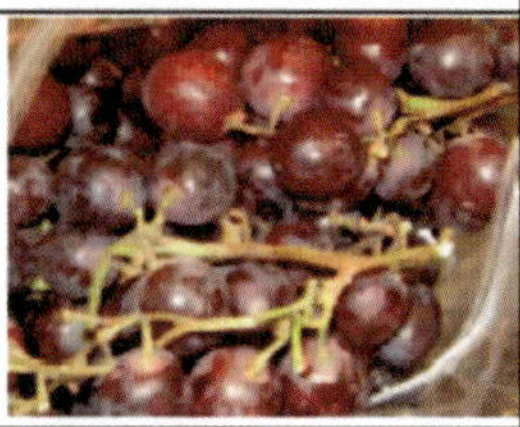	Red Grapes	
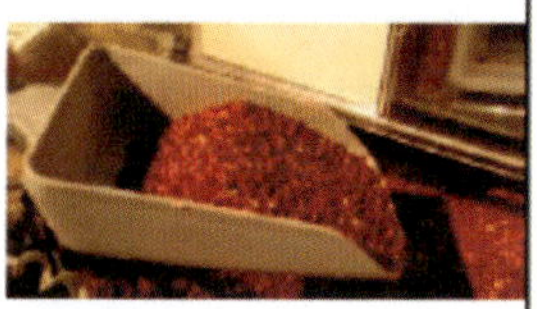	Red Quinoa	
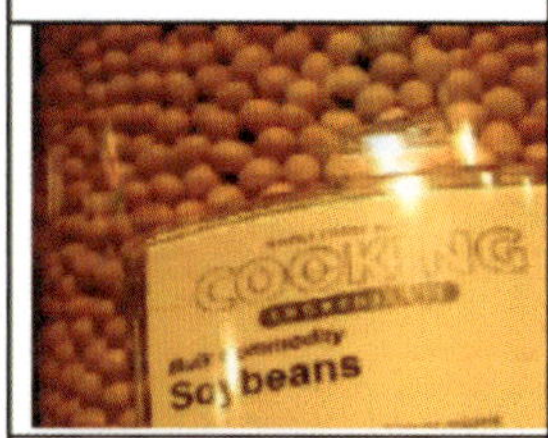	Soy Beans	
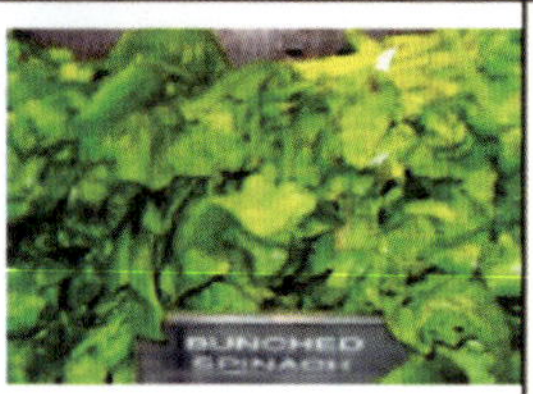	Spinach	

Test your knowledge: List the types of phytochemicals you might find in each of the following natural food products.

Products		Phytochemicals
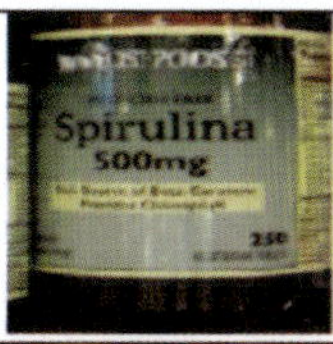	Spirulina	
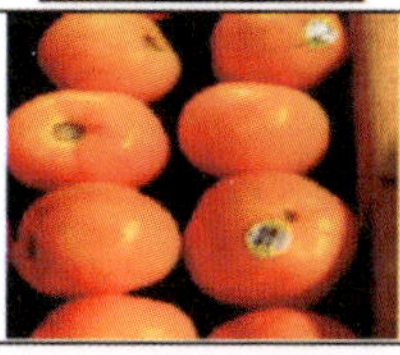	Tangerine Tomatoes	
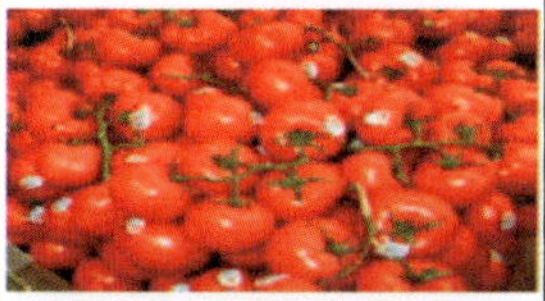	Tomatoes	
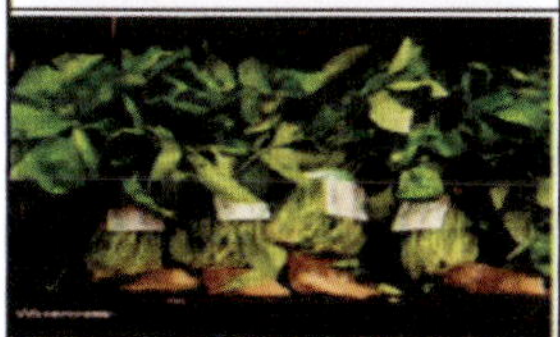	Watercress	
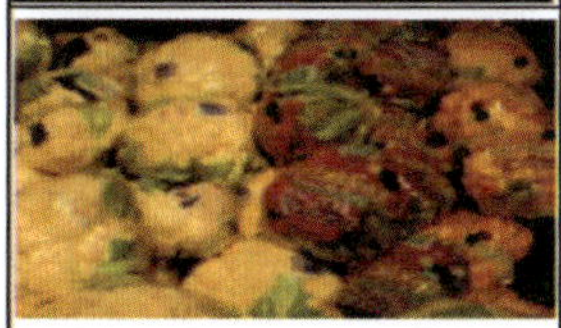	White, purple, and orange cauliflower	
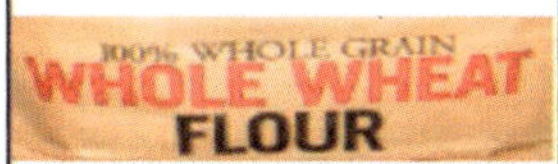	Whole Wheat Grains	
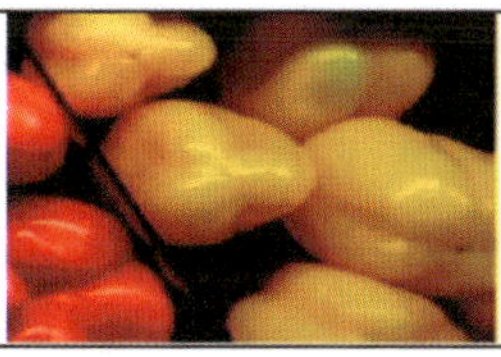	Yellow Bell Peppers	

CONFLICT OF INTEREST

The authors confirm that this chapter contents have no conflict of interest.

ACKNOWLEDGMENTS

None declared.

REFERENCES

Arias, R., Lee, T. C., Specca, D., and Janes, H. (2000). Quality comparison of hydroponic tomatoes (Lycopersicon esculentum) ripened on and off vine., *Journal of Food Science.*, p. 545–548.

Bassleer, C. T., Franchimont, P. P., Henrotin, Y. E., Franchimont, N. M., Geenen, V. G., and Reginster, J. Y. L. (1996). Effects of Ipriflavone and its metabolites on human articular chondrocytes cultivated in clusters. *Osteoarthritis and Cartilage*, p. 1–8.

Basu, T. K. and Srichamroen, A., 2010, Health Benefits of Fenugreek (Trigonella foenum-graecum leguminosse), *in* R. R. Watson, and V. R. Preedy, eds., Bioactive Foods in Promoting Health: Fruits and Vegetables: London, UK, Elsevier, p. 425–435.

Bernardo, R. R., Pinto, A. V., and Parente, J. (1996). Steroidal saponins from Smilax officinalis. *Phytochemistry*, p. 465–469.

Bhaumick, D., Acharya, S. N., and Basu, T. K. (2008). The potential benefits of saponin from Canadia-grown fenugreek (Trigonella foenum-graecum L.) in modifying cholesterol status. *World Heart Journal.*, p. 263–270.

Bialonska, D., Kasimsetty, S. G., Schrader, K. K., and Ferreira, D. (2009). The effect of pomegranate (Punica granatum L.) byproducts and ellagitannins on the growth of human gut bacteria. *Journal of Agricultural and Food Chemistry*, p. 8344–8349.

Brownmiller, C., Howard, L. R., and Prior, R. L. (2008). Processing and storage effects on monomeric anthocyanins, percent polymeric color, and antioxidant capacity of processed blackberry products. *Journal of Agricultural and Food Chemistry*, p. 689–695.

Burcelin, R., Luche, E., Serino, M., and Amar, J. (2009). The gut microbiota ecology: a new opportunity for the treatment of metabolic diseases? *Frontiers in Bioscience*, p. 5107–5117.

Cabrera-Orozco, A., Jimenez-Martinez, C., and Davila-Ortiz, G., 2013, Soybean : Non-Nutritional Factors and Their Biological Functionality, *in* H. El-Shemy, ed., Soybean - Bio-Active Compounds: Rijeka, Croatia, InTech, p. 387–410.

Cai, Q. and Wei, H. (1996). Effect of dietary genistein on antioxidant enzyme activities in SENCAR mice. *Nutrition and Cancer*, p. 1–7.

Cani, P. D., Amar, J., Iglesias, M. A., Poggi, M., Knauf, C., Bastelica, D., Neyrinck, A. M., Fava, F., Tuohy, K. M., Chabo, C., Sulpice, T., Chamontin, B., Gibson, G. R., Casteilla, L., Delzenne, N. M., Alessi, M. C., and Burcelin, R. (2007). Metabolic Endotoxemia Initiates Obesity and Insulin Resistance. *Diabetes*, p. 1761–1772.

Challinor, V. L., Parsons, P. G., Chap, S., White, E. F., Blanchfield, J. T., Lehmann, R. P., and De Voss, J. J. (2012). Steroidal saponins from the roots of Smilax sp.: structure and bioactivity. *Steroids*, p. 504–511.

Chun, O. K., Chung, S., Claycombe, K. J., and Song, W. O. (2008). Serum C-reactive protein concentrations are inversely associated with dietary flavonoid intake in U.S. adults. *The Journal of Nutrition*, p. 753–760.

Clifton, P. M., Noakes, M., Ross, D., Fassoulakis, A., Cehun, M., and Nestel, P. (2004). High dietary intake of phytosterol esters decreases carotenoids and increases plasma plant sterol levels with no additional cholesterol lowering. *Journal of Lipid Research*, p. 1493–1499.

Coleman, C. I., Hebert, J. H., and Reddy, P. (2002). The effect of phytosterols on quality of life in the treatment of benign prostatic hyperplasia. *Pharmacotherapy*, p. 1426–1432.

Denke, M. A. (2005). Reviewing your investment strategy: where does diet fit in your personal portfolio. *The American Journal of Clinical Nutrition*, p. 339–340.

Dewick, P. M., 2009, The shikimate pathway: aromatic amino acids and phenylpropanoids, *in* Medicinal Natural Products: A Biosynthetic Approach: Chichester, UK, John Wiley & Sons Ltd, p. 137–186.

DiBaise, J. K., Zhang, H., Crowell, M. D., Krajmalnik-Brown, R., Decker, G. A., and Rittmann, B. E. (2008). Gut microbiota and its possible relationship with obesity. *Mayo Clinic Proceedings*, p. 460–469.

Duffield-Lillico, A. J. and Begg, C. B. (2004). Reflections on the landmark studies of beta-carotene supplementation. *Journal of the National Cancer Institute*, p. 1729–1731.

Dwyer, J. H., Paul-Labrador, M. J., Fan, J., Shircore, A. M., Merz, C. N. B., and Dwyer, K. M., 2004, Progression of carotid intima-media thickness and plasma antioxidants: the Los Angeles Atherosclerosis Study., Arteriosclerosis, Thrombosis, and Vascular Biology., p. 313–319.

Enseleit, F., Sudano, I., Périat, D., Winnik, S., Wolfrum, M., Flammer, A. J., Fröhlich, G. M., Kaiser, P., Hirt, A., Haile, S. R., Krasniqi, N., Matter, C. M., Uhlenhut, K., Högger, P., Neidhart, M., Lüscher, T. F., Ruschitzka, F., and Noll, G. (2012). Effects of Pycnogenol on endothelial function in patients with stable coronary artery disease: a double-blind, randomized, placebo-controlled, cross-over study. *European Heart Journal*, p. 1589–1597.

Executive Summary of The Third Report of the National Cholesterol Education Program (NCEP) Expert Panel on Detection, Evaluation, and Treatment of High Blood Cholesterol in Adults (Adult Treatment Panel III). (2001). *Journal of the American Medical Associaltion*, p. 2486–2497.

Fox, D. L. (1955). Astaxanthin in the American Flamingo. *Nature*, p. 942–943.

Fox, D. L., 1976, Supplement – Carotenoids, *in* Animal Biochromes and Structural Colors: Berkeley, CA, University of California Press, p. 389–422.

Fursova, A. Z., Gesarevich, O. G., Gonchar, A. M., Trofimova, N. A., and Kolosova, N. G. (2005). [Dietary supplementation with bilberry extract prevents macular degeneration and cataracts in senesce-accelerated OXYS rats]. *Advances in Gerontology*, p. 76–79.

Gestetner, B., Birk, Y., and Tencer, Y. (1968). Soybean saponins: fate of ingested soybean saponins and the physiological aspect of their hemolytic activity. *Journal of Agricultural and Food Chemistry*, p. 1031–1035.

Giovannucci, E., Ascherio, A., Rimm, E. B., Stampfer, M. J., Colditz, G. A., and Willett, W. C. (1995). Intake of carotenoids and retinol in relation to risk of prostate cancer. *Journal of the National Cancer Institute*, p. 1767–1776.

Hammerstone, J. F., Lazarus, S. A., and Schmitz, H. H. (2000). Chocolate: modern science investigates an ancient medicine procyanidin content and variation in some commonly consumed foods. *The Journal of Nutrition*, p. 2086S–92S.

Hecht, S. S. (1995). Chemoprevention by isothiocyanates. *Journal of Cellular Biochemistry*, p. 195–209.

Higdon, J. V, Delage, B., Williams, D. E., and Dashwood, R. H. (2007). Cruciferous vegetables and human cancer risk: epidemiologic evidence and mechanistic basis. *Pharmacological Research*, p. 224–236.

Holt, E. M., Steffen, L. M., Moran, A., Basu, S., Steinberger, J., Ross, J. A., Hong, C. P., and Sinaiko, A. R. (2009). Fruit and vegetable consumption and its relation to markers of inflammation and oxidative stress in adolescents. *Journal of the American Dietetic Association*, p. 414–421.

Howell, A. B. (2007). Bioactive compounds in cranberries and their role in prevention of urinary tract infections. *Molecular Nutrition & Food Research*, p. 732–737.

Jenkins, D. J. A., Kendall, C. W. C., Marchie, A., Faulkner, D. A., Wong, J. M. W., de Souza, R., Emam, A., Parker, T. L., Vidgen, E., Trautwein, E. A., Lapsley, K. G., Josse, R. G., Leiter, L. A., Singer, W., and Connelly, P. W. (2005). Direct comparison of a dietary portfolio of cholesterol-lowering foods with a statin in hypercholesterolemic participants. *The American Journal of Clinical Nutrition*, p. 380–387.

Johns, T., Mahunnah, R. L., Sanaya, P., Chapman, L., and Ticktin, T. (1999). Saponins and phenolic content in plant dietary additives of a traditional subsistence community, the Batemi of Ngorongoro District, Tanzania. *Journal of Ethnopharmacology*, p. 1–10.

Kamel, A. and Saleh, M. (2000). Recent studies on the chemistry and biological activities of the organosulfur compounds of garlic (Allium sativum). *Studies in Natural Products Chemistry*, p. 455–485.

Kang, J., Badger, T. M., Ronis, M. J. J., and Wu, X. (2010). Non-isoflavone phytochemicals in soy and their health effects. *Journal of Agricultural and Food Chemistry*, p. 8119–8133.

Komesaroff, P. A., Black, C. V., Cable, V., and Sudhir, K. (2001). Effects of wild yam extract on menopausal symptoms, lipids and sex hormones in healthy menopausal women. *Climacteric : the Journal of the International Menopause Society*, p. 144–150.

Lagarda, M. J., García-Llatas, G., and Farré, R. (2006). Analysis of phytosterols in foods. *Journal of Pharmaceutical and Biomedical Analysis*, p. 1486–1496.

Laux, M. and Conrad, C., 1997, Natural Woman, Natural Menopause: New York, NY, Harper-Collins Publishers.

Lawson, L. D., Ransom, D. K., and Hughes, B. G., 1992, Inhibition of whole blood platelet-aggregation by compounds in garlic clove extracts and commercial garlic products., Thrombosis Research., p. 141–156.

Leela, N. K. and Shafeekh, K. M., 2008, Fenugreek, *in* V. A. Parthasarathy, B. Chempakam, and T. J. Zachariah, eds., Chemistry of Spices: Wallingford, UK, CAB International, p. 242–259.

Lerman, R. H., Minich, D. M., Darland, G., Lamb, J. J., Schiltz, B., Babish, J. G., Bland, J. S., and Tripp, M. L. (2008). Enhancement of a modified Mediterranean-style, low glycemic load diet with specific phytochemicals improves cardiometabolic risk factors in subjects with metabolic syndrome and hypercholesterolemia in a randomized trial. *Nutrition & Metabolism.*, p. 29.

Mordi, R. (1993). Carotenoids: functions and degradation. *Chemistry & Industry*, p. 79–83.

Naganawa, R., Iwata, N., Ishikawa, K., Fukuda, H., Fujino, T., and Suzuki, A. (1996). Inhibition of microbial growth by ajoene, a sulfur-containing compound derived from garlic. *Applied and Environmental Microbiology*, p. 4238–4242.

National Eye Institute (2013a). Age-related eye disease study—results. Available at: https://www.nei.nih.gov/amd (accessed: 18.02.2015.

National Eye Institute (2013b). Age-related eye disease study 2 (AREDS2). Available at: https://www.nei.nih.gov/areds2 (accessed: 18.02.2015).

Nelson-Dooley, C., Della-Fera, M. A., Hamrick, M., and Baile, A. C. (2005). Novel treatments for obesity and osteoporosis : targeting apoptotic pathways in adipocytes. *Current Medicinal Chemistry*, p. 2215–2225.

O'Donnell, G., Poeschl, R., Zimhony, O., Gunaratnam, M., Moreira, J. B. C., Neidle, S., Evangelopoulos, D., Bhakta, S., Malkinson, J. P., Boshoff, H. I., Lenaerts, A., and Gibbons, S. (2009). Bioactive Pyridine-N-Oxide Disulfides from Allium stipitatum. *Journal of Natural Products*, p. 360–365.

Ohta, R. (1999). *In vitro* inhibition of the growth of Helicobacter pylori by oil-macerated garlic constituents. *Antimicrobial Agents and Chemotherapy*, p. 1811–1812.

Osman, N., Adawi, D., Ahrné, S., Jeppsson, B., and Molin, G. (2007). Endotoxin- and D-galactosamine-induced liver injury improved by the administration of Lactobacillus, Bifidobacterium and blueberry. *Digestive and Liver Disease*: official journal of the Italian Society of Gastroenterology and the Italian Association for the Study of the Liver, p. 849–856.

Park, J. D., Rhee, D. K., and Lee, Y. H. (2005). Biological activities and chemistry of saponins from Panax ginseng C. A. Meyer. *Phytochemistry Reviews*, p. 159–175.

Petit, P. R., Sauvaire, Y. D., Hillaire-Buys, D. M., Leconte, O. M., Baissac, Y. G., Ponsin, G. R., and Ribes, G. R. (1995). Steroid saponins from fenugreek seeds: Extraction, purification, and pharmacological investigation on feeding behavior and plasma cholesterol. *Steroids*, p. 674–680.

Rahman, M. S. (2007). Allicin and other functional active components in garlic: health benefits and bioavailability. *International Journal of Food Properties*, p. 245–268.

Rayalam, S., Della-Fera, M. A., and Baile, C. A. (2008). Phytochemicals and regulation of the adipocyte life cycle. *The Journal of Nutritional Biochemistry*, p. 717–726.

Ruiz-Larrea, M. B., Mohan, A. R., Paganga, G., Miller, N. J., Bolwell, G. P., and Rice-Evans, C. A. (1997). Antioxidant activity of phytoestrogenic isoflavones. *Free Radical Research*, p. 63–70.

Sashida, Y., Kubo, S., Mimaki, Y., Nikaido, T., and Ohmoto, T. (1992). Saponins from Smilax riparia and S. china., *Phytochemistry*, p. 2439–2443.

Sautour, M., Mitaine-Offer, A. C., and Lacaille-Dubois, M. A. (2007). The Dioscorea genus: a review of bioactive steroid saponins. *Journal of Natural Medicines*, p. 91–101.

Schmidt, B., Ribnicky, D. M., Poulev, A., Logendra, S., Cefalu, W. T., and Raskin, I. (2008). A natural history of botanical therapeutics. *Metabolism*, p. S3–S9.

Scholtysek, C., Krukiewicz, A. A., Alonso, J. L., Sharma, K. P., Sharma, P. C., and Goldmann, W. H. (2009). Characterizing components of the Saw Palmetto Berry Extract (SPBE) on prostate cancer cell growth and traction. *Biochemical and Biophysical Research Communications*, p. 795–798.

Sen, S., Makkar, H. P. S., and Becker, K. (1998). Alfalfa saponins and their implication in animal nutrition. *Journal of Agricultural and Food Chemistry*, p. 131–140.

Shelef, L. A. (1984). Antimicrobial effects of spices. *Journal of Food Safety*, p. 29–44.

Shibata, S. (2001). Chemistry and cancer preventing activities of ginseng saponins and some related triterpenoid compounds. *Journal of Korean Medical Science*, p. S28–37.

Shroff, R., Vergara, F., Muck, A., Svatos, A., and Gershenzon, J. (2008). Nonuniform distribution of glucosinolates in Arabidopsis thaliana leaves has important consequences for plant defense. *Proceedings of the National Academy of Sciences of the United States of America*, p. 6196–6201.

Sidhu, G. S. and Oakenfull, D. G. (2007). A mechanism for the hypocholesterolaemic activity of saponins. *British Journal of Nutrition*, p. 643-649.

Stahl, W. and Sies, H. (1996). Lycopene: a biologically important carotenoid for humans? *Archives of Biochemistry and Biophysics*, p. 1–9.

Tantry, M. A. and Khan, I. A. (2013). Saponins from Glycine max Merrill (soybean). *Fitoterapia*, p. 49–56.

Taucher, J., Hansel, A., Jordan, A., and Lindinger, W. (1996). Analysis of compounds in human breath after ingestion of garlic using proton-transfer-reaction mass spectrometry. *Journal of Agricultural and Food Chemistry*, p. 3778–3782.

Thompson, H. J., Heimendinger, J., Diker, A., O'Neill, C., Haegele, A., Meinecke, B., Wolfe, P., Sedlacek, S., Zhu, Z., and Jiang, W. (2006). Dietary botanical diversity affects the reduction of oxidative biomarkers in women due to high vegetable and fruit intake. *The Journal of Nutrition*, p. 2207–2212.

Tosetti, F., Noonan, D. M., and Albini, A. (2009). Metabolic regulation and redox activity as mechanisms for angioprevention by dietary phytochemicals. *International Journal of Cancer*, p. 1997–2003.

Tsukamoto, C. and Yoshiki, Y., 2005, Soy Saponin, *in* M. Sugano, ed., Soy in Health and Disease Prevention: Danvers, MA, CRC Press, p. 155–172.

Vincent, H. K., Bourguignon, C. M., and Taylor, A. G. (2010). Relationship of the dietary phytochemical index to weight gain, oxidative stress and inflammation in overweight young adults. *Journal of Human Nutrition and Dietetics*: the official journal of the British Dietetic Association., p. 20–29.

Voutilainen, S., Nurmi, T., Mursu, J., and Rissanen, T. H. (2006). Carotenoids and cardiovascular health. *The American Journal of Clinical Nutrition*, p. 1265–1271.

Wang, F. Q., Yao, K., and Wei, D., 2011, From Soybean Phytosterols to Steroid Hormones, *in* H. El-Shemy, ed., Soybean and Health: Rijeka, Croatia, InTech, p. 231–252.

Wang, W., Higuchi, C. M., and Zhang, R. (1997). Individual and combinatory effects of soy isoflavones on the *in vitro* potentiation of lymphocyte activation. *Nutrition and Cancer*, p. 29–34.

Woo, H. M., Kang, J. H., Kawada, T., Yoo, H., Sung, M. K., and Yu, R. (2007). Active spice-derived components can inhibit inflammatory responses of adipose tissue in obesity by suppressing inflammatory actions of macrophages and release of monocyte chemoattractant protein-1 from adipocytes. *Life Sciences*, p. 926–931.

Woodard, G. A., Encarnacion, B., Downey, J. R., Peraza, J., Chong, K., Hernandez-Boussard, T., and Morton, J. M. (2009). Probiotics improve outcomes after Roux-en-Y gastric bypass surgery: a prospective randomized trial. *Journal of Gastrointestinal Surgery* : official journal of the Society for Surgery of the Alimentary Tract., p. 1198–1204.

Yokozawa, T., Kobayashi, T., Oura, H., and Kawashima, Y. (1985). Studies on the mechanism of the hypoglycemic activity of ginsenoside-Rb2 in streptozotocin-diabetic rats. *Chemical & Pharmaceutical Bulletin*, p. 869–872.

Zaika, L. L. (1988). Spices and herbs: their antimicrobial activity and its determination. *Journal of Food Safety*, p. 97–118.

Zhang, R., Li, Y., and Wang, W. (1997). Enhancement of immune function in mice fed high doses of soy daidzein. *Nutrition and Cancer*, p. 24–28.

Nutrition: An Approach to Good Health and Disease Management

CHAPTER 8

Influence of Socio-economic Status and Culture in Diet and Nutrition

Esperanza J. Carcache de Blanco* and Jay Mirtallo*

The Ohio State University, Columbus, Ohio, USA

Abstract: Dietary components are corner stones in having a good and balanced nutrition. Nutrition is directly correlated to health; hence, having good dietary habits will highly contribute to good health. However, there are different factors that influence good dietary patterns including socioeconomic status, income, and culture. This chapter will discuss the impact of these factors on nutrition and diet of different groups.

Keywords: Social, socioeconomic, fast food, culture, nutrition, diet, American Indian, Northern plains, Navajo, Mexican, Hispanic, African American, Asian, Chinese American, food store, convenience store, supermarket, lifestyle, income.

INTRODUCTION

A healthy diet greatly reduces risk of diseases and medical conditions because nutrition is a vital element of a healthy lifestyle. However, nutritious food is not equally available to all. Socio-economic factors shape life opportunities to the access of nutritious food.

8. SOCIO-ECONOMIC STATUS AND CULTURE IN DIET AND NUTRITION

8.1. Social and Economic Factors in Health and Nutrition

According to recent literature reports, people with low socio-economic status consume the least nutritious diets (Larsen, 2008). How and why this factor affect the level of nutritious diets in this population group will be covered in this chapter.

8.1.1. Food Store Access

Access to food stores could affect the type of diet; for instance, higher income areas have more chain supermarkets and fewer convenience stores. On the other

***Corresponding authors Esperanza J. Carcache de Blanco and Jay Mirtallo:** College of Pharmacy, The Ohio State University, Columbus, OH 43210, USA; E-mails: carcache-de-blan.1@osu.edu; mirtallo.1@osu.edu

hand, lower income areas have more convenience stores. According to literature reports; in the US, contrary to foreign countries, there is a substantial difference in access to food (Larsen and Gilliland, 2008; Powell *et al.*, 2007). For instance, African Americans have access to half the amount of chain supermarkets *versus* their white counterparts.

8.1.2. Convenience Food Stores

Convenience food stores are more widespread among areas lacking supermarkets and have less nutritionally valuable food (White, 2012). These stores sell packaged food containing high levels of sodium and refined sugars (Powell *et al.*, 2007). It is because foods made with sugars and salt are cheaper and more available within close proximity to these areas.

8.1.3. Supermarkets

Medium to high socio-economic status individuals tend to have greater access to supermarkets and stores that have a greater variety of fresh fruits and vegetables. Prices of some fruits and vegetables are significantly higher though. It has also been reported that high socio-economic status has more exotic rare produce than areas of lower economic status (White, 2012).

8.1.4. Fast Food Consumption

Fast food establishments follow an opposing pattern to supermarkets in the US. Fast food is not to provide nourishment, but to serve quickly and conveniently. Most people consume fast food because of convenience. In a recent report schools with students of lower socio-economic status have closer access to fast food restaurants. It is particularly visible in schools with a high percent of black students. In New York City, these fast food places are more concentrated around black high schools of high income than black high schools of low income (Kwate and Loh, 2010).

8.1.5. Education and Fast Food

Higher education and higher income correlate to greater access to healthier foods (Pearce *et al.*, 2007). Vocational education or no post-school qualifications are associated with an increased purchase of fast food. Particularly, "Blue collar" consume more fast food than professional workers. Based on the study, education affects knowledge about certain foods and the likelihood of purchasing them.

8.1.6. Income and Fast Food

Low income households are over four times more likely to purchase fast food as the examples presented below (Thornton *et al.*, 2011). It is particularly true for

"Blue collar" that have an irregular work schedule. They work evening or night shifts and are not at home during mealtime. The restaurant food is more expensive; hence, it is not an option. Additionally, family income directly affects food expenditures because income dictates what can and cannot be bought. Moreover, type and place of work affects food availability for lunch and the time allowed for meal preparation and consumption.

8.1.7. Overweight Prevalence and Family Income

There is a linear correlation between weight and income level, which also correlates with ethnicity (Gordon-Larsen *et al*., 2003). Overweight have also been found to correlate with education and gender. Fig. **1**. shows correlation between weight, gender, income and ethnic variation.

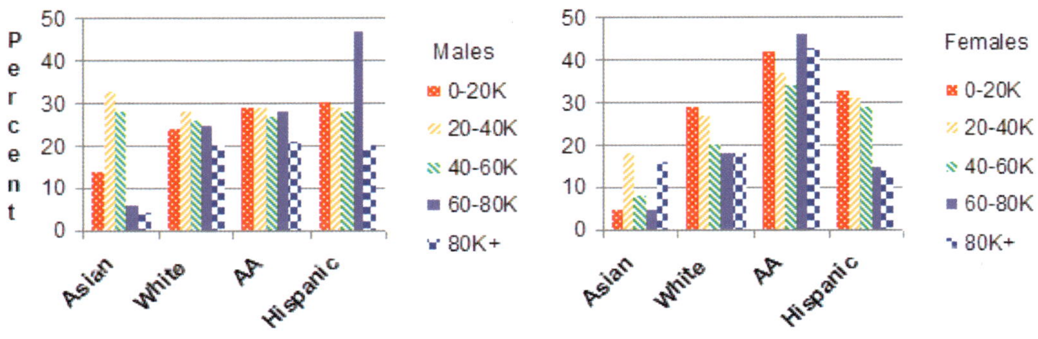

Fig. (1). Relation between overweight, income, gender, and culture. K values indicate parental income ranges. AA represents African American. Data *p* values include $p<0.05$ and $p<0.01$. Bars represent approximate values of the published data, but preserve a similar trend as in the literature. (Gordon-Larsen et al., 2003).

8.1.8. Overweight Prevalence and Parental Education

Parental education seems to have an impact on overweight prevalence (Gordon-Larsen *et al*., 2003). It is significantly higher in females than males for most cultures. Fig. **2**. shows correlation between weight, gender, education, and ethnic variation.

8.1.9. Overweight Prevalence by Ethnicity and Gender

An study by Gordon-Larsen and co-workers shows that ethnicity and gender play important roles on overweight prevalence (Gordon-Larsen *et al*., 2003). Culture, particularly, has an impact on dietary patterns, which is directly correlated to calorie intake and overweight prevalence. Fig. **2**. shows correlation between overweight prevalence, gender, and ethnic variation.

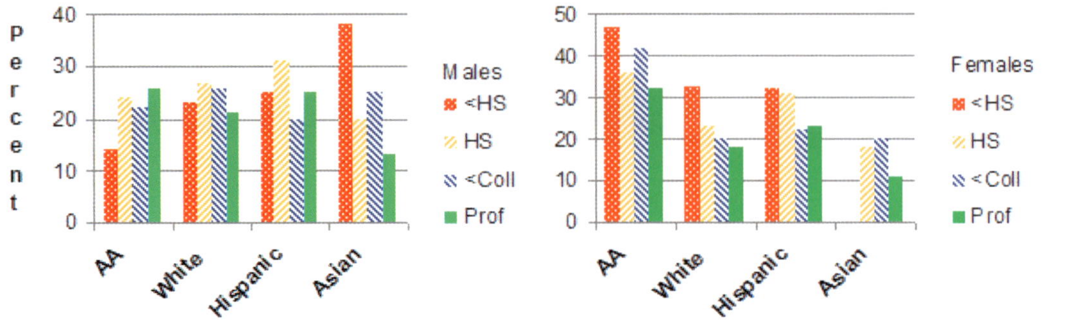

Fig. (2). Relation between overweight, education level, gender, and culture. <HS represents no or some high school; HS represents high school (or GED) diploma; <Coll represents some college; Prof represents college or professional degree. AA represents African American. Data *p* values include $p<0.05$ and $p<0.01$. Bars represent approximate values of the published data, but preserve a similar trend as in the literature. (Gordon-Larsen et al., 2003).

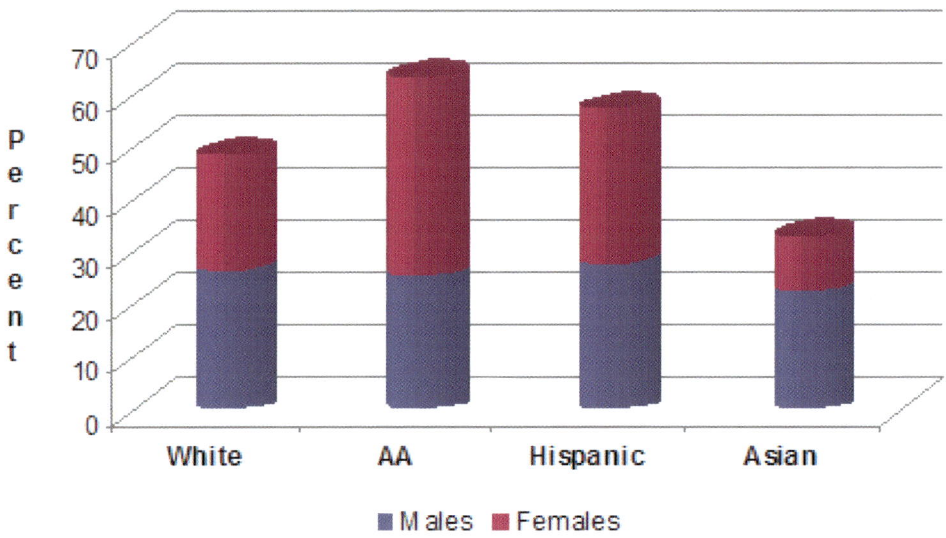

Fig. (3). Relation between overweight, gender, and ethnic group. Bars represent approximate values of the published data, but preserve a similar trend as in the literature. (Gordon-Larsen et al., 2003).

8.1.10. Overall Overweight Prevalence

According to a study, reducing disparities in income and education will not reduce disparities in overweight prevalence. Hence, what are the other factors that could play a role in a good diet? Is it culture or habits?

8.2. Culture

Ethnicity and race are key players in understanding culture. Ethnicity generates identity within and between social groups while race provide categories such as African American, Asian, Hispanic, and others. This chapter will discuss cultural aspects that affect diet in American Indians, African Americans, Chinese Americans, and Mexican Americans.

Culture goes well beyond daily sustenance because it influences choices about what, when, how, and with whom to eat (Barer-Stein, 1999). It also affects attitudes, beliefs, practices, and values about good health and disease prevention (Sucher and Kittler, 2007). Additionally, ethnicity and race is directly correlated to how to identify foods, how to prepare foods, what condiments to use, timing and frequency of meals (Barer-Stein, 1999). Hence, it is of great value to recognize that culture shapes how individuals define health, perceive illnesses and seek out treatment.

8.2.1. American Indians

In this chapter, American Indians (AI) will comprise all groups of Native Americans including Alaska Natives. AI represents 1.5-2% of the US population and is considered to be younger than the US population as a whole (Norris *et al.*, 2010). About half of this group lives on or nearby reservations. AI suffers from disproportionate rates of morbidity and mortality when compared to other Americans. Among the diseases that most affect this group include alcoholism, diabetes, homicide, suicide, and tuberculosis. Because culture has an impact on daily nourishment, good health, and prevention of certain diseases, it is of great value to look for the significance of food practices and the prevalence of certain diseases amongst different tribes of this group (Indian Health Service, 2015). Overall, AI used to have two meals, one in the morning and another later in the day. The morning meal used to be a soup of meat and broth with root vegetables or other collected wild plants. The other meal was a stew with meat, vegetables, and roots that was prepared and ready to eat. Over time AI children adapted to different foods, meal times, and holidays. Different tribes have changed in different ways.

8.2.1.1. Northern Plains Indians

Meal practices of Northern Plains Indians (NPI) have changed drastically over time as presented below (Powers, 1973). NPI used to live and hunt in the area of North and South Dakota, Wyoming, and Nebraska. The NPI diet has changed from a hunter-gatherer lifestyle with limited vegetables and roots to a meat and potatoes diet (Kindscher, 1987). They practiced communal food distribution and the meat was prepared in one of the following ways: cooked on leaf-lined pits with a fire on top simulating an oven, dried (over a fire or in the sun), or roasted over open fire. The Tables **1**, **2** and **3** below present both past and present components from different categories of the NPI diet (Colby *et al*, 2011-2012, Philips *et al*, 2014, Stang J *et al*, 2005, Taylor C *et al*, 2005 and Wiedman D, 2005). Additional, components from different categories include chokecherries, June berries, serviceberries, wild strawberries, prairie chicken, rabbit, wild turkey, ground beans, hazelnuts, and pigweed (young, tender leaves are eaten fresh or dried).

Table 1. Selected components Used in Traditional Northern Plains Indian Diet (Colby *et al*, 2011-2012, Philips *et al*, 2014).

Component	Use
Fruit Choke cherries, June berries, plums, blueberries, cranberries, strawberries, buffalo berries, gooseberries, apples, plains prickly pears	Berries used to prepare syrups, jams, pudding or pie
Vegetables Prairie turnips, squash, wild rice, potatoes, stinging nettles, corn, turnips, Cattail broadleaf nettles, spinach, asparagus, hazelnuts	Used in soups, stews, sauces, and salads
Meat Venison, buffalo, jack rabbit, pheasant, prairie chicken	Dried or used in soups or stews

*Pre-European, hunted, gathered, and traded foods

Current food choices use commodity foods such as the Special Supplemental Nutrition Program for Women, Infants, and Children (WIC) and food stamps (Goody and Drago, 2010). Current typical food for this tribe includes hamburgers, French fries, fried potatoes, commodity vegetables, gravy, large sodas, cookies, whipped topping, and “all you can eat” buffets.

The NPI are characterized by the use of Medicine wheel, herbs, and plants for health and medicinal purposes. Because the direct correlation between diet and disease risk, it is important to consider the traditional beliefs of this group regarding health.

Table 2. Components used traditionally in Northern Plains Indian Dishes and Beverages (Colby *et al*, 2011-2012, Philips *et al*, 2014).

Beverages and Dishes	
Drinks	Teas are prepared by making infusion of plant parts such as: spearmint, peppermint, bergamot, rose hips
Dishes	Wasna contains fruits and animal products, including dried meat, crushed berries, and rendered animal fat. Tipsila or washtonka soup* is rich in nutrients and include: dried meat, turnips, corn and wild onions for flavor. Ground prairie turnips used as a thickening agent. Breads made of corn or turnips and wheat (later).

*May be in combination with meats from 8.1.

Table 3. Components currently used Northern Plain Indians Diet (Stang J *et al*, 2005, Taylor C, *et al*, 2005, Wiedman D, 2005).

Contemporary Food	Comments
Fruits Gooseberries, apple, plums, raspberries, cranberries	Sugar and sugar substitutes used in preparation of core foods consist of candies, pies, cakes, and cookies. Bananas and orange juice are also sources of fruits.
Vegetables Asparagus, spinach, turnips, hazelnuts, beans, white flour	Generally, there is an absence of fruits and vegetables. French fried potatoes predominate the vegetable intake with some tomatoes, green beans, rice, and onions. Chips are also a core food in the vegetable category. Other components of core foods are white bread, butter or margarine. Fry-bread is a food common to NPI and other Indians thought to be a traditional dish; however, it was the result of assimilating 'western' or military food rations that were introduced to the Indians on reservations.
Meat Beef, chicken, bacon, salt pork	Secondary foods are ground beef and hot dogs.
Drinks Soda, coffee, tea	

Current dietary components have been compared to NHANES III diets of American public for adults aged 45-74 years (Stang *et al*, 2005). Northern Plains Indian women have a dietary composition similar to the American diet while males have minor differences to their male counterparts in the NHANES survey. This is consistent with the modernization of the NPI diet following placement on reservations and 'Westernizing' their diet with military rations. This results in food products used by NPI very similar to most Americans, with the main difference being the emphasis on certain products that may not be the most nutritious ones. The variation is with food combinations and preparation creating American Indian Foods (Wiedman D, 2005).

8.2.1.2. Navajo Indians

Diet is very important for the Navajo Indians (NI) as they perceive a direct correlation between food consumption and strength (Satterfield *et al.*, 2007). They used to have a plant-based diet with eating meat only occasionally. Food for this tribe was prepared by cooking inside a hogan, on a metal barrel, or on an adobe-type stove. Food practices are influenced by current conditions, emotions, family and friends while meal patterns depend on individual preferences, work, and daily schedule (Pelican, 1991). The Tables **4** and **5** below compare components from different categories of the traditional Navajo dietary pattern with current diet (Kopp, 1986, Wolfe and Sanjur, 1988, Ballew *et al*, 1997). Additional components from different categories include cantaloupe, watermelon, apricots, pork, beef, and beans. *Traditional foods are difficult to specify since the diet of the Navajo has been modified since the introduction of sheep into their society by the Spaniards in the 17th century. This change placed a strain on the Navajo economy because of the land needed for grazing animals displaced food usually available for their gathering practices as well as land for planting crops (Kopp, 1986). In general, traditional foods found in the contemporary Navajo diet include the following: Navajo tea, blue and yellow cornmeal mush, hominy corn, Navajo pancake, wild sumac berry pudding and goat's milk (Wolfe and Sanjur, 1988).

NI lifestyle and diet has changed in response to environmental factors. For instance, they consume more fat and sugar in food and beverages, portion sizes are larger, and they have a more sedentary lifestyle. Since they have limited traditional knowledge about local plants used by ancestors, only very few gather, hunt or cultivate for consumption (Goody and Drago, 2010). Lately, NI also eats commodity foods and other products such as apricots, beans, cantaloupe, peaches, and watermelon.

Table 4. Components Used in Traditional* Navajo Cuisine (Kopp, 1986, Wolfe and Sanjur, 1988, Ballew *et al*, 1997, Navojopeople.org).

Clay, ashes, and salts
• Clay (white, gray), Juniper ash, Rock salt, Tumbleweed (greasewood) ash
Fruits (sometimes be taken in the form of beverages with or without the addition of sugar)
• Currants, Cedar berries, Chokecherries, Rose hips, Raspberries, Sumac berries, Yucca, Prickly pear and Grapes
Meats and milk (some types are currently considered as exotic meats)
• Antelope, Elk, Deer, Mutton (all parts; boiled, roasted, dried, stew), Lamb, Praire dog, Rabbit, Rats (wood), Goat milk, and Sheep milk
Nuts and seeds (some are used in dishes and bakery as well)
• Piñon nuts, Acorns, Walnuts, Squash seed, and Hedge mustard seeds, Pigweed seed and Mountain grass seed
Vegetables (soups traditionally include vegetables)
• Non-starchy: Pigweed, Summer squash, Wild plants (such as celery, onion and spinach)
• Starchy: Corn (such as blue, sweet, yellow); Hominy, Wild potatoes, and Winter squash

Table 5: Components Currently Eaten in Navajo Culture (Wolfe and Sanjur, 1988, Ballew *et al*, 1997).

Drinks
• Coffee, Sweetened drink mixes, Juice (10%, 25%, 100%), Milk (cow, soy, rice), Powdered drink mixes, Soda soup (regular, diet), and Tea (all varieties)
Breads and grains
• Blue corn bread, Blue corn mush with blue ash, Hominy, Yellow cornmeal mush, Navajo pancake (ground cake), Pasta, White or wheat bread, and Navajo tortillas, Navajo fried bread*
Desserts
• Cakes, Cookies, Pastries, Pies, Chips and Popcorn

Table 5: contd…

Meats
• Beef, Blood sausage, Fish, Lamb (all parts), Mutton (all parts), Organ meats, Pork, Poultry, Shellfish, and Venison
Nuts and seeds
• Piñon nuts, and other nuts/seeds (salted, shelled)
Other
• Ashes, Clay, Junk food (potato chip, nachos, candy, ramen noodles), and Rock salt
Vegetables and fruits
• Apple, Corn (steamed, roasted), Potatoes (fired, boiled), Squash (winter, summer), Sumac berry pudding, and other canned, frozen, dried, juiced and fresh fruits/vegetables
Commodity Foods – made available from the USDA Food Distribution Program
• Butter and shortening, Canned meats, Canned and dry beans, Canned fruits and Fruit juices, Canned vegetables, Cheese, Cornmeal, Corn syrup, Dehydrated eggs and potatoes, Evaporated nonfat dry milk, Flour, Peanut butter, Pasta, Rice, Oats, and Raisins

*Navajo tortillas and fry bread are generally made from white wheat flour, baking powder, salt and water. On occasion, evaporated dry milk is used (Wolfe and Sanjur, 1988). Limitations on food choices occur as a result of cost (leading to Commodity foods becoming the core components and food), availability and shelf-life (many homes do not have electricity for refrigeration) (Ballew *et al*, 1997).

According to NI culture, there is a guiding principal in life and health. Illnesses are the result of imbalance between the ill person and nature (Goody and Drago, 2010). Hence, there is need for a medicine man/woman to diagnose the disease.

8.2.2. African American Diet

African American (AA) will be used in this section for individuals and groups that have origins from any of the black racial groups in Africa including descendants of African slaves and voluntary immigrants from Africa, the Caribbean, Central and South America. Overall, African Americans when compared with other American eat fewer fruits and vegetables, and less dietary fiber, calcium, and potassium (Witt, 1999). They consume excessive amounts of fatty meats, salt, and cholesterol (Goody and Drago, 2010). African American eating habits and food purchasing are associated with higher rates of hypertension, CV, and diabetes. In African American culture, socio-economic status influences meal consumption, meal planning, and nutrition (Goody and Drago, 2010). * Food and its preparation evolved from the African heritage and shaped from Southern and Caribbean cooking practices along with issues related to the acknowledgement of ethnicity and culture based on the circumstances of the AA migration to the United States. The Tables **6** and **7** below provide details of the traditional dietary patterns of the African American culture.

Table 6. Components and Food Products of the Traditional African American Diet (Burrows, 2004, Dirks and Duran, 2001, Byars, 1996).

Fats, oils, and sugars
• Bacon, Butter, Chitterlings/chitlins, Fatback, Hog/pork jowl, Lard, Molasses, Pig feet, Pork neck bones, Salt pork, Sugar, and Brown Sugar
Grains and Cereal
• Bread, Buns, Cornbread, Cornmeal, Cornstarch, Crackers, Grits, Hominy, Macaroni, Oatmeal, Pasta, Rice, and Wheat flour
Meat and Meat substitutes
• Beef, Eggs, Fish, Ham, Lamb, Pork (all parts), Pork Sausage, and Poultry
Milk and milk products
• Buttermilk, Cheese (American, cheddar), Cottage cheese, Milk (condensed, sour), and Yogurt
Nonstarchy vegetables
• Beets, Cabbage, Green/string beans, Greens (collards, mustards, turnip tops cooked with cured pork), Okra, Onions, Spinach, and Tomatoes
Starchy vegetables and beans
• Black-eyed peas, Corn, Dried beans (pinto, navy, lima, butter, kidney, garbonzo, great northern), Eddo, Pigeon pea, Sweet Potatoes, Turnips, White Potatoes, Yams, and Yautia Yuca (cassava)

AA with low socio-economic status lacks adequate access to health care for many reasons including poverty. As such, it is reported that the health care provided to AA by some doctors tends to focus on relieving immediate symptoms (Goody and Drago, 2010).

Table 7. Products Consumed in Traditional African American Dishes, Beverages and Desserts (Burrows, 2004, Dirks and Duran, 2001, Byars, 1996).

Drinks
• Lemonade, Passion Fruit, Powdered fruit-flavored drink mixes, Punch, Sun tea, and Sweet tea
Desserts
• Bread pudding, Flan, Fruits in pies and cobblers (Peach, Apple, Berry), Pecan pie, Red velvet cake (especially in Southern United States), Rice pudding, Sweet potato pie, and Yogurt
Dishes*
• Baked beans, Baked sweet potatoes, Barbecue ribs, Cabbage cooked with smoked meat, Candied sweet potatoes (or yams), Chicken and dumplings, Coleslaw, Collard, turnip or mustard greens cooked with smoked meat (ham hocks, smoked neckbones, salt pork, or bacon), Corn bread, Corn bread dressing/stuffing, Fried chicken, Fried fish, Fried green tomatoes, Fried okra, Glazed ham, Grits, Hoppin' john (beans and rice cooked with hog jawl), Macaroni and cheese, Meatloaf, Okra-tomato-and-corn-succotash, Pork chops (baked or fried), Pot likker (liquid from greens cooked with cured pork), and Red-beans-and-rice (Pigtails are commonly used to season the dish) • 'Soul food': Southern style cooking using some form of green leafy vegetable (collard, turnip tops, mustard or kale) cooked with some type of fat – usually salt pork, fat back, bacon or smoked ham hocks • Bacalao: dried salted codfish cooked with tomatoes, olives, and eggs
Fruits
• Apple, Bananas, Strawberries, Blackberries, Cantaloupe, Grapefruit, Grapes, Honeydew melon, Lemons, Oranges, Peaches, Strawberries, and Watermelon, Plantain, Breadfruit, Mango, Papaya, Persimmons, Sapodilla, Soursop, Pineapple

8.2.3. Chinese American Diet

Chinese Americans (CA) are the largest Asian American ethnic group in the United States. A large number of these CA are first generation immigrants from China, Hong Kong, Macao, and Taiwan that retain many traditional cultural values (US Census Bureau, 2015.). In general, Chinese are not concerned about the components in their diet, but about the texture, flavor, color, and aroma of the food. The main sources of protein include fish pork, and poultry. Tofu and small fish provide the calcium consumed since dairy products are not consumed in sufficient quantity, except for ice cream. Vegetables and fruits conforms a large part of the CA food intake. Rice is the pillar of the diet and is commonly consumed at every meal. Younger generations tend to disperse among the US population and adopt a more Westernized lifestyle (Chang, 2003). In Chinese culture consumption of fatty food is considered luxurious and nutritious due to history of famine. Also, affluence correlates to preference for fatty and well–marbled cuts of meat (Goody and Drago, 2010). Ethnic Chinese cooking does not include a lot of deep fried cooking. In the United States though Chinese restaurants have deep-fried dishes such as sweet and sour pork, almond fried Chicken, and deep-fried shrimp is order to promote business and to delight western tastes. Over time, CA face acculturation and American food is consumed among them even though native language is spoken at home. Moreover, sea food and duck consumption decreases as time in the US increases (Satia *et al.*, 2001; Yang and Fox, 1979). CA have a varied diet and health care practices, educational levels, lifestyle, and socio-economic status (Goody and Drago, 2010). There are different factors influencing food practices and meal patterns in the Chinese American diet, including degree of acculturation, socio-economic status, length of stay in the US, place of origin, food availability, access to food purchasing and preparation, health beliefs, and participation in government food programs (Goody and Drago, 2010). The figure below (Fig. **4**) presents a list of dietary components from different categories that are consumed with increased frequency as CA face acculturation of their diet in the United States.

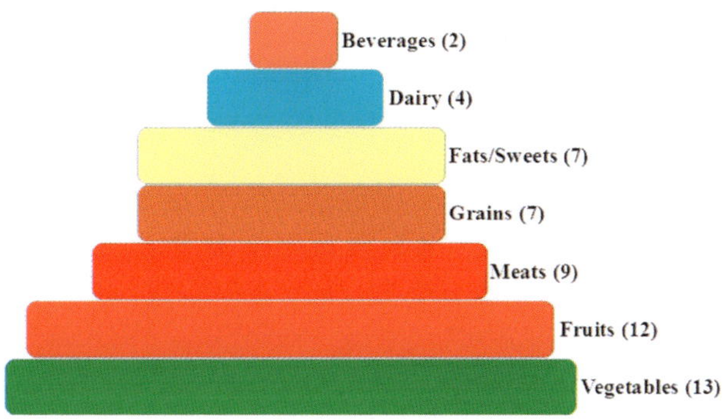

Fig. (4). Food Products with increased consumption in the Chinese American diet (Nan *et al.*, 2004).

Examples of the products in each category considered in this study are presented below from the largest to the lowest mean difference in increased consumption after immigration (Nan *et al.*, 2004). Beverages include coffee and regular sodas. Dairy products include low-fat milk, cheese, yogurt and ice cream. The group of fats and sweets include doughnuts, butter, pies, chocolate, cookies, cakes, and cooking oil (for cooking). Grains include bagels, pizza, breakfast cereal, sandwiches, pasta, bread, and tortillas. The meat group includes hamburger, hot dog, turkey meat, ham, beef, shrimp, chicken meat, bacon, and crab. Fruits include grapes, strawberries, cantaloupe, cherries, bananas, apples, grapefruit, oranges, peaches, mangoes, watermelon, and pears. The vegetable group includes broccoli, French fries, lettuce, asparagus, corn, onion, squash, carrots, potatoes, tomatoes, Snow beans (Snow peas), mushrooms, and Bell pepper (green pepper). In Fig. **5**. below, there is a list of dietary components from different categories that are consumed with decreased frequency as CA face acculturation of their diet in the United States.

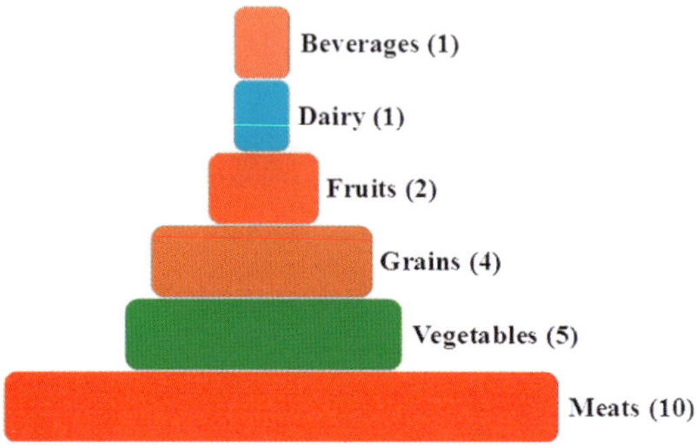

Fig. (5). Food Products with decreased consumption in the Chinese American diet (Nan *et al*., 2004).

Examples of the products in each category considered in this study are presented below from the largest to the lowest mean difference in reduced consumption after immigration (Nan *et al*., 2004). Beverages include tea as the item with reduced frequency. Dairy products include milk powder. Fruits include lychee and persimmon. Grains include steamed bun/bread, dumpling, noodles and rice. The vegetable group includes bean sprouts, bamboo shoots, eggplant, Napa cabbage, spinach. The meat group includes frog legs, soybeans, rabbit meat, Tofu (bean curd), duck meat, snake meat, dog meat, shark fin, pork, and fish.

8.2.4. Mexican American Diet

Mexico is rich in cultural heritage and regional diversity (Goody and Drago, 2010). Great diversity is also observed in food practices. Mexican cuisine use mostly ingredients native to Mexico and include some ingredients brought over by Spanish conquistadors. The staple food includes corn, beans, and chili peppers. Other native ingredients include tomatoes, squashes, avocado, and cocoa. The three primary classifications of Mexican food include *Mestizo* foods from the central plateau and the center of Oaxaca in the south, foods from the frontiers of the Maya in the southeast, and foods of the Gulf and Pacific coast. The main common characteristics of Mexican food practices are the succession of individual courses such as the consumption of rice before the main course or the beans and the use of chilies in great varieties. In the past, Mexicans enjoyed 4-5 meals per day, but today the meal pattern is three meals per day (Katz and Weaver, 2003). Fig. **6**. presents the number of foods items from each category that have the highest frequency of consumption in the Eastern Mexican diet (Barth, 2008).

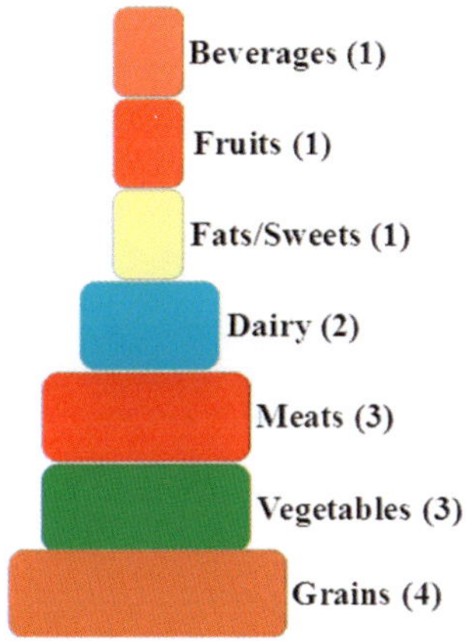

Fig. (6). Food Products Used in Traditional Mexican Cuisine (modified from Barth, 2008).

Some products in each category include more than one item. Beverages include many different types of fruits that are consumed daily as part of dink preparations. Fruits category comprise fresh fruits that are also consumed daily, but they are not consumed as part of a beverage. The fats/sweets category only includes the oil that is used in daily cooking, while dairy includes milk that is consumed daily and cheese that is consumed most days. Meats include three main sources of animal protein that are consumed most days such as beef, pork, and chicken. The vegetable category consists of fresh vegetables, peppers, and salsas. Grains includes processed and unprocessed products such as corn tortillas, cereals, and noodles that are consumed daily as well as rice that is consumed most days. (Barth, 2008).

The traditional diet is high in fruits, vegetables, and fiber as well as limited in added fat (Goody and Drago, 2010). Factors that affect current Mexican American (MA) diet include:

- Access to health care
- Chronic illnesses such as diabetes
- Degree of acculturation
- Educational background

- Family customs
- Gender
- Geographical region
- Knowledge and health beliefs
- Level of food security
- Self-efficacy
- Social support systems
- Socio-economic status including income

As a result of these factors, the current MA diet is high in fat and inadequate in fruits and vegetables (Neuhouser *et al.*, 2004). Moreover, herbal medicine and folk remedies with the use of faith or spiritual healers that focus on healing the soul in order to treat physical, mental and spiritual afflictions are popular in Mexican culture (Cotugna *et al.*, 1992). Hence, herbal products or functional foods are an integral part of the MA culture and diet.

Degree of acculturation of Mexican has a great impact on MA diet, which causes decreased consumption of traditional foods and dishes, and increased adoption of new practices with length of residency in the United States (Romero-Gwynn and Gwynn, 1997). Some of the core foods that showed decreased consumption by MA when compared to Mexicans are presented below (see Table **8**). (Romero-Gwynn and Gwynn, 1997). Only a few core foods showed an increase in consumption (see Table **8**).

8.3. The North American Diet

The cultural diversity of the United States and North America has led to interesting findings from surveys of our diet. As noted previously, cultural diets evolve as an ethnic group adapts to their new location. The North American Indian diet evolved from the tribe(s) and the geographic region they settled. As North America became settled by Europeans from England, France, Holland, and Spain, their cuisine adapted to the geography and diets of the region they settled ie, using corn learned from the Native Indians they encountered on settling the continent. As the relationship between nutrition and health and disease became more apparent, the United States government developed

Table 8. Dietary acculturation of Mexican Americans.

Core food	% Consumption	
	Mexicans	Mexican Americans
Boiled beans	84	42
Boiled rice[1]	9	32
Breakfast cereals	8	72
Cheese	85	91
Corn tortillas	98	84
Eggs	82	59
Fresh fruits and vegetables	8	92
Meat (beef, poultry, pork, and fish)	97	92
Milk	78	88
Pan dulce	84	15
Pasta	68	17
White sliced bread	15	84

[1]Consumption of rice with vegetables was reduced.

Table 9. Caloric sources of Americans NHANES 2005-2006.[a]

Caloric Source	
Breads/grains Yeast breads, Quick breads, Pizza Ready-to-eat cereals	**Desserts** Grain-based desserts Dairy desserts
Drinks Soda/energy/sports Alcoholic beverages Fruit drinks	**Dairy** Reduced fat milk Whole milk Regular cheese
Dishes Chicken and Chicken mixed Pasta Tortillas, burritos, tacos Beef and beef mixed Eggs and egg mixed Rice and rice mixed Nuts/seeds and nut/seed mixed	**Meat** Sausage, franks, bacon, and ribs Burgers Cold cuts **Snacks** Potato/corn/other chips Candy Fried white potatoes

Source: Dietary guidelines for Americans 2010.

[a]Data are drawn from analysis of usual dietary intakes conducted by the National Cancer Institute. Foods and beverages consumed were divided into 97 categories and ranked according to Calorie contribution for each age group. Additional information on Calorie contribution by age, gender, and race/ethnicity is available at http://riskfactor.cancer.gov/diet/foodsource/

an interest in the dietary habits of our society and began a survey; the National and Education Examination Survey (NHANES). This is a series of cross-sectional, nationally representative health examination surveys begun in 1960, which became a continuous survey in 1999 with data being collected on a 2-year cycle. The findings provide data concerning the prevalence of obesity (reported by State, see Chapter 9), information on the U.S diet and also comparisons of the U.S. diet to recommended intakes. The information may also be benchmarked against diets in other regions or countries where information is available (USDA and HHS, 2010).

Table **9** summarizes the most frequent sources of calories in the United States diet. (Dietary guidelines for Americans 2010). In summary, the American diet consists of grain, meat – primarily chicken, dairy, sugary drinks and for vegetables: chips or fried potatoes.

Table **10** provides the top ranked dietary sources believed to influence health and the development of disease. Yeast breads are the top ranked source of sodium and refined grain in the diet. Pasta and pasta dishes are also a high ranked source of sodium and refined grain. Grain-based desserts (ie, cookies, cake, pie) provide a significant source of nutrient types whose intake should be monitored and limited in the U.S. diet; sodium, saturated fat, solid fat, added sugar and refined grain. Pizza is also a predominant source of these nutrient types. Finally, grain and dairy-based desserts are frequent sources of added sugar to the diet.

Table 10. Top (Ranked 1-10a in body of table) sources of sodium, fat, sugar, and refined grain in the American diet.

Dietary Source	Sodium	Saturated Fat	Solid Fat	Added Sugar	Refined Grains
Pizza	3	2	2	-	2
Grain-based dessert	10	3	1	2	3
Chicken and Chicken mixed dishes	2	5	8	-	6
Tortillas, burritos, tacos	7	8	7	-	4
Pasta and pasta dishes	4	-	-	-	5
Dairy desserts	-	4	6	4	-
Sausage, franks, bacon, and ribs	8	6	4	-	-
Yeast breads	1	-	-	-	1

Adapted from Dietary guidelines for Americans 2010

[a]Not intended to provide all the ranks (1-10) of each dietary source but where the 8 dietary sources rank within the category

As noted above, NHANES information allows the U.S. to compare our diet to those of other countries or regions. Table **11** compares the usual U.S. intake to

Mediterranean patterns (Spain and Greece are countries used as examples) as well as the food pattern recommended by the USDA. The U.S. diet is below the USDA recommended intake for vegetables; including all categories of vegetables, fruits and juices, whole grains, dairy products, fish/seafood and oils. The U.S. diet exceeds USDA recommendations for solid fat, added sugar and meat. Mediterranean patterns match (*e.g.* vegetables, fruits and juices, dairy products, fish/seafood, oils and added sugar) USDA recommendations to a better extent than the U.S. diet.

Table 11. Daily adult U.S. dietary intake compared with Mediterranean and United States Department of Agriculture (USDA) recommendations.

Food Groups	**Usual U.S Intake[a]**	**Mediterranean[b] Patterns**		**USDA Food Pattern**
		Spain	Greece	
Vegetables (c)	1.6	1.2	4.1	2.5
Dark green	0.1	-	-	0.2
Beans and peas	0.1	0.4	<0.1	0.2
Red and orange	0.4	-	-	0.8
Starchy	0.5	-	0.6	0.7
Fruits and Juices (oz)	1.0	1.4	2.5	2.0
Grains, total (oz)	6.4	2.0	5.4	6.0
Whole grains	0.6	-	-	3.0
Milk and milk products (c)	1.5	2.1	1.0	3.0
Protein Foods (oz)				
Meat	2.5	3.6	3.5	1.8
Poultry	1.2	-	-	1.5
Eggs	0.4	1.9	-	0.4
Fish/Seafood	0.5	2.4	0.8	1.2
Nuts, seeds and Soy	0.5	-	-	0.6
Oils (g)	18	19	40	27
Solid fats (g)	43	-	-	16
Added Sugar (g)	79	-	24	32

[a]Source: U.S. Department of Agricultural Research Service and U.S. Department of Health and Human Services, Centers for Disease Control and Prevention. What we Eat in America, NHANES 2001-2004, 1 day mean intakes for adult males and females, adjusted to 2,000 Calories and averaged.
[b]see the DGAC report for additional information and references at www.dietaryguidelines.gov
c = cup, g = gram, oz = ounces
Adapted from www.health.gov/dietaryguidelines/dga2010/dietaryguidelines2010.pdf, accessed January 10, 2015.

In summary, the U.S. diet provides 15% of calories as protein 2/3 of which are from animal sources, 52% of calories from carbohydrate ½ of which as simple sugar, ½ as starches (pasta, bread, potatoes) and 33% as fat with the majority from animal sources (60%), the remainder is from plant origin (40%) (Wardlaw *et al.*, 2012).

CONTENT REFLECTION

1. Describe how the following factors have shaped your food preferences:

    a. Exposure to selected foods at an early age (due to culture or just trials)

    b. Advertising person to person or through the media (what is the newest food you have tried?)

    c. Eating out alone or in group

    d. Peer pressure (as a result of diversified cultures)

    e. Socio-economic factors

2. What products in your supermarket reflect the consumer demand for healthier foods? For convenience? Have you noticed a great difference between the products in your supermarket and those of other areas?

3. EF is a 37 year old single mother who has been increasingly bothered by hot flashes and was told by a friend that if she brought her diet to the pharmacist that they could help her modify it to alleviate her symptoms. She has very little time in that she just finished her job at a day-care center (which allows her to get discount day care for her young children) and is on her way to her evening job cleaning the local elementary school. EF is 5’11” and weighs 180 pounds. Her father is Caucasian and mother African-American. Her father died from cancer when she was 23 years old and her mother has diabetes. She lives in a small apartment close to the elementary school where she works and uses public transportation if she needs to travel outside the local urban area she lives.

The pharmacist makes a copy of her diet and schedules an appointment with EF the following week. After the patient leaves, the pharmacist places her diet information in the SuperTracker at myplate.gov and prints out the summary reports of her diet (build a diet using SuperTracker based on the culture related tables provided above, rich in bread, sodium, and lipids).

Based on this information, answer the following questions.

1. Look into the numbers of calories that each one of the food products she consumed generates. Compare % of calorie intake from carbohydrates, proteins, and fats to the following:

    a. Recommended calorie intake from each macronutrient.

2. Look into amount of micronutrients (vitamins and minerals) provided by each food source consumed. Based on the levels of the following:

    a. Potassium consumed vs. recommended dietary intake of potassium

        i. Is there potential risk of chronic diseases such as hypertension, why?

    b. Chromium vs. recommended dietary intake of chromium

        ii. Is there potential risk of chronic diseases such as diabetes, why?

    c. Iodine consumed vs. recommended dietary intake of iodine (Tips: How much bread does the patient eats? What dietary factor present in bread and approved by the FDA could affect the levels of iodine?)

3. Based on EF dietary record, what type (s) of phytochemicals were consumed that would potentially reduce the risk of chronic diseases (diabetes, cancer, *etc.*) in this patient?

4. Using the tips for healthy meal planning provided in class, counsel the patient on healthy food choices to improve her diet. Consider the following socioeconomic factors in your advice:

a. Job

b. Food security

c. Education

d. Cultural background

e. Food access

CONCLUDING REMARKS

This chapter has presented and applied concepts from previous chapters as well as other discussed in this chapter that have an impact on a balanced diet such as those related to socioeconomic status, income, and culture. After completing the exercises above, the reader should have understood the importance of socioeconomic status, income, and culture in the design of a healthy diet.

CONFLICT OF INTEREST

The author's confirm that this ebook contents have no conflict of interest.

ACKNOWLEDGEMENTS

The authors would like to thank you to Michelle OgavaIgual for preparing some tables.

REFERENCES

Byars, D. (1996). Traditional African American foods and African Americans. Agriculture and Human Values, 13: 74-78.

Ballew, C., White, L. L., Strauss, K. F., Benson, L. J., Mendlein, J. M. and Mokdad, A. H. (1997). Intake of nutrients and food sources of nutrients among the Navajo: findings from the Navajo Health and Nutrition Survey. Journal of Nutrition, 127: 2085S-2093S.

Barer-Stein, T. B. (1999). You Eat What You Are: People, Culture and Food Traditions. 2nd ed. Willowdale, Canada: Firefly Books. 544 pp.

Barth, M. (2008). A Nutrition Assessment of Dietary Practices of Mexicans Living in the State of Veracruz, Mexico. UW-L Journal of Undergraduate Research XI: 1-4.

Burrows, J. D. (2004). Incorporating ethnic and cultural food preferences in the renal diet. Advances in Renal Replacement Therapy, 11:97-104.

Chang, I. (2003). The Chinese in America: A Narrative History. New York, NY: Penguin Books. 496 pp.

Colby, S. E., McDonald, L. R., Adkison, G. (2011-2012). Traditional Native American foods: stories from Northern Plains elders. Journal of Ecological Anthropology, 15: 65-73.

Cotugna, N., A. Subar, J. Heimendinger, & L. Kahle. (1992). Nutrition and cancer prevention knowledge, beliefs, attitudes, and practices: the 1987 National Health Interview Survey. Journal of the American Dietetic Association. 92: 963-968.

Dirks, R. T. & Duran, N. (2001). African American dietary patterns at the beginning of the 20th Century. The Journal of Nutrition, 131:1881-1889.

Goody, C. M. & Drago, L. (2010). Cultural Food Practices. 1st ed. American Dietetic Association.

Gordon-Larsen, P., Adair, L. S. & Popkin, B. M. (2003). The Relationship of Ethnicity, Socioeconomic Factors, and Overweight in U.S. Adolescents. Obesity Research, 11: 121-129.

Indian Health Service. (2015). The IHS Gold Book: Parts 1-4. Rockville, MD: US Department of Health and Human Services. Available at: http://www.ihs.gov/scb/ (accessed 1.15.2015).

Katz, S. H., & W. W. Weaver. (2003). Encyclopedia of Food and Culture. New York, NY: Scribner Gale Group. p. 492.

Kindscher, K. (1987). Edible Wild Plants of the Prairie: An Ethnobotanical Guide. Lawrence, KS: University Press of Kansas. 276 pp.

Kopp, J. (1986). Crosscultural contacts: changes in the diet and nutrition of the Navajo Indians. American Indian Culture and Research Journal, 10: 1-30.

Kwate, N. O. A. & Loh, J. M. (2010). Separate and unequal: The influence of neighborhood and school characteristics on spatial proximity between fast food and schools. Preventive medicine, 51: 153-156.

Larsen, K. & Gilliland, J. (2008). Mapping the evolution of 'food deserts' in a Canadian city: Supermarket accessibility in London, Ontario, 1961-2005. International Journal of Health Geographics, 7: 1-16.

Carey, H. Jr. (Web Designer) (1994-2013). Navajo Food. Available at: http://navajopeople.org/navajo-food.htm (accessed August 30, 2015).

Neuhouser, M., Thompson, B., Coronado, G. & Solomon, C. (2004). Higher fat intake and lower fruit and vegetables intakes are associated with greater acculturation among Mexicans living in Washington State. Journal of American Dietetic Association, 104: 51-57.

Nan, L.V., Cason, K. L. (2004). Dietary pattern change and acculturation of Chinese Americans in Pennsylvania. Journal of American Dietetic Association, 104:771-778.

Norris, T., P. L. Vines, & E. M. Hoeffel. (2010). The American Indian and Alaska Native Population: 2010. Washington, DC: U.S. Department of Commerce Economics and Statistics Administration, U.S. Census Bureau. pp. 1-21.

Pearce, J., Blakely, T., Witten, K. & Bartie, P. (2007). Neighborhood Deprivation and Access to Fast-Food Retailing: A National Study. American Journal of Preventive Medicine, 32: 375-382.

Pelican, S. (1991). Navajo Food Practices, Customs, and Holidays. Chicago, IL: The American Dietetic Association. 26 pp.

Phillips, K. M., Pehrsson, P. R., Agnew, W. W., Scheett, A. J., Follett, J. R., Lukaski, H. C., Patterson, K. Y. (2014). Nutrient composition of selected traditional United States Northern Plains Native American plant foods. Journal of Food Composition and Analysis, 34: 136-152.

Powell, L. M., Slater, S., Mirtcheva, D., Bao, Y. & Chaloupka, F. J. (2007). Food store availability and neighborhood characteristics in the United States. Preventive medicine, 44: 189-195.

Powers, W. K. (1973). Indians of the Northern Plains. New York, NY: Capricorn Books. 256 pp.

Romero-Gwynn, E., Gwynn, D. 1997. Dietary Patterns and Acculturation Among Latinos of Mexican Descent. The Julian Samora Research Institute, Michigan State University, East Lansing, Michigan, JSRI Research Report #23:1-4.

Satia, J., Patterson, R., Kristal, A., Hislop, T., Yasui, Y. & Taylor, V. (2001). Development of scales to measure dietary acculturation among Chinese-Americans and Chinese-Canadians. Journal of American Dietetic Association, 101: 548-53.

Satterfield, D. W., Shield, J. E., Buckley, J. & Alive, S. T. (2007). So That the People May Live (Hecel Lena Oyate Ki Nipi Kte): Lakota and Dakota Elder Women as Reservoirs of Life and Keepers of Knowledge about Health Protection and Diabetes Prevention. Journal of Health Disparities Research and Practice, 1: 1–28.

Stang, J., Zephier, E. M., Story, M., Himes, J. H., Yeh, J. L., Welty, T. and Howard, B. V. (2005) Dietary intakes of nutrients thought to modify cardiovascular risk from three groups of American Indians: the Strong Heart Dietary Study, Phase II. Journal of the American Dietetic Association, 105 (12): 1895-1903.

Sucher, K. P., & P. G. Kittler. (2007). Food and Culture. 5th ed. Belmont, CA: Thompson Wadsworth. 576 pp.

Taylor, C. A., Keim, K. S., Gilmore, A. C. (2005). Impact of core and secondary foods on nutritional composition of diets in Native-American Women. Journal of the American Dietetic Association, 105 (3):413-419.

Thornton, L. E., Bentley R. J. & Kavanagh A. M. (2011). Individual and area-level socioeconomic associations with fast food purchasing. Journal of Epidemiology & Community Health, p. 873-880. doi:10.1136/jech.2009.099614

US Census Bureau. (2015). American Community Survey 1 year Estimates. Washington, DC: U.S. Consensus Bureau. Available at: http://factfinder.census.gov/faces/tableservices/jsf/pages/productview.xhtml?pid=ACS_13_1YR_S0201&prodType=table (accessed 2.4.2015).

USDA & HHS. (2010). Dietary Guidelines for Americans 2010. Washington, DC: U.S. Government Printing Office.

Wardlaw, G., A. Smith, & A. Collene. (2012). Contemporary Nutrition. New York, NY: McGraw Hill Education. 768 pp.

Wiedman, D. (2005). American Indian diets and nutritional research: implications of the Strong Heart Dietary Study, Phase II, for Cardiovascular Disease and Diabetes, Journal of the American Dietetic Association, 105 (12): 1874-1880.

White, R. (2012) Examining the Effect of Socioeconomic Status on Access to Nutritional Food. Perspectives (University of New Hampshire). pp. 114-120.

Witt, D. (1999). Black Hunger: Food and the Politics of U.S. Identity. New York, NY: Oxford University Press. 304 pp.

Wolfe, W.S. and Sanju, D. (1988). Contemporary diet and body weight of Navajo women receiving food assistance. An ethnographic and nutritional investigation. Journal of the American Dietetic Association 88 (7): 822-827.

Yang, G. & Fox, H. (1979). Food habit changes of Chinese persons living in Lincoln, Nebraska. Journal of American Dietetic Association, 75: 420-424.

CHAPTER 9

Factors Contributing to Health and Disease

Jay M. Mirtallo* **and Esperanza J. Carcache de Blanco**

The Ohio State University, Columbus, Ohio, USA

Abstract: There are many aspects of the American diet that should be improved in order to promote health and prevent disease. The United States Departments of Agriculture and Health and Human Services are responsible for developing and updating guides to educate the public and professionals on nutritional health. The current guide: Dietary Guidelines for Americans, 2010 provides a wealth of ideas in simple, actionable health messages to improve the diet. This chapter reviews many of these principles for good nutrition health in addition to dietary reference intakes (DRI) important to assess the adequacy of specific nutrients in the diet as well as activity, a lifestyle that facilitates nutritional health.

Keywords: Dietary reference intakes, empty calories, estimated average requirement, food groups, healthy diet, MyPlate, nutrition health, physical activity and exercise, recommended dietary allowance, tolerable upper limits.

INTRODUCTION

There are fundamental improvements in the American diet that are necessary to improve health and minimize the development of disease. The 'Dietary Guidelines for Americans 2010' provide a wealth of information on methods to improve the nutrition health of the American society. As covered in Chapter 8 there are nutrients that are deficient in the diet as well as those that are excessive for Americans. In order to understand the consequences of continual, long-term deficient or excessive intake, it is important to understand Dietary Reference Intakes (Institute of Medicine, 2005). This chapter will provide a description of Dietary Reference Intakes as well as review tips to improve the diet. Important messages provided in the 'My Plate' website will be reviewed along with methods to initiate and improve physical activity and exercise in our society.

DIETARY REFERENCE INTAKES

Important definitions for Dietary Reference Intakes are provided in the Glossary and will be reviewed in this section.

***Corresponding author Jay Mirtallo:** College of Pharmacy, The Ohio State University, Columbus, OH 43210, USA; E-mail: mirtallo.1@osu.edu

Dietary reference intakes (DRI) are a set of values for specific nutrients that provide the criteria for adequacy of the diet. The Recommended Dietary Allowance (RDA) is the most well-known DRI and is the amount in the diet where there is a very small probability or risk of inadequacy (2-3 percent). The level of intake between the RDA and the Tolerable Upper Limit (UL) is the amount where the risk of inadequacy or excess is close to 0.0 percent (Institute of Medicine 2005). At nutrient levels above the UL, the risk of adverse events is likely to increase. This is demonstrated in Fig. **1** The EAR (Estimated Average Requirement) is the intake level that the risk of inadequacy is about 50% (Institute of Medicine, 2005).

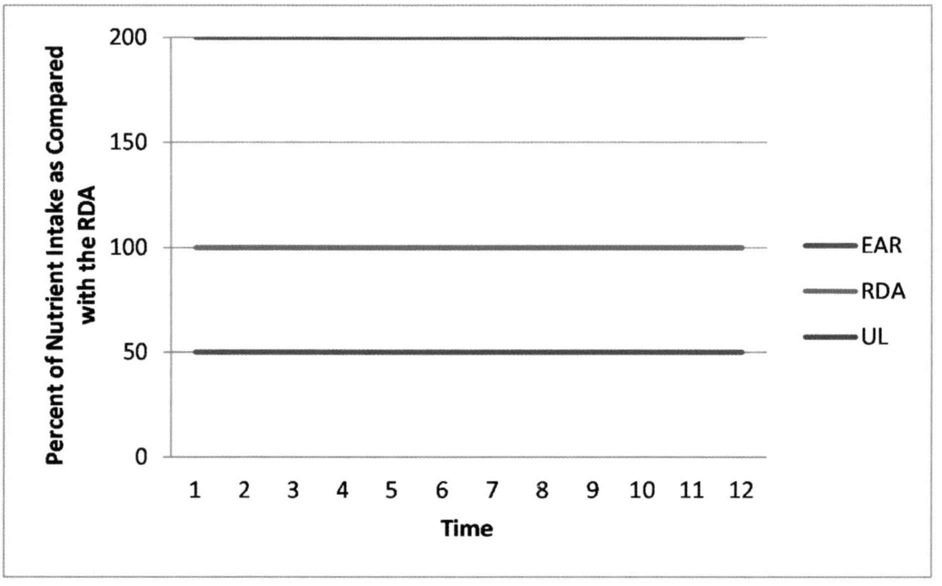

Figure 1: Dietary reference intakes for nutrients. EAR = estimated average requirement, RDA = recommended daily allowance, UL = tolerable upper limit. The risk for inadequacy (or nutrient deficiency) increases when intake is < 100 % of the RDA for prolonged periods of time whereas the potential for nutrient toxicity increases when intake continually exceeds the UL set here at an arbitrary value of 200% of the RDA. The UL value will depend on the nutrient in question as well as other hereditary and environmental factors.

It is important to consider adequate *versus* inadequate nutrient intake. For example, if energy intake over time is below the EAR, an individual may have difficulty maintaining a healthy weight or if weight loss is also associated with inadequate protein, develop a loss in lean body mass which leads to aberrations in cellular function. At a very basic level, this is the definition of malnutrition. Types of malnutrition described by the World Health Organization are marasmus – a depletion of both energy and protein and kwashiorkor – protein depletion with minimal or no energy deficit. On the contrary, excess energy intake is associated with weight gain and increase in the fat mass of the body. This form of malnutrition is termed obesity which will be covered in more detail in Chapter 10. For the most part, maintaining a diet that meets the RDA will promote health and minimize the development of disease.

Exercise 9.1: Determining Body Composition and Energy Requirements for Males and Females (Refer to Body Composition section in Chapter 1)

1. An adult Male weighs 150 pounds and is 6 feet 2 inches tall. Calculate this individual's ideal body weight in kilograms and his percent ideal body weight

Ideal Body Weight kg

% Ideal Body Weight %

Determine his Body Mass Index (BMI) and classify his body composition according to the criteria in Table **3** of Chapter 1.

BMI: kg/m^2

BMI Classification:

Determine the energy requirements for this individual using the RDA provided in Table **1**

Energy requirement: Calories

Table 1: Recommended Dietary Intake for Calories/Energy based on Age

Life Stage Group	Kcal/kg
0-6 months	75-100
6-12 months	60-80
1-12 years	50-75
>12-18 yrs	30-50
Adults	27-28

2. An adult Female weighs 200 pounds and is 5 feet 1 inch tall. Calculate her weight in kilograms (kg) and her percent ideal body weight (%).

Determine her Body Mass Index (BMI) and classify her body composition according to the criteria in Table 3 of Chapter 1.

BMI: kg/m^2

BMI Classification:

Determine the energy requirements for this individual using the RDA provided in Table **1**

Energy requirement: Calories

Note: there is a continual debate in the field of nutrition on which body weight to use to calculate energy requirements. This is dependent on the body composition of the individual whereas, it is believed that energy expenditure is derived mostly from the lean body mass. A person who is underweight, and therefore a low lean body mass will have an energy expenditure lower than that calculated using their ideal body weight whereas an overweight or obese individual will have an energy expenditure which may be normal or elevated depending on the proportion weight gain that is lean body mass as compared with fat mass. Therefore it is not likely the energy expenditure would be as great as would be calculated using their actual body weight for the calculation since the lean body mass does not increase in the same proportion as the amount of fat mass in obese individuals. It may be suggested then to use the actual body weight for calculation of energy requirements (RDA) for underweight and normal weight individuals and use the ideal body weight for overweight or obese individuals. However, other variables influence these estimates of energy expenditure (RDA) such as height, weight, sex, activity level, growth and disease. Therefore, caloric intake should be monitored by measuring a daily weight to assess the adequacy of energy intake (RDA) calculated using the criteria in Table **1**

MyPlate: Messages Concerning a Healthy Diet

You were introduced to the United States Department of Agriculture's (USDA) food guides in Chapter 1. In previous other chapters, content specific to macro- and micronutrients have been covered in addition to their dietary sources. Exercises were provided to determine the amount of nutrients consumed in the diet. Chapter 8 included a review of the typical American diet. According to NHANES surveys, the American diet is low in vegetables, including all types, fruits and juices, whole grains, dairy products, fish/seafood and oils. Amounts for solid fat, added sugar and meat exceed the RDA. MyPlate (www.choosemyplate.gov) builds on the principles for nutrition health presented in MyPyramid with a focus on simpler and clearer messages for the public and educators. This section will cover more specifics related to the USDA recommendations and messages for improving the diet. The basis for this discussion is from Dietary Guidelines for Americans 2010 (USDA, 2010).

MyPyramid has completely transtioned to MyPlate so the websites are no longer available (www.mypyramid.gov/downloads/MyPyramid_Anatomy.pdf, www.my-pyramid.gov/downloads/MiniPoster.pdf) however, concepts that remain current should be considered when using MyPlate. The MyPyramid (Fig. **2**) had a specific anatomy used to visualize the approach to nutrition health. The approach included six subject areas outlined below:

1. Personalization: the adequacy of the diet is dependent on the population, their body composition as well as genetic, environmental and cultural factors inherent to the individual. No one approach is successful in all individuals.

2. Proportionality: as noted by the colors in the pyramid, the diet should be balanced with the proper proportion of each nutrient to promote and maintain health

3. Variety: as noted, the colored sections of the pyramid are for each of the five food groups: orange – grains, green – vegetables, red – fruits, yellow – oils, blue – dairy, purple – meat and /or beans.

4. Steps to a healthier you: successful change in dietary and lifestyle habits come from gradual, incremental changes using small rather than large steps. Therefore, the change is likely to be sustained for a lifetime with minimal risk of falling back to previous unhealthy actions.

5. Moderation: the broad bands at the base of the pyramid represent the proportion of healthier foods as the foundation of nutrient intake. In contrast, rather than total elimination of other less healthy options such as solid fat or added sugars, these are represented in the narrower sections of the bands representing their less frequent inclusion in the diet.

6. Activity: a factor not considered in previous food guides is the importance of daily physical activity as a part of a healthy diet.

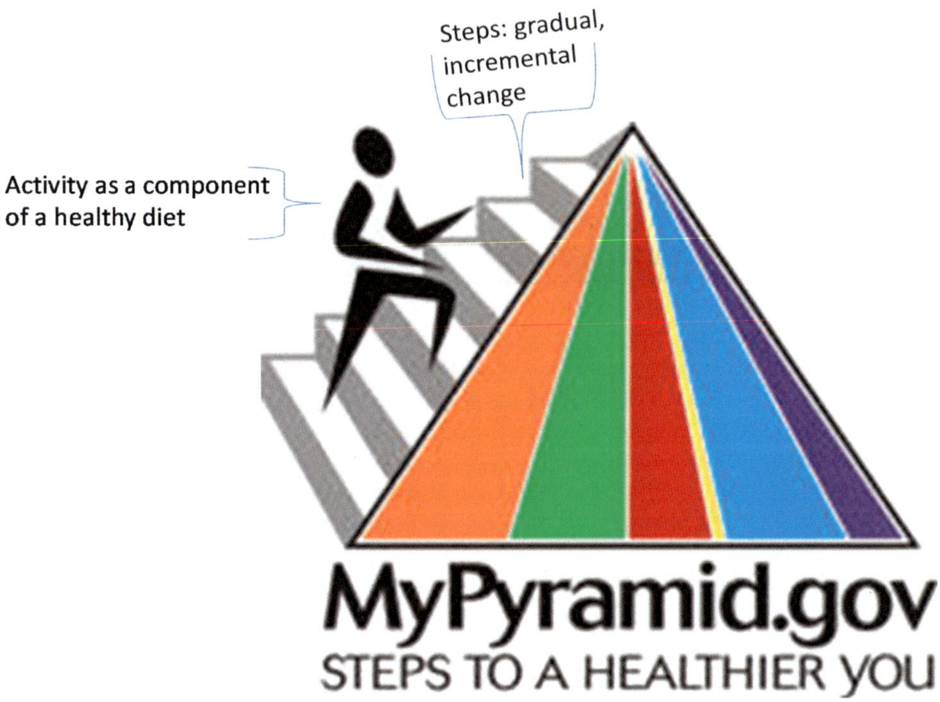

Figure 2: MyPyramid: Steps to a Healthier You.

As an example, the following table (Table **2**) provides the amounts of nutrients in each food group and some direction for healthier choices to put the MyPyramid concepts into practice.

Of note, it is important to maintain a balance between food and physical activity. Physical activity allows for more variation in the proportion of foods selected from each food group and is important to preventing weight gain and sustaining weight loss achieved. To summarize healthy food choices provided in MyPyramid that have translated to MyPlate, their should be a limit on fats, sugars and salt (sodium) in the American diet. Fish, nuts and vegetable oils are suggested sources of fat. However there should be a limit of solid fat such as butter, margarine, shortening and lard. The amount of saturated and trans fat should be monitored and limited in the diet. Understanding and using food labels to monitor the nutrient content of foods is an essential activity in understanding and choosing a healthier diet. Finally, food and beverages low in added sugars should be chosen.

Table 2: Food Groups and Considerations for a Healthy Diet

Food Group	Proportion[1]	Message	Comments
Grains	6 ounces	Make half your grains whole	Whole grain cereals, breads, crackers, rice or pasta 1 ounce ≈ 1 slice bread, 1 cup cereal, ½ cup cooked rice
Vegetables	2 ½ cups	Vary your veggies	Eat more: Dark green – broccoli, spinach, leafy greens Orange – carrots, sweet potatoes Dry beans and peas – pinto and kidney beans, lentil
Fruits	2 cups	Focus on fruits	Eat a variety Source: fresh, frozen, canned or dried Caution with fruit juices (added sugar)
Milk	3 cups	Get your calcium-rich foods	Choose low-fat or fat-free dairy products If milk is not chosen or an intolerance occurs, choose other sources of calcium such as fortified foods or beverages
Meat & Beans	5 ½ ounces	Go lean with protein	Choose low-fat or lean meats and/or poultry Preparation: bake, broil or grill Vary protein: include fish 1-2 times per week

Source: U.S. Department of Agriculture

MyPlate. The current evolution of USDA food guides focuses on the delivery of the message(s) important to nutritional health. The icon (MyPlate, Fig. **3**) shows the food choices as a meal (plate) to assist with visualizing your choices.

As such, MyPlate is intended to provide consumers with information about their nutritional health as simple, actionable health messages. For example, selected messages for consumers (http://www.choosemyplate.gov/print-materials-ordering/selected-message.html) that complement the MyPlate icon are outlined below (choosemyplate.gov):

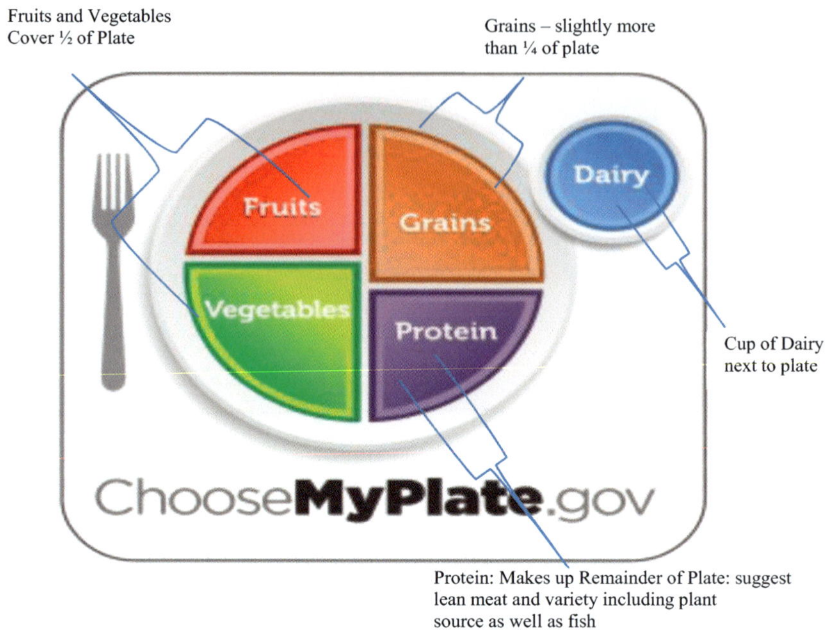

Figure 3: MyPlate icon Source: U.S. Department of Agriculture) with Descriptions of Recommended Food Choices. There is no separate group for fats and oils; these are to be incorporated into other foods. Messages are available to reinforce the limits on solid fats and suggestion for inclusion of plant oils rich in essential fatty acids. Adapted from MyPlate.com icon found at ChooseMyPlate.gov.

Balancing Calories

- Enjoy your food, but eat less.
- Avoid oversized portions.

Foods to Increase

- Make half your plate fruits and vegetables.
- Make at least half your grains whole grains.
- Switch to fat-free or low-fat (1%) milk.

Foods to Reduce

- Compare sodium in foods like soup, bread, and frozen meals and choose the foods with lower numbers.

- Drink water instead of sugary drinks.

The 10 Tips Nutrition Education Series can be found on the ChooseMyPlate website (www.choosemyplate.gov). Each topic provides 10 tips to assist with food choices and actions used to achieve the goals. Topics are provided for each food group. More detail is provided for each of the general concepts already discussed. Lifestyle such as food choices at school, for snacks and improving the health of celebrations are available as well as specific content for males including adults and teens in addition to females. A wealth of ideas is presented to improve the health of the diet in a high quality, easy-to-follow format. The discussion that follows provides examples for food groups as well as other messages that may be useful in choosing a healthy diet.

Specific messages for the five basic food groups covered in the 10 Tips Nutrition Education Series are provided in Table **3** This provides a summary of selected tips, more details are provided at the website including other of the 10 tips that are not presented here.

These are just a few examples of how an individual may alter their diet and make healthier food choices. A variety of tips are provided so the individual may choose an option that is of interest to them either because it is preferred or it may functionally be easier to incorporate into their daily life. For fruits, the idea that they can be used to sweeten a meal (rather than dairy desserts or cookies), are a great source of fiber and have sources other than fresh fruits available for lunches, snacks and dinner can facilitate this food group replacing unhealthy food choices. Vegetables are also a source of fiber as well as vitamins and minerals but to meet the RDA of all of these micronutrients, a variety of vegetables are needed.

Table 3: Selected Tips for a Healthy Diet with a Focus on the 5 Basic Food Groups

Food Groups	MyPlate Message	Selected Tips to Improve Nutrition Health
Fruits	Focus on fruits	Keep visible reminders: have a bowl of fruit on the counter, table or refrigerator Experiment with fruit at dinner: include orange sections, dried cranberries, grapes to salads Think about variety: buy dried, frozen or canned (in 100% juice) so a supply is always available
Vegetables	Add more Vegetables to your Day	Discover fast ways to cook: use microwave for fresh or frozen vegetables. Frozen vegetables are available in microwavable bags in portions sufficient for family meals. Steam green beans, carrots or broccoli in small amounts of water in the microwave.

Table 3: contd...

		Choose vegetables rich in color: vegetables that are red, orange or dark green provide different amounts of essential micronutrients especially vitamins and minerals. Examples include acorn squash, cherry tomatoes, sweet potatoes or colored greens
Grains	Make Half your Grains Whole	Try whole-wheat versions of brown-rice, pasta. Examples include brown-rice stuffing in baked green peppers or tomatoes and whole wheat macaroni in macaroni and cheese Know what to look for on the food label (ingredient list): choose products that name a whole-grain ingredient ('whole wheat', 'brown rice', 'bulgur', 'whole oats') first on the list
Protein	With Protein Foods, Variety is Key	Choose seafood twice a week: select a variety of seafood including those higher in oils and lower in mercury such as salmon, trout and herring Eat plant protein more often: these are naturally low in saturated fat and high in fiber. Examples include beans – kidney, pinto, black, white and peas – split and chickpeas. Also includes hummus, soy products, nuts and seeds
Dairy	Got your Dairy Today?	'Skim' the fat: drink fat-free or low fat to lower saturated fat intake and calories. Gradually reduce from whole milk to lower fat versions to cut calories but maintain calcium and other nutrient intake What about cream cheese? Regular cream cheese, cream and butter are not part of the dairy food group. They are high in saturated fat and have little or no calcium

Source: U.S. Department of Agriculture

This is easy to implement by considering vegetables in a different way: a variety of colors offers a more reliable source and variety of nutrients. Americans consume a large amount of grain. Processed grain is useful in shelf-life especially during transportation but this processing removes healthy nutrients. If just part of the grains consumed were as 'whole' grains, the American diet would be healthier. Use caution with this food group though and know what to look for on labels, its easy to be fooled into thinking you are purchasing a product that is a whole grain but is not. Animal sources are the major contributor to saturated fat intake. Using lean cuts of meat and adjusting to plant and seafood sources of protein increases the variety of fat sources to the diet. The goal is to move to unsaturated fatty acids and get the benefit of fish oils in the diet so a better balance of fat sources is achieved. Dairy provides a reliable source of calcium however, it is derived from animal sources so the fat content is a source of saturated fat and extra calories from the fat that is not needed. Adjusting to a lower fat dairy product makes sense for the move to a healthier diet.

Remember that foods may be sources of multiple nutrients (Table **4**, USDA, 2010). The foods selected for the table are foods commonly found in the American diet.

Interesting that the foods consistently provide grains to the diet, occasionally they provide a source of vegetable or protein and very rarely provide a healthy source of fruit. Finally, cheese is the primary source of dairy in the foods.

Whether you eat your meals at home or in a restaurant, tips to a great plate may be used to improve the nutritional content. Using smaller plates or bowls help reduce the portion size which is big for Americans as compared with other cultures. Also, the size of the drink container may significantly contribute to caloric intake, especially if your beverage is refillable. Transitioning to water or unsweetened beverages may make a significant change in your daily caloric intake. It is interesting to think of celebrations as another opportunity to make healthy choices. Being active and decreasing the focus on food and beverages while enjoying other traditions will lead to healthier nutritional intakes. Eating out, because of portion sizes, menu choices that include unhealthy fats and added sugars as well as the amount of added sodium in the prepared meal will adversely affect your health over time. Avoiding fried food in favor of grilled, broiled or steamed menu items as well as avoiding added salt are choices that improve the health of the diet.

Table 4: Foods providing Multiple Nutrients

Food and sample portion	Grains Group (oz)	Vegetable Group (cups)	Fruit Group (cups)	Dairy Group (cups)	Protein Group (oz)	Estimated Total Calories
Pizza with cheese and extra vegetables, thick crust (1 piece)	3	½	0	¾	0	380
Burrito with beaf, beans, rice, cheese (1 large)	4 ½	¼	0	½	3	840
Breakfast sandwich: egg, cheese, and sausage on English muffin (1 sandwich)	2	0	0	½	1 ½	455
Chicken vegetable soup with rice, chunky style (1 cup)	½	¼	0	0	1	130
Cherry cobbler (1/2 cup)	1	0	¼	0	0	210

Source: U.S. Department of Agriculture

Table **5** (www.choosemyplate.gov) includes a variety of topics covered by the 10Tips Nutrition Education Series not related to the food groups.

Table 5: Selected 10Tips Nutrition Education Series Topics to Improve Nutrition Health

Topic	MyPlate Message	Selected Tips to Improve Nutrition Health
Choose MyPlate	Tips to a Great Plate	Avoid oversized portions: use smaller plate, bowl or glass. Portion out foods prior to eating
		Balance your calories: being physically active helps you balance calories
		Eat desserts and treats less often, not everyday
Beverages	Make Better Beverage Choices	Enjoy your beverage but cut back
		Check the serving size and number of servings in the container
		Select smaller cans, cups or glasses and avoid supersizing
		Manage your calories by drinking water with and between meals
Celebrations	Make Celebrations Fun, Healthy and Active	Try out some healthier recipes: reduce sugar, salt and fat. Adults that participate set an example for children
		Create healthy habits by having activities that get people up and moving. Avoid food and drinks being the primary focus of the party.
		Be creative with including whole grains such as crackers and switch from meat snacks to vegetable sources of protein such as a bean dip
Eating Out	Tips for Eating Healthy when Eating Out	Ask for water or unsweetened tea for a beverage. Avoid drinks with added sugar
		Start with salad and dressing on the side
		Select steamed, grilled or broiled dishes
		Order appetizer or lunch size of main dish
Salt and Sodium	Tips to Help you Cut Back	Eat at home – you are in control of what's in your food, especially the sodium content
		Fill up on vegetables and fruit – foods naturally low in sodium
		Pay attention to condiments – ketchup, salad dressings and seasoning packets are high in sodium
		Boost your potassium intake. Foods high in potassium: potatoes, tomato juice, sweet potatoes, beans and bananas. Also found in yogurt, clams, halibut, orange juice and milk

Source: U.S. Department of Agriculture

Exercise 9.2: MyPlate: A Guide to Better Nutritional Health

The nutrient content of a food diary has been determined and reported in the tables below. The menu items ingested during the day are as follows:

Breakfast: Low-fat berry smoothie with blueberry muffin

Lunch: garden salad with ranch dressing, a cup of bean soup and 2 biscuits with butter and a soft drink that was refilled twice

Dinner: ravioli with meat sauce, 2 breadsticks with garlic butter, a garden-fresh salad with italian dressing and lemonade including 1 refill

Nutrient Intake Summary as Compared with Recommended Daily Allowance (RDA)

	Carbohydrate Content			Protein Content	
	Grams	Calories	%Total	Grams	Grams/kg
RDA	180-330	26-28/kg	45-65	56	0.8
Daily intake	508	1990	64	66	

Calculated total calories: 3127 (RDA 2000-2400)

	Fat Content			Type of Fat Content	
	Grams	% Total	Cholesterol	Saturated Fat	Trans Fat
Healthy diet*	44-78	20-35	<300 mg	15.5 G or < 7% of Total Calories	<1% of Total Calories
Daily Intake	103	29	34	30 (8.5%)	0

*Based on a 2000 Calorie diet

Using the 10Tips Nutrition Education Series select strategies you would use to address the following issues to overcome on the way to a healthier diet than presented in the food diary above.

1. Add more vegetables
2. Focus on fruit
3. Make half your grains whole
4. Got your dairy today?
5. With protein, variety is the key
6. Salt and sodium
7. Make better food choices

Empty Calories. Caloric sources originated from solid fats or added sugars are considered empty calories. This is because these caloric sources provide calories but few if any other necessary nutrients. Solid fats are solid at room temperature and are found in natural food but are also added during the processing and preparation of food. Added sugars are sugars or syrups added to foods or beverages as they are prepared. Empty calories may make food appealing but add an excessive amount of calories. Since they contribute very little other essential nutrients it is best to minimize this source of calories or look for other caloric sources that offer a better balance of other essential nutrients. The most frequent sources of empty calories in the American diet may be presented in a manner based on which empty calorie they include; added sugar, solid fat or both (Table **6**).

Table 6: Predominant Sources of Empty Calories in the American Diet

Empty Calorie	Solid Fat	Added Sugar	Both Solid Fat and Added Sugar (SoFas)
Food	Cheese Pizza Sausages, Hot Dogs, Bacon, Ribs	Sodas Energy Drinks Sport Drinks Fruit Drinks	Cakes Cookies Pastries Donuts Ice Cream

Source: U.S. Department of Agriculture

There are some foods that ALL the calories are empty such as some candies and soda. However, empty calories are also found in other foods that do provide important nutrients (Table **7**).

Table 7: Foods with Some Empty Calories with Healthy Alternative

Empty Calorie	Food	Healthy Alternative
Added Sugar	Sweetened apple sauce Sugar-sweetened cereal	Unsweetened Apple Sauce Unsweetened cereal
Solid Fats	Regular Ground Beef (75% Lean) Fried Chicken Whole Milk	Lean Ground Beef (95% Lean) Baked Chicken without the skin Fat-free milk

Source: U.S. Department of Agriculture

Ingestion of small amounts of empty calories is acceptable but Americans tend to eat an excessive amount. Limits for empty calories as a portion of total have been established to assist Americans in their food choices. For example, an adult male requiring 2200 Calories has a daily limit of empty calories of 265. An adult female has a limit of 160 empty calories based on a requirement of 1800 Calories (www.choosemyplate.gov). Examples of foods with empty calories as they relate to the total Calories in the food are provided in Table **8**.

Table 8: Empty Calorie Content of Common Foods in Relation to Total Estimated Calories Provided by a Specified Portion Size

Food	Amount	Estimated Total Calories	Estimated Empty Calories
Dairy Group			
Whole Milk	1 cup	149	63
1% Milk (low-fat)	1 cup	102	18
Ice Cream, vanilla	1 cup	275	210
Fruit flavored low-fat yogurt	1 cup (8 fl. Ounces)	250	152
Protein Group			
Beef Sausage, pre-cooked	3 ounces, cooked	345	172
Grains			
Whole bread	1 slice, (1 ounce)	69	0
Biscuit, plain	1 medium (2.5" diameter)	186	71
Chocolate Chip Cookies	2 large	161	109
Other			
Pepperoni Pizza	1 slice of a 14" pizza, regular crust	340	139
Regular soda	1 can (12 fl ounces)	136	136

Source: U.S. Department of Agriculture

The foods in Table **8** are commonly found in the American diet and provide a range of empty calorie sources ranging from 0% for whole bread to 100% (regular soda) of total calories. It is interesting to note both the total calories per serving size as well as amount of total calories. Interesting in the sense that these are small serving sizes compared to what is usually chosen in the American society. Finally, empty calorie limits are based on limited physical activity (< 30 minutes per day). These limits may be increased for those individuals that consistently perform exercise in excess of 30 minutes per day.

Physical Activity and Exercise. To complete the approach to improving your nutritional health, physical activity and exercise provides an important health benefit the extent of which relates to the amount and vigor of the activity performed. Physical activity is movement of the body that uses energy. This can be walking, gardening, climbing stairs or dancing. For health purposes, activity should be of either moderate to vigorous intensity. Intensity relates to the extent in which the activity increases your breathing or heart rate. At moderate levels of intensity you breath harder and have an increased heart rate and you may talk while exercising but not sing. At vigorous levels you may say only a few words before needing to catch your breath. You may achieve similar health benefits to moderate intensive activity with vigorous intensity activity in half the time.

The amount of exercices recommended is dependent on age (www.choosemyplate.gov). For adult males, it is recommended to perform 2 hours and 30 minutes per week of moderate intensity and 1 hour 15 minutes for vigorous intensity activity. For optimal health benefits, there should be 5 or more hours per week of exercise, the time of which should be spread out over at least 3 days. Each session should have a duration of at least 10 minutes. Other than the aerobic exercise (those that increase both respiratory and heart rate) described above adults should perform strengthening exercises to maintain optimal bone function. Strengthening exercises are those that produce a force on the bones like jumping. These should be done 2 times per week.

Examples of moderate and vigorous activity derived from MyPlate.com (www.choosemyplate.gov) are tabulated below:

Intensity	Activity
Moderate	Walking briskly (about 3 ½ miles per hour) Bicycling (less that 10 miles per hour) Gardening (raking leaves, trimming shrubs) Dancing Golf (walking and carrying clubs) Water aerobics
Vigorous	Running/jogging (5 miles per hour) Walking very fast (4 ½ miles per hour) Bicycling (greater than 10 miles per hour) Heavy Yard Work (planting trees, chopping wood) Swimming (free style laps) Aerobics Soccer (Competitive)

The amount of calories burned while performing moderate or vigorous intensity activities depends on the activity. A table of commonly performed activities may be found at MyPlate.com in the physical activity section. Common examples are provided below:

Intensity of Activity	Activity	Calories Expended per hour
Moderate	Walking	280
	Stretching	180
Vigorous	Bicycling	590
	Running/Jogging	590
	Walking	460

Some examples of exercise based on location are also provided. Ideas for activities at home would be clean the house or wash the car; at work – replace a coffee break with a 10 minute walk and at play – take a nature walk or play golf. What is important is to make a choice you enjoy.

Physical Activity as a Contributing Factor for Health and Disease

Physical activity was not considered as a contibuting factor for health and disease. It was not included as part of the models in the United States created to promote a healthy diet. Recently, the models have improved founded on better understanding of nutritional concepts and include physical activity as a key element (Fig. **4**). In this chapter, sedentary lifestyle and physically active life styles are included as two main categories of physical activities. Some of the clear benefits of physical activities are included below with many of other benefits not being mentioned, but having great impact on human health.

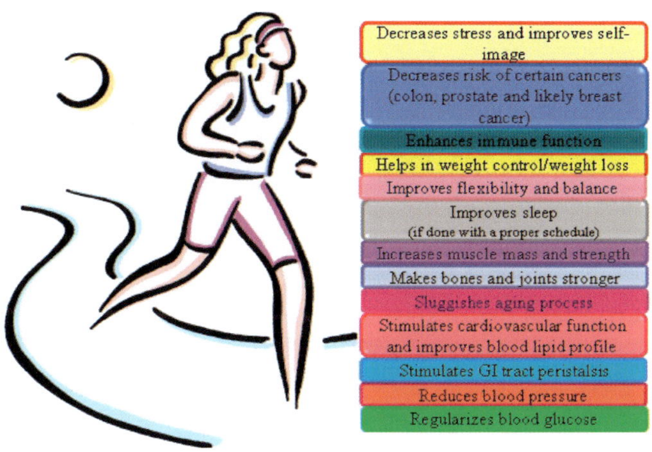
Decreases stress and improves self-image
Decreases risk of certain cancers (colon, prostate and likely breast cancer)
Enhances immune function
Helps in weight control/weight loss
Improves flexibility and balance
Improves sleep
(if done with a proper schedule)
Increases muscle mass and strength
Makes bones and joints stronger
Sluggishes aging process
Stimulates cardiovascular function and improves blood lipid profile
Stimulates GI tract peristalsis
Reduces blood pressure
Regularizes blood glucose

Figure 4: Potential benefits of physical activity.

A sedentary lifestyle is a style of living in which an individual does not participate in enough physical activity or exercise to have a healthy living. The intense use of computers and mobile devices, HDTV and video games, food delivery and instant microwavable meals, along with the use of endless transportation options make seems a nice lifestyle; however, it can also be risky. Many people are living less active lifestyles. Sedentary lifestyles have been correlated with some chronic disease and studies show that these individuals are experiencing serious health issues. In the past, our ancestors had physically active lifestyles hunting, building and migrating. Staying sedentary or at rest for too long is contrary to human nature. The body receives extra energy from the diet that is not burned off, and it is stored; making fat out of calories. Hence, the body becomes obese. But obesity is not the only problem with a sedentary lifestyle. Sedentary lifestyles are more prone to overall poor nutrition. Whether poor nutrition leads to obesity or not, it will still ultimately put you at risk for many chronic diseases.

Among the diseases correlated to a sedentary lifestyle include cancer, gout, heart diseases, mood disorders, muscle loss, obesity, skin problems, type-2 diabetes, and vitamin deficiencies.

- Heart Disease/Stroke

  Less active individuals are far more likely to develop heart disease or blood clots. Cholesterol settles around the arteries more readily in people having sedentary lifestyles.

- Type-2 Diabetes

  A lack of physical activity put you at risk of type-2 diabetes. Heart diseases and diabetes are highly correlated.

- Obesity

  Lack of enough exercise increases the risk of becoming obese.

- Cancer

  Physical activity has been correlated with the production of free radicals. Free radicals have been directly correlated with the development of cancer.

- Skin Problems.

  Sedentary lifestyle puts you at risk of developing skin problems and suffering from hair loss.

- Vitamin Deficiencies.

  Sedentary lifestyle can put you at risk of vitamin D deficiency due to lack of sunlight.

- Muscle Loss.

- Not exercising your muscles for long period of time will result in muscle loss.

Determine Level of Physical Activity

How do you know if you have a sedentary or a physically active lifestyle? Many factors are involved, but first and foremost a little bit of math is needed. First, the number of calories will determine the amount of energy generated; hence, the individual needs to find out the number of calories he burns to plan accordingly. The number of calories needed can be determined by using factors such as age, height, and weight. This will allow calculation of total calorie expenditure for the day. Daily calorie expenditure is a crucial factor in predicting weight loss rate. Second, the individual should find out his basal metabolic rate (BMR) (McNab, 1997). BMR is essentially the minimum number of calories needed to burn each day in order to stay alive. This value is identified as the calorie expenditure rate when the individual is not performing any activity at all (including the digestion of food). The BMR assumes that the individual is not burning calories to cool or heat the body either. Third, the individual should know how to determine the activity factor. The activity factor is a number used to convert BMR into daily calorie expenditure rate. BMR has usually an activity factor of 1. In general, the activity factor of a person with a sedentary lifestyle is 1.2. A person with a physically vigorous job has an activity factor of 1.9. The units used in the calorie expenditure equations are: height in centimeters and weight in kilograms.

<u>Equation</u>

The Harris-Benedict equations calculate the BMR for both genders.

Men use the formulae: BMR = (Weight x 13.75) + (Height x 5.003) - (Age x 6.775) + 66.5.

Women use the formulae: BMR = (Weight x 9.563) + (Height x 1.850) - (Age x 4.676) + 655.1.

Multiply the BMR value by the activity factor 1.2 to obtain the daily calorie expenditure for a sedentary lifestyle.

Health condition of an individual is a key factor in determining how much, how intense, and the type of exercise he needs. The type of aerobic activity can be determined by determining the *"Target Zone"*. The *"Target Zone"* is very important to avoid overdoing physical activity and then becoming scared or hesitant. Hence, an individual should plan doing exercise based on the maximum heart rate (MHR) the individual can tolerate. The MHR is determined as follow (American Heart Association, 2014):

- MHR is calculated by subtracting the age of the individual from 220.
- MHR is then multiplied by 0.60 and 0.90 to obtain a range of heart rates, sometimes called the "*Target Zone*".

Measuring heart rate (pulse) is easy. The individual only needs to stop and count his pulse for 10 seconds and then multiply that number by 6 to determine his heart rate for one minute. Some exercise equipment and watches/timers have heart rate monitors. At the beginning of an exercise program, the individual should aim for the lower end of the target zone. For instance, medications may impact heart rate; hence, the individual should consult his physician to personalize his target zone.

Exercise 9.3: Physical Activity

Test your knowledge

1- Mention a health risk factor associated to sedentary lifestyle and reason on why a sedentary lifestyle increases this risk.

____
____
____
____
____
____
____
____

2- Mention health benefits of regular/moderate physical activity and exercise.

____
____
____
____
____
____
____
____

Case I

A 44-year-old man visits the clinic to perform his annual check-up. He has a weight of 72 kg and a height of 181cm.

a) Calculate his BMR.

b) What is this individual daily calorie expenditure if he has a sedentary lifestyle?

Case II

An individual would like to start an exercise program. Determine the MHR of a 20-year-old person using the MHR formulae:

The values obtained from the applications above can be used by an individual to:

- Compare the values with his daily consumption
- Check the requirements of all dietary components (carbohydrates, proteins, lipids, *etc*.) and see how he is doing
- Find out what he needs to improve as sedentary lifestyle will require less amount of some nutrients than a physically active lifestyle

CONCLUSION

There are many areas where the American diet can be improved. To take action, health messages need to be delivered in a simple, easy to understand manner. There also needs to be a variety of actions or choices available to match the interest and potential of the diverse cultural and regional settings from which

Americans derive their culinary preferences. Lifestyles choices can also be improved by taking into account the most appropriate levels of physical activity. Educating the public and professionals that are responsible for their health on basic principles of a healthy diet with a suitable lifestyle is essential to promoting health and preventing diseases in Americans.

CONFLICT OF INTEREST

The authors confirm that this chapter contents have no conflict of interest.

ACKNOWLEDGEMENTS

Declared None.

REFERENCES

American Heart Association. (2014). Target Heart Rates. Dallas, TX: American Heart Association. Available at: http://www.heart.org/HEARTORG/GettingHealthy/PhysicalActivity/FitnessBasics/Target-Heart-Rates_UCM_434341_Article.jsp (Accessed: 8.26.2014).

Food and Nutrition Board, I. O. M. (2005). *Introduction to dietary reference intakes*. Washington, D.C.: National Academy Press.

McNab, B. K. (1997). On the Utility of Uniformity in the Definition of Basal Rate of Metabolism. *Physiol Zool*, 70, 718–720.

U.S. Department of Agriculture and U.S. Department of Health and Human Services (2010). Dietary Guidelines for Americans 2010. Available at: http://www.health.gov/dietaryguidelines/dga2010/DietaryGuidelines2010.pdf (accessed 12.12.2014).

CHAPTER 10

The Role of Nutrition in Disease Management

Jay M. Mirtallo*, Nicole A. Eggers and Esperanza J. Carcache de Blanco

The Ohio State University, Columbus, Ohio, USA

Abstract: There are many nutrition and lifestyle actions that Americans should consider that will influence the risk of developing disease. Cardiovascular disease, diabetes, osteoporosis and cancer have many risk factors that are both modifiable and non-modifiable. This chapter reviews these diseases and nutritional strategies and lifestyle changes that are useful in reducing the risk for developing disease. Since disease is frequently associated with malnutrition it is essential for health professionals to be able to screen for the risk of malnutrition and understand the criteria for its diagnosis.

Keywords: Atherosclerosis, atherosclerosis, cardiovascular disease, cholesterol, diabetes, disease-related malnutrition, glucose load, glycemic index, Heart-check mark, hypertension, inflammation, metabolic syndrome, modifiable risk factors, obesity, osteopenia, osteoporosis, pre-diabetes, the DASH eating plan.

INTRODUCTION

Previous chapters discussed the importance of nutrition and exercise in maintaining or improving the health of an individual. It is also important to consider good nutritional principles important to preventing disease. This chapter will discuss the dietary modifications to prevent specific diseases such as cardiovascular disease and hypertension, diabetes, osteoporosis, cancer and obesity (as a component of malnutrition). Nutritional aspects of each disease will be discussed along with risk factors for the disease. A focus will be on modifiable or preventable risk factors since dietary modifications or lifestyle changes may be directed at these risks to prevent individuals from developing disease. Finally, malnutrition will be defined and content specific to screening individuals at nutritional risk and understanding the criteria for diagnosis of malnutrition will establish the basis for future applications of nutritional principles in managing and treating disease.

***Corresponding author Jay Mirtallo:** College of Pharmacy, The Ohio State University, Columbus, OH 43210, USA; E-mail: mirtallo.1@osu.edu

Esperanza J. Carcache de Blanco and Jay Mirtallo (Eds)

CARDIOVASCULAR DISEASE AND HYPERTENSION

Cardiovascular disease (CVD) is a general term that refers to any disease (any condition that impairs normal function) of the heart and circulating system. This includes conditions such as heart failure, heart attack, arrhythmias and stroke. Pre-existing disorders that are closely associated with CVD are hyperlipidemia (cholesterol) and hypertension (HBP). CVD is the main killer of North Americans including about 500,000 people per year (or more than 1 million if deaths from stroke and other circulatory diseases are included). Heart disease and stroke account for more than $500 billion in healthcare expenditures. (HealthyPeople.gov, 2012) CVD mortality has fallen 50% over the past 50 to 60 years with preventive efforts accounting for over ½ of the decline. Primary contributors to this effect are associated with a decline in average cholesterol concentration, mean blood pressure levels, and tobacco use rates. (Gidding SS *et al.*, 2009) However, the increased prevalence of obesity and diabetes has dramatically slowed this rate. Therefore, preventing CV disease continues to be a challenge. Nutrition is the cornerstone of strategies used to prevent CV disease.

The cardiovascular system is responsible for delivering nutrients and oxygen to tissues as well as removing cellular wastes and delivering them to the body's excretory organs. The cardiovascular system also serves to deliver hormones to target organs, maintain a constant body temperature and distribute white blood cells throughout the body (facilitating the body's immune response). The capillaries are where the cardiovascular system connects with cells and the fluids surrounding them (Fig. **1**).

Observe the delivery of amino acids; oxygen, water and glucose from the arteriole side while water, carbon dioxide, and other waste molecules are picked up in the venous circulation for transport to the liver and/or kidneys for excretion.

Risk Factor is a term used frequently when discussing factors that contribute to the development of disease. A risk factor is an aspect of our lives – such as heredity, lifestyle choices (*e.g.* smoking) or nutritional habits. Risk factors for cardiovascular disease are listed below:

- Total blood cholesterol > 200 mg/dl
- Smoking
- Hypertension

- Diabetes
- HDL cholesterol < 40 mg/dl
    - Total:HDL cholesterol ratio > 4:1
- Age: Men > 45, Women >55
- Family history of CVD
- Blood triglyceride > 200 mg/dl
- Obesity
- Inactivity
    - Exercise conditions the arteries and improves insulin action

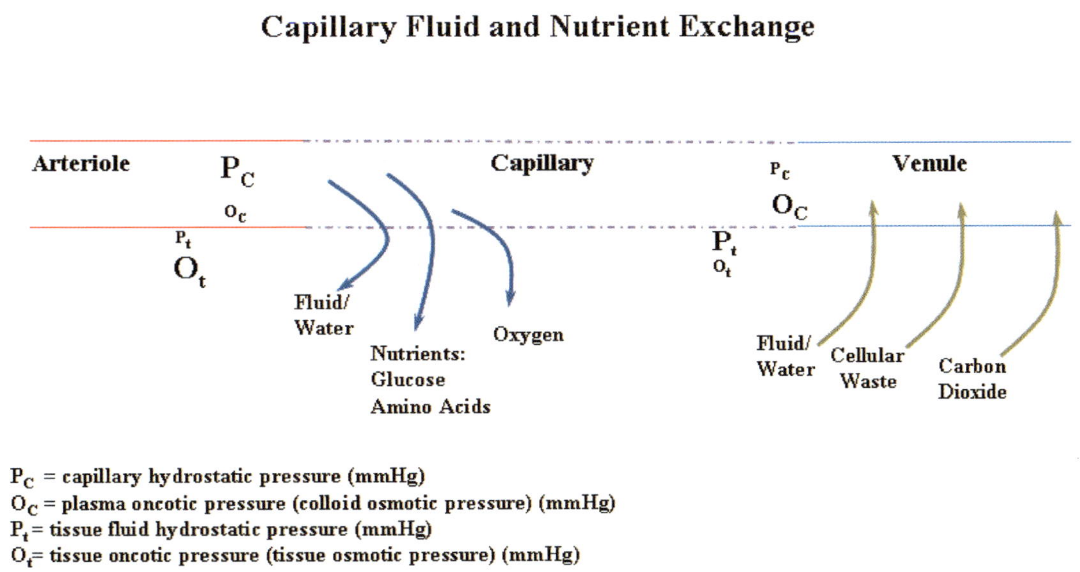

Figure 1: Capillary exchange depicting the delivery of nutrients, fluid and hormones while receiving cellular waste to be delivered to the body's excretory organs. In the arterioles, hydrostatic pressure in the capillary exceeds capillary and tissue hydrostatic pressure creating a net movement of fluid out of the capillary into the fluid surrounding the tissues (interstitial fluid) and thereby delivering water, nutrients and oxygen to tissues. On the venule side, tissue oncotic pressure is lower and tissue hydrostatic pressure pushes fluid back into the capillary for delivery to the venous system. The fluid pulled in from the interstitial space contains waste, carbon dioxide as well as water.

"The leading modifiable (controllable) risk factors to heart disease and stroke are: high blood pressure, high cholesterol, cigarette smoking, diabetes, poor diet and physical activity and overweight and obesity"(https://www.healthypeople.gov/2020/topics-objectives/topic/heart-disease-and-stroke).

Cardiovascular disease is generally characterized by the deposition of fatty material in the blood vessels (Fig. **2**) a process frequently termed; hardening of the arteries. CVD is also known as coronary artery disease (CHD), as the vessels of the heart are the primary sites of the disease.

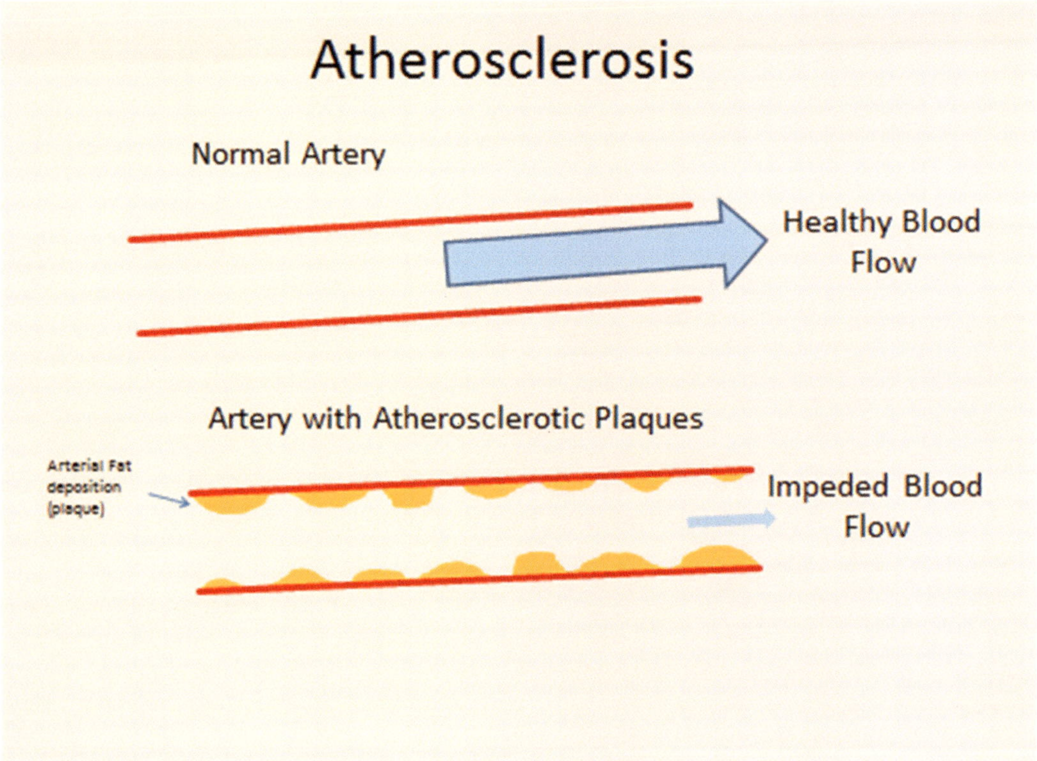

Figure 2: Atherosclerosis comparing a normal artery with an artery containing atherosclerotic plaque. Accumulation of fatty deposits (plaque) creates an impediment to blood flow and initiates an inflammatory process characteristic of cardiovascular diseases.

Atherosclerosis develops as a result of damage to the blood vessel lining. Damage can be associated with smoking, diabetes, hypertension, LDL cholesterol and viral and bacterial infections. The atherosclerotic plaque that builds up in the vessel leads to hardening of arteries and veins and low elasticity. Typical forms of CVD are associated with inadequate blood circulation due to the buildup of this plaque, which if combined with blood clots could cause complete blockage of the vessel. The complete blockage of blood vessels results in the following serious, life-threatening conditions:

- Myocardial infarction: death of a part of the heart muscle, also known as heart attack.

- Cerebrovascular accident: death of a part of the brain tissue due to a blood clot. Also termed a stroke.

Cholesterol. Cholesterol is a waxy lipid found in all body cells. It comes from 2 sources; about 75% is produced in the liver and other body cells while 25% comes from dietary sources. The two types of cholesterol 'good' or 'bad' are measured in cholesterol screening. The good cholesterol is HDL which helps keep the bad 'LDL' cholesterol from depositing in artery walls. A healthy level of HDL may also protect against heart attacks and stroke while low levels are associated with cardiac risk. Regular physical activity may improve HDL levels. Reducing *trans* fats and eating a balanced nutritious diet may also increase HDL. LDL is produced in the body and some people inherit genes that cause them to make too much. Eating *trans* fats, saturated fats, and cholesterol also increase LDL. New approaches to managing atherosclerosis are focusing on oxidized LDL as a major contributor to the disease and use of phytochemicals (antioxidants) in the prevention of CVD.

The case for Fiber in Controlling Cholesterol:

- High intake of viscous fiber – inhibits absorption of cholesterol and cholesterol-rich bile acids from the small intestine.

- Bacteria in large intestine degrade soluble fiber and produce fatty acids which may reduce cholesterol synthesis in the liver.

- Viscous fiber slows glucose absorption which decreases insulin release. Insulin stimulates cholesterol synthesis in the liver.

How do I know if my cholesterol and triglyceride levels are optimal? See Table **1** below for desirable levels of lipoproteins.

Table 1: Classification for various levels of cholesterol, LDL and HDL cholesterol as well as triglycerides

Total Cholesterol Level	**Classification**
< 200 mg/dL	Desirable
200-239 mg/dL	Borderline-high risk
240 mg/dL and above	Very high risk
LDL Cholesterol Level	**Classification**
< 100 mg/dL	Desirable
100-129 mg/dL	Near optimal/above optimal
130-159 mg/dL	Borderline high
160-189 mg/dL	High risk
190 mg/dL and above	Very High Risk
HDL Cholesterol Level	**Classification**
< 40 mg/dL for men, < 50 mg/dL for women	Major heart disease risk factor
60 mg/dL or higher	Gives some protection against heart disease
Triglyceride Level	**Classification**
<150 mg/dL	Desirable
150-199 mg/dL	Borderline-high risk
200-499 mg/dL	High risk
500 mg/dL or higher	Very high risk

Source: National Heart, Lung, and Blood Institute, National Institutes of Health

Hypertension is usually defined by persistent elevation of normal blood pressure 120/80 to more than 140/90. This level of blood pressure is often associated with serious cardiovascular diseases. The numbers 140/90 reflect Systolic/Diastolic blood pressure.

Systolic blood pressure: represent the pressure in the arteries when the heart is contracting.

Diastolic blood pressure: represent artery pressure when the heart is relaxed.

Ninety-five percent of hypertensive patients have no clear cause and are diagnosed as essential hypertension. Secondary hypertension has a cause that is usually amenable to treatment *i.e.*; kidney disease, structural abnormality of the aorta, narrowing of the arteries.

Health consequences of hypertension are listed below:

- "Damage to the heart and coronary arteries
- Stroke
- Kidney damage
- Vision loss
- Memory loss
- Fluid in the lungs
- Angina
- Peripheral artery disease

Risk factors for developing high blood pressure

- Family history
- Advanced age
- Gender-related
    - Men age >45, same for men and women age 55-64, women > age 65
- Lack of physical activity
- Poor diet, especially one that includes too much salt
- Overweight and obesity
- Drinking too much alcohol"

The DASH (Dietary Approaches to Stop Hypertension) Eating Plan is a diet rich in calcium, phosphorus, and magnesium and low in salt. It adds 2 extra vegetable and fruit servings and a serving of nuts, seeds or legumes (beans) 4-5 days per week to the MYPLATE food plan. It limits sodium intake to no more than 3 grams per day and alcoholic drinks are restricted to 1-2 drinks per day (Table **2**). Study of a DASH 2 diet varying sodium intake from 3300 to 2400 and 1500 mg/d found a steady decline in blood pressure but all levels were associated with lower blood pressure than controls. Overall the DASH diet lowers blood pressure, improves blood lipids and reduces cardiovascular risk compared with typical American diets.

Table 2: The Number of Daily Servings for a 1800 Calorie Diet according to the DASH Eating Plan

Food Group	Servings, N	Serving Sizes
Grains	6	1 slice bread 1 oz dry cereal ½ cup cooked rice, pasta, or cereal
Vegetables	4-5	1 cup raw leafy vegetable ½ cup-cut-up raw or cooked vegetable ½ cup vegetable juice
Fruits	4-5	1 medium fruit ¼ cup dried fruit ½ cup fresh, frozen, or canned fruit ½ cup fruit juice
Fat-free or low-fat milk and milk producst	2-3	1 cup milk or yogurt 1 ½ oz cheese
Lean meats, poultry, and fish	6 or less	1 oz cooked meats, poultry, or fish 1 egg
Nuts, seeds, and legumes	4 per week	1/3 cup or 1 ½ oz nuts 2 Tbsp peanut butter 2 Tbsp or ½ oz seeds ½ cup cooked legumes (dried beans, peas)
Fats and oils	2-3	1 tsp soft margarine 1 tsp vegetable oil 1 Tbsp mayonnaise 1 Tbsp salad dressing
Sweets and added sugars	5 or less per week	1 Tbsp sugar 1 Tbsp jelly or jam ½ cup sorbet, gelatin dessert 1 cup lemonade
Maximum sodium limit	2300 mg/day	

Source: U.S. Department of Agriculture

Lifestyle changes may also have a positive effect on blood pressure. Table **3** provides a few examples of lifestyle changes that result in a drop in systolic blood pressure.

Table 3: Lifestyle Changes that Lower Systolic Blood Pressure

Lifestyle Change	Details	Drop in Systolic Blood Pressure
Lose excess weight	For every 20 pounds lost	5-20 points
Follow a DASH diet	Eat a low fat diet rich in vegetables, fruits and low fat dairy products	8-14 points
Exercise daily	Get 30' a day of aerobic exercise (brisk walking)	4-9 points
Limit sodium	Eat no more than 2400 mg/day or better 1500 mg/day	2-8 points
Limit alcohol	No more than 2 drinks per day for men; 1 per day for women	2-4 points

The American Heart Association has established healthy diet goals suggesting lifestyle changes and improving healthy diet choices as major factors that will assist in achieving the goals. The national goal is that by 2020, "the cardiovascular health of all Americans will improve by 20 percent and deaths from cardiovascular disease and stroke will decrease by 20 percent. The health and behavior factors that impact health and quality of life are listed as follows:

- Don't smoke
- Maintain a healthy weight
- Engage in regular physical activity
- Eat a healthy diet
- Manage blood pressure
- Take charge of cholesterol
- Keep blood sugar, or glucose at healthy levels

To assist with choosing a heart healthy diet, looking for the American Heart Association (AHA) heart check mark" (Heart-Check Mark Certificate, found at the American Heart Association website: www.heart.org) in the grocery is a first step to a sensible eating plan. It certifies that the product meets specific nutritional levels based on a single serving size (as specified by the FDA).

Guidelines for a standard certification FDA-regulated product are outlined below:

- Total fat <6.5 g
- Saturated fat 1 g or less and 15% or less calories from saturated fat
- Trans fat < 0.5 g (and per label serving)
- Cholesterol: 20 mg or less
- Sodium: 480 mg or less (and per label serving)
- Beneficial nutrients: 10% or more of the Daily Value of 1 of 6 nutrients (vitamin A, vitamin C, iron, calcium, protein or dietary fiber)

Notes concerning select food products: "Unsweetened popcorn is the only certifiable product in the snack category. No desserts are eligible for certification. Beverage certification is limited to milk, dairy alternatives (*i.e.* soy milk, rice milk and nut milk), drinkable yogurts, fruit juices and vegetable juices".

To assess the heart health of a meal, the AHA has established a heart check mark below for meals (Heart-Check Mark Certificate, found at the American Heart Association website: www.heart.org). This takes the confusion out of spotting heart healthy options when eating out. Categories for certified meals include the following: calories, total fat, saturated fat, *trans* fat, cholesterol, sodium, beneficial nutrients. A heart healthy meal certified with an AHA certified check mark meets all the criteria outlined below:

> "Calories: 700 or less for the entire meal.
>
> Total fat: 3 grams or less total fat per 100 grams, and 30% or less calories from total fat in the meal and 26 grams or less total fat per the entire meal.
>
> Saturated fat: 1 gram or less saturate fat per 100 grams, and < 10% calories from saturated fat in the meal and 5 grams or less saturated fat per the entire meal.
>
> Cholesterol: 20 mg or less cholesterol per 100 grams and 105 milligrams or less cholesterol per the entire meal.

Trans fat: less than 0.5 grams *trans* fat per the entire meal.

Sodium: 900 milligrams or less sodium per the entire meal decreasing to 800 mg or less starting July 1, 2013.

Beneficial nutrient: 10 percent or more of the Daily Value of the following nutrients per the entire meal: vitamin A, vitamin C, calcium, iron, dietary fiber or protein."

Exercise 10.1 Pharmaconutrition Application Scenario: Cardiovascular Disease

A 56 year old male enters your pharmacy and has just been told by his physician that he needs to make lifestyle and dietary changes to avoid the development of hypertension and cardiovascular disease. He has a strong family history of cardiovascular disease; his grandfather expired 30 years ago from a heart attack and both his mother and father have hypertension and atherosclerosis. His physician has said that he has pre-hypertension and abnormalities in his lipid profile.

The individual shows the pharmacist the report of his lipid profile which is outlined below:

Total Cholesterol Level	**220 mg/dl**
LDL Cholesterol Level	161 mg/dl
HDL Cholesterol Level	38 mg/dl
Triglyceride Level	148 mg/dl

He is 6 feet tall and weighs 206 pounds (BMI = 28). He works as a manager in an accounting firm and spends most of his time at his desk on the computer. On weekends he sleeps in and reads the paper occasionally driving to the store. He loves sports and watches sports most Saturday afternoon and evenings. Frequently, he and his wife dine out at sports bars. His favorite meal is steak and salad (with blue cheese dressing). During the week, he typically has a Specialty coffee with a pastry for breakfast, and hamburger and french fries for lunch and for dinner he has meat (over ½ of meal), potatoes and a small portion of vegetables (he only likes corn).

He has several questions

1. What are my risk factors for cardiovascular disease?

    a. Which of these risk factors are ones that I can control (modifiable)?

2. What is my healthy weight? (see BMI table)

    b. Would I have to reduce my weight to my healthy weight to achieve a reduction of my cardiovascular risk?

3. What are some other simple lifestyle/diet changes that I can make to improve my risk of developing cardiovascular disease?

4. How do I know if my cholesterol and triglyceride levels are optimal?

5. What are the current recommendations for a heart healthy diet? How does my diet compare?

6. What tips do you have for me to begin eating healthy? Is there a special diet I can follow that would help?

    c. Has this diet been proven to help people achieve their goals?

7. When I eat out, is there any help choosing heart healthy meals?

Diabetes

Diabetes is a group of diseases characterized by high blood glucose. There are 3 types of diabetes which will be described in this section; Type1, Type 2 and Gestational diabetes. Type1 diabetes is also known as insulin dependent or juvenile onset and is characterized by insufficient or impaired release of insulin from the pancreas. Adult onset or non-insulin dependent diabetes is Type 2. This type is characterized by the inability to act on certain body cells (muscle). Gestational diabetes is high blood glucose during pregnancy. The incidence of diabetes has been increasing in the U.S. population and is currently at 8.3% (25.8 million). The incidence is expected to increase and reach 15% of the population by 2020. Diabetes is the 7th leading cause of death involving about 200,000 deaths per year. Table **4** provides a comparative chart of Type 1 and Type 2 diabetes.

Table 4: Characteristics of Type 1 as compared with Type 2 diabetes

Characteristic	Type 1 Diabetes	Type 2 Diabetes
Prevalence	5-10% of diabetes cases	90% of diabetes cases
Cause	Autoimmune	Insulin resistance
Risk Factors	Genetics (moderate)	Genetics (strong) obesity inactivity ethnicity metabolic syndrome prediabetes
Characteristics	Overt symptoms: excessive thirst, hunger, urination ketosis (Type 1) Unexplained weight loss exhaustion blurred vision frequent urination poor wound healing	
Treatment	Insulin Diet Exercise	Diet Exercise Oral hypoglycemics Insulin (advanced cases)
Complications	Cardiovascular disease Kidney disease Nerve disease Blindness Infection	

Overt symptoms of diabetes are similar for both types except ketosis is more likely to appear in Type 1 disease. Also, irrespective of type, diabetes over time will impair function of the heart, kidney, nervous system, vision and immune system.

There are both non-modifiable and modifiable risk factors for diabetes. The non-modifiable risk factors include family history (genetics), race/ethnicity, age>40, history of gestational diabetes or infant > 9 pounds at birth. Certain minority populations have a higher prevalence of diabetes: african-american, latino/hispanic, native americans, asian americans and pacific islanders. Modifiable risk factors for diabetes are listed below:

- Obesity

- poor diet
- lack of physical activity
- medication
- smoking

There are specific criteria related to blood glucose to be diagnosed with diabetes. The primary determinant is a fasting (have not ingested any food or sugary drinks >6 hours) blood glucose that is $\geq$ 126 mg/dL. Another test used to diagnose diabetes is the 2 hr glucose tolerance test which measures the highest glucose in the blood stream of an individual that has consumed a specific gram quantity of sugar. Finally, glycosylated hemoglobin (also know as hemoglobin A_{1c}) measures the percent of glucose that is attached to hemoglobin. This value is dependent on the average glucose in the blood stream over time. As such, glycosylated hemoglobin is a reliable measure of average glucose levels in the blood stream for the past several days. The tests used for diagnosing diabetes are also used to establish goals for managing diabetic patients. It is important to note that there is a new category of diabetes, pre-diabetes which occurs when blood glucose is drifting above normal but has not reached the criteria for diagnosis of diabetes. Pre-diabetics are at risk of developing diabetes and are targeted particularly with dietary strategies and lifestyle changes to prevent the disease. For clarity, Table **5** outlines the criteria for diabetes, pre-diabetes and normal glucose individuals.

Table 5: Diagnostic criteria for diabetes, pre-diabetes and normal glucose values

Conditions	**Fasting Glucose, mg/dL**	**2 hr Glucose Tolerance, mg/dL**	**HgA1c, %**
Diabetes	$\geq$ 126	$\geq$ 200	$\geq$ 6.5
Pre-Diabetes	100-125	140-190	5.7-6.4
Normal	< 100	< 140	< 5.7

It is important to note the strong association of pre-diabetes to the development of the disease. An individual with pre-diabetes is 5 to 15 times more likely to develop Type 2 diabetes. This 'elevated' glucose is also associated with a syndrome linked to both diabetes and heart disease. The metabolic syndrome (also known as Syndrome 'X') is a group of several risk factors that are highly associated with disease (Table **6**).

Table 6: Parameters and criteria for Metabolic Syndrome

Parameter	Criteria
Waist Circumference	≥ 40 in (102 cm) males ≥ 35 in (85 cm) females
Fasting Triglycerides	≥ 150 mg/dL (>1.7 mmol/L)
HDL Cholesterol	< 40 mg/dL males < 50 mg/dL females
Blood Pressure	Systolic ≥ 130 and/or diastolic ≥ 85 mm Hg and/or use of medications for hypertension
Fasting Glucose	≥ 100 mg/dL and/or use of medication for hyperglycemia

Lifestyle and Dietary Strategies to prevent Diabetes.

Choose healthy, unsaturated fats and limit total fat intake: this helps to improve the lipid profile (cholesterol).

Increase physical activity: exercise improves insulin action to deliver glucose into cells thereby reducing glucose levels in the bloodstream. The pancreas releases insulin more efficiently.

If overweight, lose 10% or more of your body weight. Weight loss reduces the stress on the pancreas to produce enough insulin to meet the demands of a larger body. This also will reduce fasting plasma glucose by about 50% in 2 weeks.

Evenly distribute carbohydrate calories and high and low glycemic index foods throughout the day: this helps minimize insulin swings and thus carbohydrate cravings and stress on the pancreas for insulin production.

Reduce the size of meals rich in simple sugars and starch: this will reduce the production of triglycerides.

Eat plenty of anti-oxidant rich fruits and vegetables: this helps reduce the damage to blood vessels by LDL cholesterol.

Gycemic Index (GI). This is the blood glucose response of a food compared to a standard (typically glucose or white bread). This is used as a measure to objectively assess one's diet related to its effect on blood glucose. The higher the glycemic index, the more likely the food will cause an increase in blood glucose. The criteria compared to reference glucose are outlined below:

Reference food glucose = 100

- Low GI food is < 55%
- Intermediate GI food is between 55 and 70
- High GI food is > 70

Glucose Load is the amount of carbohydrate in a serving of food multiplied by the glycemic index of the carbohydrate. The result is divided by 100

Glucose load food descriptors

- Low GL food < 15
- Intermediate GL food is between 15 and 20
- High GL food > 20

Examples of the glycemic index and glucose load of common foods is provided in Table **7**.

Table 7: Glycemic index and Glucose Load of Common Foods

Food	Serving Size	Glycemic Index	Carbohydrates (Grams)	Glucose Load
Pasta/Grains				
White, long grain rice	1 cup	56	45	25
Spaghetti	1 cup	41	40	16
Vegetables				
Sweet corn	I cup	49	39	22
Potato, Baked	1 cup	85	57	48
Dairy Food				
Yogurt, low fat	1 cup	33	17	6
Ice Cream	1 cup	62	31	19
Legumes				
Baked beans	1 cup	48	54	26
Navy beans	1 cup	38	54	21
Sugars				
Honey	1 tsp	75	6	4
Sucrose	1 tsp	65	5	3

Breads/Muffins				
Bagel	1 small	72	10	22
Whole-wheat bread	1 slice	69	13	9
White bread	1 slice	70	10	7
Fruits				
Apple	1 medium	38	22	8
Banana	1 medium	55	29	16
Orange	1 medium	44	15	7
Beverages				
Orange juice	1 cup	46	26	13
Gatorade	1 cup	78	15	12
Coca-cola	1 cup	63	26	16
Snack Foods				
Potato chips	1 oz	54	15	8
Vanilla wafers	5 cookies	77	15	12
Jelly beans	1 oz	80	26	21

Source: U.S. Department of Agriculture

In general, low glycemic index and glucose load foods include yogurt and fruit. Intermediate level foods include ice cream. Potatoes are high glycemic index and glucose load foods. It is important to note serving size in this evaluation. Some very high index glycemic index foods provide low glucose loads based on their serving size (honey and snack foods). Learning the glycemic index and glucose load (based on the serving size you select) will assist in your making food choices that minimize the effect on blood sugar and development of diabetes.

Exercise 10.2 Pharmaconutrition Application Scenario: Diabetes

A female individual who is picking up her prescription for blood pressure medication states that her physician is concerned that she is predisposed to type-2 diabetes. She is 45 years old, is 5'2"tall and weighs 169 pounds. Her waist inseam is 37" and she recently had a glucose tolerance test while fasting of 112 mg/dl. She is relatively sedentary, picking up her prescription at the drive-up window and spends most of the day watching TV, doing light housework ie, washing dishes and dusting. She loves to read and is especially excited to use her Kindle to download and read books. She rarely travels to the library or bookstore like she had a few years ago. Her diet usually consists of oatmeal with whole milk, brown sugar and raisons along with white toast and butter for breakfast, for lunch she usually has a salad with Italian dressing and several slices of bread and for dinner she usually eats out with friends and choses a full meal consisting of either beef or chicken portions with mashed potatoes and gravy along with either green beans, corn, broccoli and biscuits or bread and butter. She orders dessert with her evening meal 4-5 times a week. Her usual fluids are soft drinks (2-3 16 ounce servings per day). She wants to know what lifestyle and diet changes she can make to reduce her risk of diabetes.

1. What factors predispose her to type-2 diabetes? What variables contribute to her having metabolic syndrome?

2. What components of her diet have a high glycemic index? Glycemic load?

3. What tips do you have for her to reduce her caloric intake? Added sugars? Refined grains?

4. Is there an easy way for her to increase her activity without joining a health club?

Osteoporosis

Osteoporosis is decreased bone mass related to the effects of aging, including estrogen loss during menopause in women, genetic background and poor diet. By 2020, half of all Americans over age 50 are expected to have low bone density or osteoporosis. Decreased bone mass alone does not confirm the diagnosis of osteoporosis. Low bone mass is termed, osteopenia. The T-score is used to determine bone density as it compares to normal. Using DEXA to measure bone density, the T-score is calculated from the measured density as it compares with the density of a person at an age of peak bone strength (*i.e.* 30 years old). A T-score that ranges between -1.0 to +1.0 is normal. A T-score of -1.0 to -2.5 is low bone density and a T-score < -2.5 is usually associated with the presence of osteoporosis. The other variable leading to the diagnosis of Osteoporosis is low bone density associated with one or more bone fractures. Osteopenia is not just a disease for women. As many as 1 in 4 men over 50 will have a bone fracture due to osteoporosis (http://www.nof.org/learn/detection). At older ages, men may break bones in the spine or break a hip but usually at an older age than women. Another consideration for age and osteoporosis is bone mass or density over our lifetime is dependent on the peak bone mass we achieve at a young age. From a different perspective, osteoporosis could be considered a 'pediatric' disease with geriatric consequences. Adolescence is a critical time for optimal nutrition and facilitating the development of quality bone. Subsequently, the bone consolidates over time to reach peak bone mass between age 20 and 30 years. Bone loss or decrease in bone mass begins at age 30. If the bone mass reaches a critical point to cause fractures, the individual has osteoporosis.

Fortunately, there are several strategies one may use to assist in building strong bones and reaching an appropriate bone mass and then slowing the breakdown or loss of bone mass over time. Nutrition plays an essential role in the prevention and management of osteoporosis.

Risk factors for osteoporosis are provided in Table **8**.

Table 8: Risk Factors for Osteoporosis

Non-Modifiable Risk Factors	Modifiable Risk Factors
Gender	Obesity
Race/ethnicity	Poor diet
Age	Medications
Genetics	Alcohol
Skeletal Frame Size	Smoking
	Hormonal abnormalities
	Weight-bearing Activity

This discussion will focus on nutrition and bone health. There is a continual process for synthesis and breakdown of bone mediated by the parathyroid gland. Nutritional factors may facilitate or impede this process over time. Those factors that improve bone growth and maintain bone mass are adequate amounts of dietary: protein, calcium, phosphorus, magnesium, potassium, vitamins A, D and K, iron, copper, fluoride, manganes and boron. Foods that provide these nutrients include the following: fruit, vegetables, dairy and foods fortified with vitamin D and calcium. A fortified food is a food that has extra nutrients added to it or has nutrients added that are not normally found in the food. It has been a government policy since the 1940's to fortify foods with nutrients where deficiency is common for Americans. Examples of fortified foods are milk with vitamin D, salt with iodine, orange juice with calcium and almond milk with vitamin D. Vitamin D is necessary for calcium absorption. Children need vitamin D to build strong bones and adults need vitamin D to keep bones strong and healthy. Most Americans are deficient in vitamin D. Another strategy to improve bone health is to make choices that decrease bone loss. Certain foods have nutrients that may facilitate the breakdown of bone. For example, soda (phosphorus) if taken in excess will facilitate the leaching of calcium from bone. Soda also decreases bone growth by replacing an important source of calcium (milk) in the diet. Alcohol simlarly can reduce bone health by replacing milk in the diet. Other nutrients that may be harmful to bone mass are, sodium, caffeine and wheat bran.

The most important dietary consideration to prevent osteoporosis is to ingest enough calcium and vitamin D. The RDA for calcium is 1000 mg/day and vitamin D is 800 IU/day.

A lifestyle activity that enhances bone health is weight-bearing and muscle strengthening exercise. Examples of these exercises are outlined below:

Weight-Bearing Exercise	**Muscle Strengthening Exercise (Provides Balance and Tension on Bone)**
Dancing, hiking, jogging/running Jumping rope Stair climbing Tennis Elliptical training machines Low-impact aerobics Stair-step machines Fast walking	Weight lifting Elastic exercise bands/weight machines Lifting your own body weight Functional movements such as standing and rising upon your toes

<u>Designing a bone-building dinner for a carnivore.</u>

Entrée: Salmon patties with cheese (made with canned salmon with bone)

Sides: Spinach salad with almonds, shredded Swiss cheese, sliced hard boiled egg and tomato slices

Drink: Perrier mineral water

Dessert: Frozen yogurt

Eat your meal in the afternoon sun!!

Note: sunscreen is very useful in protecting the skin from the harmful effects of the sun. However, the sun is very useful in activing vitamin D to a form that is necessary to help with the absorption of dietary calcium from the diet. Therefore some sun is healthy for your bones.

Exercise 10.3. Pharmaconutrition Application Scenario: Osteoporosis

A new clinic is opening next to your pharmacy that is going to include a specialty in bone disorders – osteoporosis. Your pharmacy has decided to develop an awareness campaign for osteoporosis and asks you to be responsible for the content of the material that will go into the posters, brochures and pamphlets. The following content should be included:

1. What is the difference between osteopenia and osteoporosis?
2. Who is at risk of developing osteoporosis?
3. What are dietary strategies that can improve bone health? What are good dietary sources of calcium and vitamin D?
4. When would dietary supplements of vitamin D and Calcium be indicated?
5. Are there any lifestyle changes that can improve bone health?

Obesity - Malnutrition

Obesity is a form of malnutrition that is becoming increasingly prevalent in the United States affecting children, adolescents as well as adults. The NHANES survey has provided information concerning the rates of obesity since before 1990. As a refresher, body mass index (BMI) criteria for overweight (>25), obese (>30) and morbidly obese (>40) were provided in Chapter 1. Table **9** provides obesity trends determined in the NHANES surveys since 1976 (http://www.cdc.gov/obesity/data/adult.html).

Table 9: Trends in Obesity in the United States (1976-2010)

BMI Classification	2009-2010	2007-2008	1999-2000	1988-1994	1976-1980
Overweight		34.1	34.1	32.8	32.3
Obesity	35.7	33.9	31.1	23.3	15.1
Morbid Obesity		5.7	4.9	2.9	
Total*		68	65.2	56	47.4

* Total prevalence of overweight and obese (morbidly obese is a subsection of the obese population) at each time interval.

The important information to glean from this table is the continual increase in prevalence in the obese and morbidly obese categories since 1976. From 1976-

2010, the prevalence of obesity increased from 15.1 to 34.7 percent of the American population; a 236% change. Also, morbidly obese were not present until 1988 and now are 5.7 percent of the population. Obesity is a disease of energy balance. When energy intake exceeds the amount of energy expended, an individual gains weight. In a report from the United Kingdom (Lean M *et al.*, 2006), adults on average consume 20 kcal per day more than they expend. This results in weight gain of 1 kg (2.2 pounds) per year. Obese individuals consume 100 kcal per day or more in excess of what is used leading to more weight gain (10 kg or 11 pounds) per year (Lean M *et al.*, 2006). There are several factors that are believed to contribute to obesity. In the food supply, there is an abundance of low cost, palatable, high caloric density foods. On average the daily calories have increased by about 600 Calories and include added fats and oils, grains, milk and milk products as well as caloric sweeteners. Portion sizes have also increased. Caloric intake is increased with increases in portion size and this correlates with weight gain. A 'toxic environment' has been described noting the increase appearance of fast food or quick-service restaurants, a higher proportion of caloric intake coming from foods eaten away from home and a preponderance of food commercials for candy, fast food, soft drinks and sugared cereals. A sedentary lifestyle is also thought to contribute to the obesity epidemic. A lack of sidewalks or parks as well as safety issues from being outdoors are barriers to an active lifestyle. Fewer adults participate in leisure time physical activity and labor saving transportation and technology reduces the requirement for physical activity.

Obesity is the second leading preventable cause of deaths (Table **10**).

Table 10: Disease prevalence attributable to obesity

Disease	% Attributable to Obesity
Type 2 diabetes	90
Gallbladder disease	30
Hypertension	75
Coronary heart disease	17
Osteoarthritis	14
Breast cancer	11
Uterine cancer	11
Colon cancer	11

An important consideration to strategies used to manage obesity is that weight loss of just 5-10% of body weight greatly reduces an individual's risk of many diseases.

Healthy People 2020 provides useful advice for those at risk of obesity. The focus is on promoting health and reducing chronic disease risk through the consumption of healthful diets and achievement and maintenance of healthy body weights (http://www.healthypeople.gov/2020/topics-objectives/topic/nutrition-and-weight-status). As noted in the website, Americans that consume a healthful diet:

- "Consume a variety of nutrient-dense foods within and across the food groups, especially whole grains, fruits, vegetables, low-fat or fat-free milk or milk products, and lean meats and other protein sources.
- Limit the intake of saturated and trans fats, cholesterol, added sugars, sodium (salt) and alcohol.
- Limit caloric intake to meet caloric needs."

Physical activity (http://www.CDC.gov/physicalactivity/everyone/guidelines/index.html) is an important component to achieving and maintaining a healthy weight. Physical exercise increases the number of calories used for energy and is useful in creating a 'caloric deficit' favoring weight loss. Even though most weight loss occurs as a result of decreased caloric intake, physical activity is necessary to maintain the weight loss. The benefits of weight loss may be outlined as follows:

- "Maintain weight
- Reduce high blood pressure
- Reduce risk for type 2 diabetes, heart attack, stroke, and several types of cancer
- Reduce arthritis pain and associated disability
- Reduce risk for osteoporosis and falls
- Reduce symptoms of depression and anxiety"

It is important to note the body composition of weight loss. Fat (adipose tissue) contains about 3500 Calories per pound. Weight loss may come from the adipose, lean body or water mass of the body. For example, if you kept your caloric intake the same and increased your physical activity by walking 30 minutes a day (expends an additional 140 Calories per activity), you would lose 1.2 pounds in 1 month. Any greater weight loss would likely be from the fluid or lean body compartment of the body which if prolonged for long periods of time could adversely affect your health.

Maintenance of a healthy weight is a challenge in our society. Understanding that weight is the net result of the balance between Caloric intake and energy expenditure assists with developing useful strategies to achieve our goals for a healthy weight.

Malnutrition is an acute, sub-acute or chronic state of nutrition associated with varying degrees of under- or over nutrition with or without inflammatory activity that leads to a change in body composition and diminished function (Soeters PB and AM, 2009). There are 3 etiology-based diagnosis in disease-related malnutrition (Jensen GL *et al.*, 2010):

- Starvation-related malnutrition described as chronic malnutrition due to altered nutrient intake with no inflammatory activity.
- Chronic disease-related malnutrition involves chronic inflammation of mild to moderate intensity. This type is usually associated with diseases such as renal or liver failure or rheumatoid arthritis.
- Acute disease-related malnutrition occurs in individuals that have acute and severe inflammation as occurs in critical illness or trauma.

Inflammation is a key component of malnutrition resulting from disease. The inflammatory process influences nutritional status in several ways:

- Increases energy expenditure
- Favors a rapid turnover of protein and increases protein breakdown (catabolism) that mobilizes protein substrate to be used in the production of immune proteins and protein to repair injured tissue all at the expense of the lean body mass
- Fat oxidation is dramatically increased as an energy source
- Altered metabolism continues while infammation persists and may be of mild, moderate or severe intensity

These processes lead to both energy and protein deficits and acute or chronic depletion of the lean body mass.

The symptoms of malnutrition are difficult to distinguish from symptoms of other diseases. Many organ systems are involved. Examples of the symptoms of malnutrition are listed below:

- Psychlogical and mental: depression, hysteria and hypochondriasis, preoccupation with food, social withdrawal and isolation, decline in concentration and judgment capabilities.
- Physiologic processes (starvation alone, if inflammation is present these parameters will change in response to the inflammatory condition): decreased energy expenditure, body temperature, respiration, heart rate and edema in extremities.
- Other conditions associated with malnutrition include immunologic dysfunction and infections, anemia, poor wound healing, more frequent complications of surgery, longer recovery and poorer outcomes from illness, infertility, tiredness, fatigue and apathy, diminished organ function – renal, liver, pulmonary and heart.
- Individual nutrient deficiencies are the result of improper balance of nutrients in the diet due to poor food selection, food security or poverty. The most frequent nutrient deficiencies in Americans include iron, vitamin A, iodide, zinc, various B vitamins (folate), selenium and vitamin C.

The prevalence of disease-related malnutrition is high. Malnutrition is present in 40-60% of hospitalized patients, 40-65% of nursing home and 20-60% of patients at home. Since malnutrition is difficult to distinguish from other diseases it is important for health professionals to be able to identify individuals who are at nutrition risk.

Determine Nutritional Health (Nutrition Screening Initiative, 1991)

Tool to assess nutrition risk that can be administered by any level of healthcare professional. Based on the Warning Signs described below:

> "**Disease**: any illness that changes the way you eat, or makes it hard for you to eat. Four of five adults have chronic diseases that are affected by diet. Confusion or memory loss that continues to get worse affects 1 in 5 older adults.

Eating poorly: too little or too much is not healthy. Poor variety and diet low in vegetables and fruits will cause poor nutritional health.

Tooth loss/mouth pain: missing, loose or rotten teeth or dentures which don't fit well, or mouth sores make it hard to eat.

Economic hardship: as many as 40% of older Americans have low incomes resulting in less to spend on food.

Reduced social contact: 1/3 of all older people live alone. Being with people daily has a positive effect on morale, well-being and eating.

Multiple medicines: the greater the number the more chance of side effects, alterations in appetite, taste or symptoms such as weakness, drowsiness, nausea or GI distress. Vitamins or minerals taken in large doses, act like drugs and can cause harm.

Involuntary weight loss/gain: losing or gaining weight when not trying to is an important warning sign that should not be ignored.

Needs assistance in self care: 1 of 5 older adults has trouble walking, shopping, buying and cooking food.

Elderly years above age 80: risk of frailty and health problems increase."

Characteristics Recommended for the Identification of Malnutrition

Characteristics are according to the etiology-based malnutrition definitions: starvation-related malnutrition, chronic disease-related malnutrition and acute injury-related malnutrition (White JV *et al.*, 2012). The identification of 2 or more of the following 6 characteristics is recommended for diagnosis of malnutrition:

- "Insufficient energy intake
- Weight loss
- Loss of muscle mass
- Loss of subcutaneous fat

- Localized or generalized fluid accumulation that may mask weight loss
- Diminished functional status as measured by hand-grip strength."

Clinical Characteristic	MN in Acute Injury		MN in Chronic Illness		MN in Social or Environment	
	Moderate	Severe	Moderate	Severe	Moderate	Severe
Energy Intake	<75%, > 7d	<50%, > 5 d	<75%, > 1 mo	< 75%, > 1 mo	< 75%, > 3 mo	< 50%, > 1 mo
Weight loss	1-2%, 1 wk 5%, 1 mo 7.5%, 3 mo	> 2%, 1 wk >5%, 1 mo >7.5%, 3 mo	5%, 1 mo 7.5%, 3 mo 10%, 6 mo 20%, 1 y	>5%, 1 mo >7.5%, 3 mo >10%, 6 mo >20%, 1 y	5%, 1 mo 7.5%, 3 mo 10%, 6 mo 20%, 1 y	>5%, 1 mo >7.5%, 3 mo >10%, 6 mo >20%, 1 y
Physical findings: changes in physical exam						
Body fat	Mild	Moderate	Mild	Severe	Mild	Severe
Muscle mass	Mild	Moderate	Mild	Severe	Mild	Severe
Fluid accumulation	Mild	Moderate to severe	Mild	Severe	Mild	Severe
Reduced grip strength	NA	Measurably reduced	NA	Measurably reduced	NA	Measurably reduced

Malnutrition occurs in healthy individuals when there are inadequate resources to obtain healthy nutrients or when food choices by individuals lead to a poorly balanced diet that may include nutrients in toxic amounts or be inadequate in healthy nutrients such as vitamins, minerals and healthy fats. The prevalence of malnutrition increases when an individual develops a chronic or acute disease. Unfortunately, the symptoms of malnutrition are often confused with the symptoms of disease and often go unrecognized. The diagnosis of malnutrition is not often done leaving this important disease untreated. Malnutrition affects every organ and cell system in the body and is often associated with poor response to disease, increased complications of disease, increased length of stay in health institutions and mortality. It is imperative that health professionals understand malnutrition and have knowledge of clinical characteristics common to malnutrition so it is appropriately diagnosed and managed.

Exercise 10.4. Pharmaconutrition Application Scenario: Malnutrition

"A 26 year-old woman was admitted to the hospital with a diagnosis of anorexia nervosa and a longstanding history of restrictive eating behavior. She had lost one-third of her body weight over 6 months. Upon admission, the individual was 5'6" (167.6 cm) in height and weighed 82 pounds (37.2 kg)". (Jensen GL, *et al.* 2012) Her resting heart rate was 50 beats per minute. She was afebrile. Laboratory values (Normal values in parenthesis) included the following:

Laboratory	Measured Value	Normal Value
C-reactive protein, mg/dl	0.7	< 10
WBC, $/mm^3$	6200	4500-10,000
Serum albumin, g/dL	4.0	3.5-5.5
Prealbumin, mg/dL	25	18-45
Fasting blood glucose, mg/dL	75	(80-120)

"She exhibited generalized loss of muscle and subcutaneous fat. Marked underweight status was evident with weight loss of 42 pounds (19.1 kg) over 6 months. Mid-arm muscle circumference measurement was below the fifth percentile."

1. Calculate her BMR

   Women: BMR= 655 + 9.6 (wt in kg) + 1.8 (ht cm) – 4.7 (age)

2. Determine her BMI

   Identify (if possible) any of the 6 characteristics used to determine malnutrition

3. Energy intake (% of estimated, duration)

4. Interpretation of weight loss (% of original, duration)

5. Body fat

6. Muscle mass

7. Fluid accumulation

8. Reduced grip strength

Is there evidence of inflammation? (Chronic disease, organ failure, infection)?

What malnutrition syndrome would you give this woman? Why?

Starvation-associated

Chronic Disease-associated

Acute Disease-associated

10.5. PHYTOCHEMICALS AS CANCER CHEMOPREVENTATIVE AND CHEMOTHERAPEUTIC AGENTS

10.5.1. Introduction to Phytochemicals in Cancer Chemoprevention and Chemotherapy

Cancer is a complicated group of diseases that acts in multiple stages to affect the proliferation process of normal cells (Greenwald, 2002). Through the multistage process, genetic alterations from DNA-damaging agents transform normal cells into neoplastic cells, which divide without control and may invade other tissues (National Cancer Institute, 2015a). The development of malignant tumors may involve the interplay between both, exogenous and endogenous factors, such as environmental, genetic, hormonal, and immunological factors (Alberts *et al.*, 1999; Desphande *et al.*, 1996; Weinstein, 1988). It is not uncommon for 10-20 years to pass between exposure to harmful environmental factors and development of detectable cancer.

There are several modern approaches for combatting the uncontrolled growth of tissue invasion and metastasis: surgical removal of a solid mass, radiation to induce double stranded DNA breakage, induction of apoptosis through application of chemotherapy, or personalized treatment targeting specific molecular markers that have become misregulated through the development of cancer. Physicians often use two or more of these modern approaches in combination to treat cancer. Chemotherapy is commonly used as part of the combination approach, and many chemotherapeutic agents are natural products or derivatives thereof (Cragg *et al.*, 2009). Some of the most important chemotherapeutic agents that were either isolated from plants or are derivatives of phytochemicals include the Vinca alkaloids, etoposide, paclitaxel and docetaxel, and two camptothecin derivatives.

Since cancer continues as a major public health problem, and the above treatment approaches have not been able to control the incidence of most cancer types, cancer chemoprevention is an active line of research that utilizes the principle of Pharmaconutrition. Unlike chemotherapy, chemopreventative agents are taken only on a voluntary and precautionary basis, so they must be more palatable or tolerable with fewer side effects and less toxicity. Therefore, nutritious foods, containing phytochemicals with chemopreventative properties, are often great candidates for cancer chemoprevention. Before learning specifically about such foods, individuals interested in the cancer chemoprevention approach should learn a little about carcinogenesis, or the multistage process of developing of cancer.

10.5.2. The Process of Carcinogenesis

Carcinogenesis is a multistage process that comprises three overlapping stages: initiation, promotion, and progression. Initiation is an irreversible event. It begins when cells in normal tissues are exposed to a carcinogen that damages their genomic DNA to an unrepairable state (or the DNA remains mis-repaired) (Surh, 1999). Initiation typically only takes a few hours to a couple days. In promotion, damaged cells multiply to form a premalignant population of mutated cells. The promotion phase is a long, slow process that takes place over the course 10-40 years. Progression is also an irreversible process that produces clones of mutated cells that have increased potential to proliferate, invade, or metastasize. Due to the rapid, uncontrolled or misregulated growth rate of neoplastic cells, progression often takes only 1-2 years (Surh, 1999). The chronic nature of the carcinogenesis process permits numerous opportunities for intervention at different stages (Fig. **5**), including the use dietary components (Greenwald, 2002). Selected dietary plants, rich in phytochemicals, macro- and micro-nutrients, may be of great value in controlling or preventing the initiation or promotion phases of carcinogenesis.

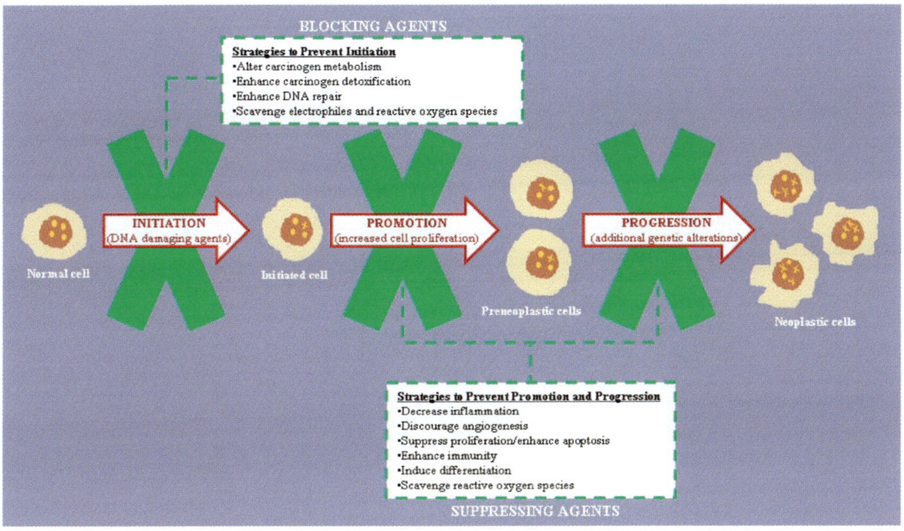

Figure 3: Prevention strategies for the multistage process of carcinogenesis. (Greenwald, 2002).

Potential cancer chemopreventative agents have been subdivided in blocking agents and suppressing agents (Surh, 1999), depending on the mechanisms by which an agent may exert protective effects in a specific stage of the carcinogenesis process. Blocking agents "block" or prevent initiation by inhibiting carcinogen formation, facilitating carcinogen detoxification, or stimulating DNA repair enzymes. The facilitation of carcinogen detoxification is achieved through two related mechanisms within xenobiotic metabolism, which will be discussed below. Suppressing agents act in the promotion and progression stages to inhibit the malignant expression of initiated cells through numerous different mechanisms (Surh, 1999). Many of the known cancer chemopreventative agents act through more than one mechanism of action and may belong to both categories (Morse and Stoner, 1993).

To understand how blocking agents prevent initiation, it is important to think about phase I and phase II xenobiotic metabolism (Fig. **6**). A xenobiotic is a non-endogenous chemical substance that is introduced to an organism (*e.g.*, phytochemicals or pharmaceutical drugs that are consumed by humans). The human body metabolizes these xenobiotic compounds with phase I enzymes and phase II enzymes such as cytochrome P450 isozymes and glutathione S-transferase, respectively. A xenobiotic, which may or may not be a carcinogen or pro- carcinogen, is metabolized by a phase I enzyme. The compound may undergo an oxidation, reduction, or hydrolysis reaction with the help of the phase I enzyme, producing one of two things: an activated (or ultimate) carcinogen or a harmless metabolite. An activated carcinogen may then cause DNA damage or ideally, go through phase II metabolism. Phase II enzymes conjugate a functional group to the activated carcinogen to deactivate it, allowing for safe excretion. Blocking agents may be taken simultaneously with pro-carcinogens to inhibit phase I enzymes, thereby preventing the formation of ultimate carcinogens. Consumption of blocking agents alongside carcinogens or pro-carcinogens works by inducing phase II enzymes to detoxify the carcinogen or ultimate carcinogen.

Natural food sources such as tea, garlic, and onion (in the form of extracts) have been shown to cause phase I inhibition. Extracts of fruits and vegetables such as broccoli, cauliflower, grapes, and kale stimulate phase II induction. (Cragg and Newman, 2000; Paolini and Nestle, 2003; Park and Pezzuto, 2002)

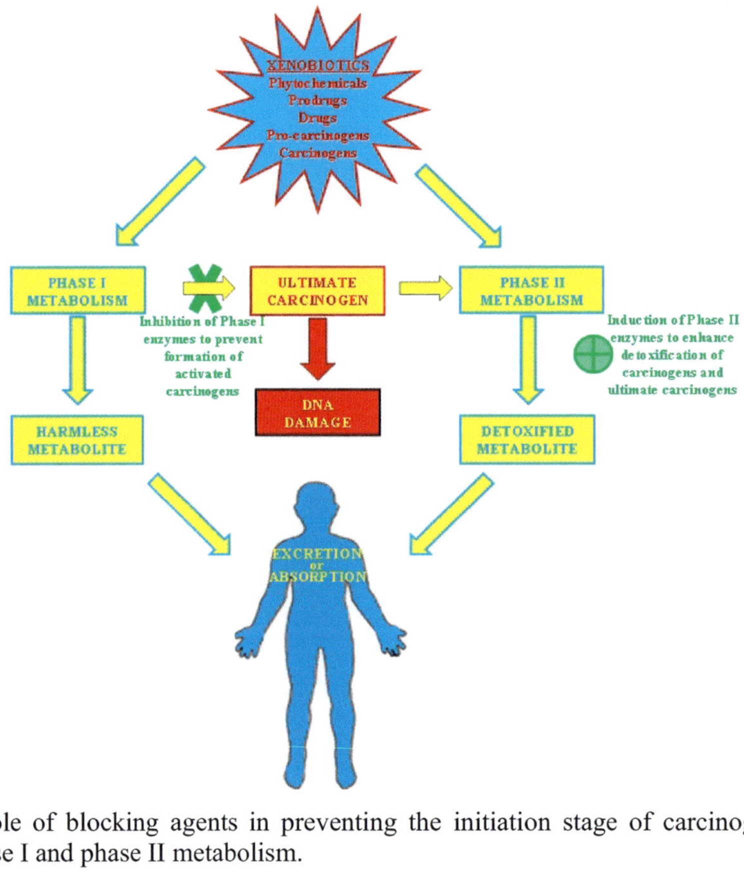

Figure 4: Role of blocking agents in preventing the initiation stage of carcinogenesis through affecting phase I and phase II metabolism.

10.5.3. Risk Factors and Realities of Cancer and Nutrition

Cancer is classified as a genetic disease since mutations in genes cause cancer and control the way cells replicate and grow. However, only five to ten percent of cancer types are hereditarily passed to an individual from his or her parents (National Cancer Institute, 2014a). The majority of cancers are acquired through enduring harmful environmental factors such as tobacco smoke, asbestos, or radiation.

10.5.3.1. Risk Factors

Since most people have not had their genetic makeup analyzed, how can an individual know if he or she is at risk of developing cancer? There are several risk factors that indicate the likelihood of developing cancer (Table **11**), however, many of these risk factors are also indicators of other diseases or of generally poor health conditions. In addition, having any or all of these risk factors does not mean a patient will undoubtedly develop cancer, but rather that the individual has a higher risk or probability of developing cancer.

Table 11: Risk factors that increase the likelihood of an individual developing cancer (National Cancer Institute, 2014b)

CANCER RISK FACTORS	
Smoking Tobacco	Second-Hand Smoke
Environmental Pollution	Extensive Exposure to Pesticides
Certain Viral Infections (*e.g.*, Hepatitis B and C, Human papillomavirus, Epstein-Barr)	Certain Bacterial Infections (*e.g.*, *Helicobacter pylori*)
Consuming High Levels of Arsenic	Exposure to Radon
Immunosuppressive Medications	Exposure to Asbestos
Alcohol Use	Unbalanced and Unhealthy Diets
Lack of Physical Activity	Obesity (gain of > 30 pounds since 30 years of age, or BMI ≥ 30)
Ultraviolet Radiation (*e.g.*, UVA and UVB Rays)	Radiation from Certain Medical Diagnostic Tests
Diabetes or High Fasting Blood Glucose Levels	Genetics and Family History

10.5.3.2. Myths and Realities

In addition to the risk presented above, there are also several myths and controversies about practices thought (or once thought) to cause or prevent cancer.

- Some people believe that artificial sweeteners cause cancer. The artificial sweetener saccharin, at high doses, was shown to increase the incidence of bladder cancer in rats. However, no association between saccharin consumption and bladder cancer has been observed in humans, and mechanistic studies indicated that the cancer-causing effect was specific only to rats (National Cancer Institute, 2009). Cyclamate is another artificial sweetener that was banned by the FDA in 1969. The FDA has since concluded that cyclamate is not a carcinogen, but the substance has not been reapproved due to other non-cancer related concerns. The artificial sweetener aspartame, in one study with doses equivalent to drinking 8 to 2083 cans of diet soda per day, indicated an increased rate of lymphoma and leukemia in rats (Soffritti *et al.*, 2005). The FDA found that the results of the study were inconsistent and not dose-dependent (FDA, 2006). Acesulfame potassium, aspartame, neotame, saccharin, and sucralose are all FDA approved as general purpose sweeteners; and to achieve this status, numerous safety studies were conducted with no evidence that the compounds cause cancer in humans or are harmful to human health (National Cancer Institute, 2009).

- Another commonly held myth is that sugar feeds cancer. Indeed, cancer cells consume more glucose than non-cancerous cells, but there is no evidence that eating sugary foods will accelerate the spread of cancer. However, eating foods high in sugar will contribute to weight gain and eventually obesity, and obesity increases the risk of developing cancer (National Cancer Institute, 2014a).

- Some claim that eating red meat causes cancer. In fact, an association between consumption of red meat and increased risk of cancer is not clear, but numerous epidemiological studies have connected high consumption of well-done, fried, and barbecued meats with increased risk of prostate, pancreatic, and colorectal cancers. From experimental evidence, meats that contain creatine (any muscle meat including beef, fish, pork, and poultry), when cooked over an open flame or at very high temperatures may form compounds that cause changes or damage to DNA. Foods that are charred also contain these DNA-damaging compounds, increasing the risk of developing cancer. There are several studies of these compounds in animal models that indicate carcinogenic activity, but the doses used in the studies were thousands of times greater than the dosage a person would consume on a typical diet. Although there are no guidelines or limits for the consumption of muscle meats or the compounds in question, concerned individuals can cook at lower temperatures or reduce cooking times, use a microwave to partially cook the meat to reduce the amount of time that high heat levels are necessary, continuously turn the meat while cooking on a high heat source, remove the charred parts before eating the product, and avoid the use of drippings to make gravies or dipping sauces (National Cancer Institute, 2010).

- There is some controversy surrounding whether dietary supplements are helpful or harmful in the prevention and/or treatment of cancer. While dietary supplements and herbal products do not cure cancer, they may relieve some of the side effects of cancer treatment. However, some of these alternative or complementary therapies are actually counter-productive when they interact with chemotherapy or radiation treatments. Cancer patients should consult with their doctor about taking any vitamin, mineral, or herbal supplements. In addition to counteracting chemotherapies, there are a few substances once thought to prevent or treat cancer, which now appear to increase the risk of developing cancer in certain individuals. Vitamin A, vitamin E, and vitamin A precursor beta-carotene, are three such examples of agents that were hypothesized to prevent cancer. Unfortunately, large clinical studies showed that these compounds actually increase the lung cancer incidence rate among smokers who were on the intervention agents compared to those on controls. More information regarding these clinical trials can be found in chapter 7 about phytochemicals. In general when undergoing cancer treatment, it is better to take in vitamins, minerals, and phytochemicals at dietary levels rather than as mega-doses or supplements, which may cause significant interference with treatment.

Among all these myths and controversies, there are also a few solid realities that are supported with research data.

- Cancer cells are not normal cells, they learn how to avoid apoptosis and repair, and some methods available are not able to detect them.

- Over 350 mutations have been identified among the different types of cancer cells, indicating the enormous complexity of the cancer disease state.
- Large-scale studies support a link between obesity and cancer.
- There is also an evidence-based link between higher fat intake and the incidence of pancreatic cancer.
- Several studies support and guidelines suggest daily intake of 5-9 servings of fruits and vegetables, as a protective approach against cancer.

10.5.4. Folkloric and Popular Alternative Therapies

Cancer is a heartbreaking and physically painful disease. Many patients seek alternative treatments when modern approaches fail or when the side effects are unacceptable to the patient. As some of these alternative treatments have been proven ineffective or even harmful, it is important to gather all evidence and to talk to a doctor before pursuing alternative treatments. Seeking alternative treatment that is ineffective may delay the use of proven treatment methods and raises ethicality concerns. It is thus important to classify each popular folkloric or alternative therapy as having varying levels of safety and efficacy. Detailed below are one or more examples of ineffective, dangerous, questionably beneficial, popular to Europe, or beneficial complementary alternative therapies. These and further examples that are continuously updated can be found on the National Cancer Institute Physician Data Query comprehensive cancer database (National Cancer Institute, 2013).

10.5.4.1. Potentially Dangerous or Ineffective Alternative Therapies

Shark cartilage and bovine cartilage have been investigated as cancer treatment options. The notion that shark cartilage may be effective against cancer originates in the misconception that sharks, whose skeletons are composed primarily of cartilage, are not affected by cancer. It was also hypothesized that because cartilage is one of the few tissues that do not have blood vessels, that cartilage must have some substance that inhibits the formation of blood vessels. In researching cancer treatments, many scientists look for agents that inhibit blood vessel formation, or angiogenesis, because cancer cells need increased resources delivered by the blood in order to grow at such a fast rate. Although a few compounds that inhibit angiogenesis have been isolated from bovine and shark cartilage, there is still no indisputable evidence that administration of bovine or shark cartilage products prevents or treats cancer in humans (National Cancer Institute, 2015b).

The Hoxsey treatment was first formulated in the 1920s by John Hoxsey, who observed that his horse developed a tumor that disappeared after eating wild plants in the meadow. John's son, a veterinarian, later treated people with a mixture of those plants and household cancer remedies. John's grandson, who had no medical or scientific training, then marketed the product and opened numerous cancer treatment centers. Hoxsey was developed into an herbal treatment regimen with two formulations: a tonic and a topical cream. The main ingredients consist of barberry, buckthorn bark, burdock root, cascara, licorice, pokeweed, potassium iodide, prickly ash bark, red clover, and stillingia root. In addition to the two herbal products, the use of laxatives and douches are encouraged, and a restricted diet is also part of the treatment. Hoxsey is said to remove toxins, boost the immune system, and augment the ability of the body to rid and stop the spread of tumors. However, both formulations are caustic and may burn or scar skin. Many of the individual plants that make up Hoxsey are poisonous, cause diarrhea or vomiting, or interact with pharmaceutical drugs. There is no clinical evidence that Hoxsey cures cancer; in fact many patients who were said to be "cured" of cancer through the use of Hoxsey were never confirmed to have cancer or were also treated by conventional means. The FDA banned the Hoxsey treatment and forced the closure of the Hoxsey cancer clinics in the United States. Hoxsey is still available in Tijuana, Mexico at a clinic run by relatives of the grandson (American Cancer Society, 2008).

Amygdalin is found in the seed pits of many fruits, and a pill form was used to treat cancer in Russia and eventually in the United States. However, the pill formulation was too toxic, so an intravenous formulation was introduced and called laetrile. The main anticancer constituent of amygdalin or laetrile is cyanide. Cyanide poisoning (nausea, dizziness, oxygen deprivation, liver damage, coma, and death) is always a threat when taking laetrile, or especially amygdalin. In addition to its high toxicity, laetrile has very little evidence of anticancer activity in animal studies and no evidence in human trials; thus, laetrile is no longer FDA approved (National Cancer Institute, 2014c).

10.5.4.2. Alternative Therapies with Questionable Benefits

Essiac is an herbal tea that contains burdock root, Indian rhubarb root, sheep sorrel, and the inner bark of slippery elm. Flor Essence is another herbal tea that contains all of the Essiac ingredients as well as blessed thistle, kelp, red clover, and watercress. Both herbal products are claimed to detoxify the body, boost the immune system, relieve pain, reduce side effects, and possibly reduce tumor size and prolong the life of an individual with cancer. Neither product is FDA approved for treating cancer, but both are sold in the United States as dietary supplements. Some proponents suggest using the herbal teas alone while others suggest a complementary, conventional anticancer treatment. There is no reputable evidence that Essiac or Flor Essence is an effective anticancer treatment (National Cancer Institute, 2015c).

Gerson therapy is a strict organic, vegetarian-based diet with additional administration of vitamin and mineral supplements, pancreatic enzymes, liver extracts or coenzyme Q_{10}, and regular coffee enemas. The Gerson therapy regimen is said to detoxify the body and boost the immune system. Dr. Max Gerson believed that cancer is a symptom of a diseased organism, and that restoration of the normal metabolic state would rid the body of toxic substances and cancer. The pancreatic enzymes, live extracts, and coffee enemas were incorporated into the treatment in order to aid the liver in detoxification. Both the American Chemical Society and the National Cancer Institute concluded that the Gerson therapy lacked scientific evidence and demonstrated no benefit (National Cancer Institute, 2015d).

10.5.4.3. Other Popular Alternative Therapies Practiced in Europe Involving Phytochemicals

Mistletoe is a semiparasitic plant that grows on host trees. Mistletoe extracts have been formulated in Europe for injectable administration routes. *In vitro* and *in vivo* studies have indicated that mistletoe extracts are cytotoxic to cancer cells and stimulate immune cells. However, there have not been any well-designed and executed clinical studies to demonstrate efficacy in humans. In addition, the extracts vary among manufacturers and lots because the natural products produced by mistletoe are different depending on the type of host tree, the harvest season, and the growing conditions. Therefore the FDA does not allow the importation or distribution of injectable mistletoe preparation outside of clinical research (National Cancer Institute, 2015e).

The Budwig diet was developed by Johanna Budwig to incorporate fruits, vegetables, and fiber into the diet. The most notable part of the diet is the consumption of flaxseed mixed with cottage cheese or milk. Flaxseed is very high in fiber, vitamins, and minerals. Avoiding sugar, solid fats, salad oil, and meat is also part of the diet. Although a diet regimen is difficult to apply to *in vitro* or animal models, flaxseed oil alone appeared to have a cytostatic effect on several different types of cancer cells *in vitro*. There was also a small trial in men with prostate cancer where flaxseed reduced testosterone levels and tumor size. However, larger randomized controlled trials remain necessary before flaxseed can be recommended as a cancer treatment in humans (Cancer Research UK, 2013).

10.5.5. Nutrition Guidelines for Cancer Prevention

Given that the above alternative or complementary treatments are not FDA approved and many of the conventional cancer treatments have undesirable side effects, what can one do to prevent the development of cancer? Aside from working to avoid or limit the risk factors listed in Table **11**, nutrition is a modifiable factor that can have a great impact. Some studies have shown that some dietary components can even affect DNA methylation patterns as potential cancer chemopreventives. (Zorko *et al*., 2010)

What types of substances should be included in a diet designed for cancer chemoprevention? There are three very important categories of phytochemicals that should be included: antioxidants, anti-inflammatory agents, and anticarcinogens.

10.5.5.1. Antioxidants

Antioxidants reduce oxidation at the cellular level and prevent free radical formation and thus DNA damage. Natural food sources with antioxidant phytochemicals include:

- Coenzyme Q_{10} in fish, broccoli, wheat, eggs, and spinach
- Vitamin E found in avocado, nuts, seeds, wheat germ, and whole grains
- Vitamin C found in fruits and vegetables, especially bell peppers, berries, citrus, and kiwi
- Polyphenols from cocoa and tea
- Carotenoids from yellow to red fruits and vegetables
- Flavonoids ubiquitous to most fruits and vegetables

- Sulfur-containing compounds from garlic and onion

10.5.5.2. Anti-inflammatory Agents

Anti-inflammatory agents reduce inflammation, preventing metabolic mistakes that may lead to elevated rates of cell division and cancer. Food-source anti-inflammatory agents include:

- Salicylate rich-food such as apricots and broccoli, and dishes high in salicylates such as those made with the culinary herbs turmeric, rosemary, and thyme
- Cyclooxygenase inhibitors including green tea, cocoa, and red wine
- Omega-3 fatty acids, eicosapentaenoic acid, and docosahexaenoic acid found in fish oil, salmon, pine nuts, sardines, and walnuts
- Alpha- and gamma-linolenic acids found in borage, blackcurrant seed oils, and flaxseed

There is a recommended balance of oils and fats for optimal cancer chemoprevention effects. Most individuals consuming a Western diet take in too many omega-6 fats and too few omega-3 fats. The appropriate ratio of omega-6 to omega-3 is around 15:1 (Simopoulos, 2002). In addition, a ratio of one part omega-3 to 3 parts monounsaturated fats to 1 part saturated fat is recommended.

10.5.5.3. Anticarcinogens

Anticarcinogens encourage damaged cells to undergo apoptosis instead of continuing to replicate, and they prevent and help repair DNA damage. Natural food sources of anticarcinogens include:

- Tannins and anthocyanidins in berries
- Turmeric, cumin, and other phytochemicals found in curry powder
- Flavonoids in citrus, especially naringenin and limonene
- Epigallocatechin gallate and other components from green tea
- Pomegranate seeds
- Brazil nuts, which are rich in selenium

- Lycopene from tomatoes and other sources
- Vitamin D in seafood, eggs, milk, and liver

For additional information regarding phytochemicals with preliminary data supporting their use as anticancer agents or cancer chemopreventative agents, read about cruciferous vegetables and the *Allium* species in chapter 7 on phytochemicals.

Chapter 7 also discussed soy isoflavones as phytoestrogens. As a reminder, soy isoflavones can act mechanistically in four distinct ways: as estrogens and antioxidants, immune enhancers, estrogens and antiestrogens, and cancer enzyme inhibitors. The former two were discussed in detail in chapter 7, and the latter two are mechanisms specific to cancer and will be discussed here.

Antiestrogens are compounds that structurally resemble estrogen, but act in an opposite manner. Estrogen signals cells to proliferate, which can contribute to carcinogenicity. As antiestrogens then, isoflavones compete with natural estrogen for binding to estrogen receptors, limiting the number of estrogens that can bind and send the proliferation signal. Since antiestrogens such as genistein bind with only one thousandth of the affinity or hormonal activity of estrogen, they blunt the estrogen effect without causing severe side effects from an imbalanced ratio.

Phytoestrogens can also act as cancer enzyme inhibitors. Isoflavones inhibit enzymes that promote cancer cell growth such as the activity of tyrosine kinase. Genistein in particular blocks the growth of blood vessels, or angiogenesis, that tumor cells rely upon to grow and replicate.

There are also several other foods with possible cancer chemopreventative activity, but their efficacy has not been tested in clinical trials. Lemon grass, for example, is a rich source of citral, which induces cancer cell death *in vitro* (Dudai *et al.*, 2005; Kumar *et al.*, 2008). Mushrooms, which are rich in potassium and beta-glucans, can induce natural killer cells (Akramien *et al.*, 2007). Guava is a great source of lycopene, and lycopene has been shown in numerous studies to reduce tumor size in prostate cancer (Barber and Barber, 2002). Concentrated (lyophilized) black raspberries can modify the expression of hundreds of human genes and are highly effective at inducing apoptosis of cancer cells *in vitro* and in animal studies (Chen *et al.*, 2006; Kresty *et al.*, 2001; The Ohio State University, 2008; Zikri *et al.*, 2009). Pomegranate is rich in all "3A's" (antioxidants, anti-inflammatory agents, and anticarcinogens) (Zarfeshany *et al.*, 2014).

10.5.6. Suggestions for Individuals Already Diagnosed with Cancer

Today is the dawn of personalized treatment, which is based upon the specific characteristics of a single patient's cancer cells and how they depend on certain processes for survival. Gaining knowledge of the cancer cell characteristics allows treatment approaches that inhibit the delivery of nutrients to the cancerous cells, inhibit the formation of new blood vessels, stimulate apoptosis, or facilitate recognition of the cancer cells by the immune system for targeted destruction. In addition to cancer chemotherapeutic approaches such as personalized treatment, having supportive nutrition during treatment is extremely important.

When diagnosed with cancer and/or when receiving cancer chemotherapy, there may be several barriers to eating healthier. Many individuals experience a sore mouth or painful swallowing as a side effect of chemotherapy treatments. For the most comfortable eating experience, those individuals should eat soft-textured, non-acidic, room temperature foods. Creamy textures such as custard, ice cream, Greek yogurt, and pasta with cream sauce are great options. An alcohol-free mouthwash will also be more tolerable than the more astringent rinses.

Hence, if diagnosed with cancer, an individual should carefully look into his diet and make an effort to improve his diet including changes such as the following:

- Having a diet rich in colorful fruits and vegetables
- Eating smaller and more frequent meals or snacks
- Increasing the amount of protein consumed; most need an extra amount of protein (*e.g.*, 15g of proteins in the afternoon and again before bed). To add more protein, here are some suggestions:
    - Adding milk, Greek yogurt, or whey protein to soups or sauces
    - Including a protein shake or smoothie with meals or as a snack
    - Keeping hard boiled eggs in the refrigerator for quick snacks or salad toppings
    - Using nut butters and spreads, almonds, peanuts, walnuts, pine nuts, pistachios, pecans, *etc*.

  - Improving appetizers such as on low-fat cottage cheese and whey or string cheese
  - Including tofu and other fermented bean products in the diet
  - Eating more fish
- Eat foods with soft textures if the diagnosed individual is experiencing pain or sensitivity of the mouth or GI tract as side effects of chemotherapy
- Avoid spicy and highly acidic foods (*e.g.*, chemotherapy can cause stomach irritation or heartburn)

Some also have poor appetites or feel nauseated from anticancer treatments; in this case, ginger tea or crystallized ginger may settle the stomach. If the individual feels full very quickly, calorie-dense foods such as protein smoothies, egg custards, avocados, or eating very frequent but small meals may be more tolerable.

For those who experience diarrhea, following the BRAT diet is often helpful. The BRAT diet is made up of bananas, rice, apple sauce, and toast. Another option is to try a liquid-only diet for one day, followed by white rice and baked potatoes. It is also advisable to avoid high fiber foods such as iceberg lettuce, wheat germ, whole grain bread, and crackers. As with any condition that causes diarrhea, one should be careful to stay hydrated with water and electrolytes, especially potassium (Mayo Clinic, 2012; National Cancer Institute, 2014d). Additionally, breads may have high content of bromide, which has been approved by the FDA to be used in bakery. Bromide can compete with iodide absorption and with long-term consumption or large amount consumption of bread rich in bromide the levels of iodide can be affected as well as the production of hormones related to the absorption of iodide. This, in turn, may increase the risk of developing certain chronic diseases related to the metabolism of iodide and the production of hormones.

It is common for individuals with cancer to feel depressed. In this case, look for counselling or help if the individual's mood prevents him or her from making self-supportive actions. Surround the individual with love and use dark chocolate, it is as a tasty mood modifier. For individuals experiencing insomnia, limit or exclude coffee, tea, and other caffeinated products from the diet.

Content Reflection

Match Puzzle 1: Disease States

Match each item with the correct description or definition.

Term	Description Definition
1. Cardiovascular Disease	A. State in which energy intake matches the energy expended
2. Fiber	B. Contains about 3500 Kcal per pound
3. Adipose tissue	C. Disease associated w/ increased fat mass, decrease in residual lung volume, increased pressure on diaphragm
4. Pickwickian Syndrome	D. Inhibits absorption of cholesterol & cholesterol-rich bile acids in small intestine
5. Energy Expenditure	E. Condition that develops when body does not receive right amount of vitamins, minerals, & other nutrients needed to maintain healthy tissues and organ function
6. Energy balance	F. Composed of basal metabolic rate, thermogenic effect of digestion, physical activity & growth
7. Malnutrition	G. Any disease of the heart and circulating system

Match Puzzle 2: Disease States

Match each item with the correct description or definition.

Term	Description Definition
8. Kwashiorkor	H. Cancer that begins in skin or tissues that line or cover internal organs
9. Type 1 Diabetes	I. Disease characterized by inability of insulin to act on certain body cells (muscle)
10. Type 2 Diabetes	J. Consuming fair or adequate calories but diet has inadequate amount of protein
11. Carcinoma	K. Daily caloric expenditure (Cal/day) for a 68 kg and 72 in, 24 year old man living a sedentary lifestyle
12. Sarcoma	L. Protein need (mg/day) for a 121 lb and 67 in, 20 year old woman performing moderate intensity endurance activities daily
13. 2.099	M. Cancer that starts in bone, cartilage, fat, muscle, blood vessels, or other connective or supportive tissue
14. 66,000	N. Disease characterized by insufficient or impaired release by the pancreas of insulin

Harris Benedict Equation:

Men: BMR = (weight x 13.75) + (Height x 5.003) – (Age x 6.775) + 66.5

Women: BMR = (weight x 9.563) + (Height x 1.85) – (Age x 4.676) + 655.1

<u>Case I</u> (Using a similar scenario as in chapter 8)

NE is a 45 year old single mother who has been increasingly bothered by hot flashes and was told by a friend that if she brought her diet to the pharmacist that they could help her modify it to alleviate her symptoms. She has very little time in that she just finished her job at a day-care center (which allows her to get discount day care for her young children) and is on her way to her evening job cleaning the local elementary school. NE is 5'11" and weighs 180 pounds. Her father is African-American and mother Chinese-American. Her father has diabetes and her mother died from cancer when she was 23 years old. She lives in a small apartment close to the elementary school where she works and uses public transportation if she needs to travel outside the local urban area she lives.

The pharmacist makes a copy of her diet and schedules an appointment with NE the following week. After the patient leaves, the pharmacist places her diet information in the SuperTracker at myplate.gov and prints out the summary reports of her diet (build a diet using SuperTracker based on the culture related tables provided chapter 8, rich in rice, bread, sodium, and lipids).

Based on this information, answer the following questions.

1. Look into the numbers of calories that each one of the food products she consumed generates. Compare % of calorie intake from carbohydrates, proteins, and fats to the following:

    a. Recommended calorie intake from each macronutrient.

2. Look into amount of micronutrients (vitamins and minerals) provided by each food source consumed. Based on the levels of the following:

    a. Potassium consumed *vs.* recommended dietary intake of potassium

        i. What is the risk of hypertension

    b. Chromium *vs.* recommended dietary intake of chromium

        ii. What is the risk of diabetes

    c. Iodine consumed *vs.* recommended dietary intake of iodine (Tips: How much bread does the patient eats? What dietary factor present in bread and approved by the FDA could affect the levels of iodine?)

iii. What is the risk of hormone related diseases such as breast cancer?

3. Based on NE dietary record, what type (s) of phytochemicals were ingested that would potentially reduce her risk of diabetes or cancer in this patient?

4. To reduce the risk of the following: diabetes, cancer, and hypertension:

   a. What foods could be added to this patient's diet?

   b. What foods will be

      i. Removed and replaced from her diet? or

      ii. Reduced to avoid surpassing her dietary requirements?

5. How would you counsel the patient on healthy food choices to improve her diet. Consider the following socioeconomic factors in your advice:

   a. Job

   b. Food security

   c. Education

   d. Cultural background

   e. Food access

CASE II

Using the information gathered in chapter 4, practice session VI and chapter 6, practice session III respond to the case questions below in order to summarize the content assembled in all ten chapters.

Put all of the different reports from the SupperTracker project so that you can use the data in answering the following questions.

1. Look into the numbers of calories that each one of the food products you consumed generates. Compare % of calorie intake from carbohydrates, proteins, and fats to the following:

    a. usual or customary North American diet

    b. recommended calorie intake from each macronutrient

2. Look into amount of micronutrients (vitamins and minerals) provided by each food source consumed. Based on the levels of the following:

    a. Vitamin D and calcium

        i. What is the risk of osteopenia or osteoporosis

    b. Sodium consumed in your record,

        ii. How is the sodium intake compared with the recommended intake?

        iii. Does this intake pose a health related risk for the development of diseases? If yes, mention examples of disease states.

3. Look into the type of phytochemicals provided from each dietary source.

    c. Depending on the type and amounts, how could these phytochemicals have health benefits for you in regards to cancer chemoprevention, cholesterol and heart related diseases?

4. To reduce the risk of the following: osteopenia/osteoporosis, hypertension, and high cholesterol?

    d. What foods could be added to your diet?

    e. What foods will be

        iv. Removed and replaced with your choices? or

        v. Reduced to avoid surpassing your dietary requirements?

Using the 'myplate' approach, design a healthy diet for one day consumption (three meals and two snacks) by modifying the original record.

CONCLUSION

Nutrition and lifestyle changes are important factors that improve the risk of developing diseases. To be effective, one must understand the underling basis of the disease and identify those modifiable risk factors to the disease that nutrition and lifestyle strategies may be applied. Various government agencies and professional organizations (*e.g.*, American Heart Association) have organized the most current consensus recommendations for nutrition to prevent diseases such as cancer, diabetes, hypertension and heart related diseases. The principles presented in this chapter are intended to provide health professionals a comprehensive, yet concise approach to nutrition for maintenance of health and preventing disease.

CONFLICT OF INTEREST

The authors confirm that this chapter contents have no conflict of interest.

ACKNOWLEDGEMENTS

I would like to acknowledge the work of Amy Arnholt, PharmD for researching and organizing the diabetes and osteoporosis content of this chapter.

REFERENCES

Akramien, D., Kondrotas, A., Did, J., and Egidijus, K., 2007, Effects of β-glucans on the immune system., Medicina (Kaunas)., p. 597–606.

Alberts, A. S., Colvin, O. M., Conney, A. H., Emster, V. L., Garber, E. J., Grenwald, P., Gudas, L. J., Hong, W. K., Kelloff, G. J., Kramer, R. A., Leman, C. E., Mangelsdorf, D. J., Matter, A., Minna, J. D., Nelson, W. G., Pezzuto, J. M., Prendergast, F., Rusch, V. W., Sporn, M. B., Wattenberg, L. W., and Weinstein, I. B., 1999,

Prevention of cancer in the next millennium: report of the chemoprevention working group to the American Association for Cancer Research., Cancer Research., p. 4743–4758.

American Cancer Society (2008). Hoxsey herbal treatment. Available at: http://www.cancer.org/treatment/treatmentsandsideeffects/complementaryandalternativemedicine/herbsvitaminsandminerals/hoxsey-herbal-treatment (accessed 22.02.2015).

Barber, N. J. and Barber, J., 2002, Lycopene and prostate cancer., Prostate Cancer and Prostatic Diseases., p. 6–12.

Cancer Research UK (2013). What is the Budwig diet? Available at: http://www.cancerresearchuk.org/about-cancer/cancers-in-general/cancer-questions/what-is-the-budwig-diet (accessed 22.02.2015).

Chen, T., Hwang, H., Rose, M. E., Nines, R. G., and Stoner, G. D., 2006, Chemopreventative properties of black raspberries in N-nitrosomethylbenzylamine-induced rat esophageal tumorigenesis: down-regulation of cyclooxygenase-2, inducible nitric oxide synthase, and c-Jun., Cancer Research., p. 2853–2859.

Cragg, G. and Newman, D., 2000, Antineoplastic agents from natural sources: achievements and future directions., Expert Opinion on Investigational Drugs., p. 2783-2797.

Cragg, G. M., Grothaus, P. G., and Newman, D. J., 2009, Impact of natural products on developing new anti-cancer agents., Chemical Reviews., p. 3012–3043.

Desphande, S. S., Desphande, U. S., and Salunkhe, D. K., 1996, Cancer, *in* D. L. Madhavi, S. S. Desphande, and D. K. Slunkhe, eds., Food Antioxidants: New York, NY, Marcel Dekker, p. 431–435.

Dudai, N., Weinstein, Y., Krup, M., Rabinski, T., and Ofir, R., 2005, Citral is a new inducer of caspase-3 in tumor cell lines., Planta Medica., p. 484–488.

FDA (2006). FDA Statement on European aspartame study. Available at: http://www.fda.gov/NewsEvents/Newsroom/PressAnnouncements/2006/ucm108650.htm (accessed 20.02.2015).

Gidding, S. S., Lichtenstein, A. H., Faith, M. S., Karpyn, A., Mennella, J. A., Popkin, B., Rowe, B., Vanhorn, L. & L, W. 2009. Implementing American Heart Association Pediatric and Adult Nutrition Guidelines: A Scientific Statement From the American Heart Association Nutrition Committee of the Council on Nutrition, Physical Activity and Metabolism, Council on Cardiovascular Disease in the Young, Council on Arteriosclerosis, Thrombosis and Vascular Biology, Council on Cardiovascular Nursing, Council on Epidemiology and Prevention, and Council for High Blood Pressure Research Circulation. *Circulation,* 119, 1161-1175.

Greenwald, P., 2002, Cancer chemoprevention., British Medical Journal, p. 714–718.

Healthypeople.gov. 2012. *Heart disease and stroke National snapshot.* Healthy People.gov. Available at: http://www.healthypeople.gov/2020/topics-objectives/topic/heart-disease-and-stroke/national-snapshot [Accessed September 23 2012].

Jensen, G.L., Hsiao, P.Y., Wheeler D., (2012)., Adult nutrition assessment tutorial. *J Parenter Enter Nutr* 36: 267-274.

Jensen, G. L., Mirtallo, J. M., Compher, C., Dhaliwal, R., Forbes, A., Grijalba, R. F., Hardy, G., Kondrop, J., Labadarios, D., Nyulasi, I., Pineda, J. C. C., & Waitzberg, D., 2010., Adult starvation and disease-related malnutrition: a proposal for etiology-based diagnosis in the clinical practice setting from the International Consensus Guideline Committee. *J Parenter Enter Nutr,* 34, 156-159.

Kresty, L. A., Morse, M. A., Morgan, C., Carlton, P. S., Lu, J., Gupta, A., Blackwood, M., and Stoner, G. D., 2001, Chemoprevention of esophageal tumorigenesis by dietary administration of lyophilized black raspberries., Cancer Research., p. 6112–6119.

Kumar, A., Malik, F., Bhushan, S., Sethi, V. K., Shahi, A. K., Kaur, J., Taneja, S. C., Qazi, G. N., and Singh, J., 2008, An essential oil and its major constituent isointermedeol induce apoptosis by increased expression of mitochondrial cytochrome c and apical death receptors in human leukaemia HL-60 cells., Chemico-Biological Interactions., p. 332–347.

Lean, M, Lara, J & Jo, H. 2006. ABC of obesity: strategies to preventing obesity. *BMJ,* 333, 959-962.

Mayo Clinic (2012). Diarrhea: cancer-related causes and how to cope. Available at: http://www.mayoclinic.org/diseases-conditions/cancer/in-depth/diarrhea/art-20044799 (accessed 20.02.2015).

Morse, M. A. and Stoner, G. D., 1993, Cancer chemoprevention: principles and prospects., Carcinogenesis., p. 1737–1746.

National Cancer Institute (2009). Artificial sweeteners and cancer. Available at: http://www.cancer.gov/cancertopics/factsheet/Risk/artificial-sweeteners (accessed 20.02.2015).

National Cancer Institute (2010). Chemicals in meat cooked at high temperatures and cancer risk. Available at: http://www.cancer.gov/cancertopics/factsheet/Risk/cooked-meats (accessed 20.02.2015).

National Cancer Institute (2013). PDQ® NCI's comprehensive database. Available at: http://www.cancer.gov/cancertopics/pdq

National Cancer Institute (2014a). Common cancer myths and misconceptions. Available at: http://www.cancer.gov/cancertopics/causes-prevention/risk-factors/myths (accessed 20.02.2015).

National Cancer Institute (2014b). Cancer prevention overview. Available at: http://www.cancer.gov/cancertopics/pdq/cam/laetrile/HealthProfessional/page1/AllPages (accessed 22.02.2015).

National Cancer Institute (2014c). Laetrile/amygdalin (PDQ®). Available at: http://www.cancer.gov/cancertopics/pdq/cam/laetrile/HealthProfessional/page1/AllPages (accessed 22.02.2015).

National Cancer Institute (2014d). Gastrointestinal complications (PDQ®). Available at: http://www.cancer.gov/cancertopics/pdq/supportivecare/gastrointestinalcomplications/HealthProfessional/page1/AllPages (accessed 20.02.2015).

National Cancer Institute (2015a). What is cancer? Available at: http://www.cancer.gov/cancertopics/what-is-cancer (accessed 20.02.2015).

National Cancer Institute (2015b). Cartilage (bovine and shark) (PDQ®). Available at: http://www.cancer.gov/cancertopics/pdq/cam/cartilage/HealthProfessional/page1/AllPages (accessed 22.02.2015).

National Cancer Institute (2015c). Essiac/Flor Essence (PDQ ®). Available at: http://www.cancer.gov/cancertopics/pdq/cam/essiac/HealthProfessional/page1/AllPages#_1_toc (accessed 22.02.2015).

National Cancer Institute (2015d). Gerson therapy (PDQ®). Available at: http://www.cancer.gov/cancertopics/pdq/cam/gerson/healthprofessional/page1/AllPages (accessed 22.02.2015).

National Cancer Institute (2015e). Mistletoe extracts (PDQ®). Available at: http://www.cancer.gov/cancertopics/pdq/cam/mistletoe/HealthProfessional/page1/AllPages (accessed 22.02.2015).

Nutrition Screening Initiative. 1991. Determine your nutritional health. Washington, D.C.: Nutrition Screening Initiative.

Paolini, M. and Nestle, M., 2003, Pitfalls of enzyme-based molecular anticancer dietary manipulations: food for thought., Mutation Research., p. 181–189.

Park, E. J. and Pezzuto, J. M., 2002, Botanicals in cancer chemoprevention., Cancer and Metastasis Reviews., p. 231 255.

Simopoulos, A. P., 2002, The importance of the ratio of omega-6/omega-3 essential fatty acids., Biomedicine and Pharmacotherapy., p. 365–379.

Soeters, P. B. & Schols, A. M. 2009. Advances in understanding and assessing malnutrition. *Curr Opin Clin Nutr Metab Care,* 12, 487-484.

Soffritti, M., Belpoggi, F., Esposti, D. D., and Lambertini, L., 2005, Aspartame induces lymphomas and leukaemias in rats., European Journal of Oncology., p. 107–116.

Surh, Y. J., 1999, Molecular mechanisms of chemopreventive effects of selected dietary and medicinal phenolic substances., Mutation Research., p. 305–327.

The Ohio State University (2008). Black raspberries slow cancer by altering hundreds of genes. Research Communications. Available at: http://researchnews.osu.edu/archive/berrygene.htm (accessed 20.02.2015).

Weinstein, I. B., 1988, The origins of human cancer: molecular mechanisms of carcinogenesis and their implications for cancer prevention and treatment., Cancer Research., p. 4135–4143.

White, J. V., Guenter, P., Jensen, G., Malone, A., Schofield, M. & Academy Nutrition Work Group., 2012. Consensus statement: Academy of Nutrition and Dietetics and American Society for Parenteral and Enteral Nutrition: Characteristics recommended for the identification and documentation of adult malnutrition. *J Parenter Enter Nutr,* 36, 275-283.

Zarfeshany, A., Asgary, S., and Javanmard, S. H., 2014, Potent health effects of pomegranate., Advanced Biomedical Research., p. 100–114.

Zikri, N. N., Riedl, K. M., Wang, L. S., Lechner, J. F., Schwartz, S. J., and Stoner, G. D., 2009, Black raspberry components inhibit proliferation, induce apoptosis and modulate gene expression in rat esophageal epithelial cells., Nutrition and Cancer., p. 816–826.

Zorko, B., Bueno Perez, L. & Carcache de Blanco, E. 2010. Effects of ILTG on DAPK1 promoter methylation in colon and leukemia cancer cell lines. *Anticancer Res*, 30, 3945-3950.

Nutrition: An Approach to Good Health and Disease Management

Glossary

TERMINOLOGY

Adequate Intake (AI) - the recommended average daily intake level based on observed or experimentally determined approximations or estimates of nutrient intake by a group (or groups) of apparently healthy people that are assumed to be adequate—used when an RDA cannot be determined.

Adipocytes – Fat cells.

Adipogenesis – The growth of new fat cells.

Age-Related Macular Degeneration – Age-related macular degeneration or AMD, a progressive disease of the eye that results in blindness. It is usually diagnosed later in life, and the macular degeneration progresses along with the age of the patient. The disease is caused by exposure of the retina to damaging blue light.

Aglycone – Any molecule which has had its sugar moeity cleaved. An anthocyanidin would be an aglycone of a corresponding anthocyanin.

AHA - American Heart Association

AI - adequate intake

Amylase – starch digesting enzyme found in the saliva.

Anthocyanidins – Flavonoids with a positive charge on the oxygen atom of the heterocyclic ring (ring C). Anthocyanidins are natural plant pigments, often with blue or purple color due to the electric charge.

Anthocyanins – Anthocyanidins with sugar molecules attached.

Anthropometrics - Dealing with determining the size, weight, and properties of the human body.

Antioxidant – Chemical compounds that have the ability to donate or receive an extra electron in order to stabilize or neutralize damaging free radicals.

Apoptosis – Programmed cell death; the apoptotic process often occurs when the cell is too old or damaged to safely and accurately perform all of its cellular duties. When a cell adapts or learns to avoid apoptosis, cancer becomes a concern.

Esperanza J. Carcache de Blanco and Jay Mirtallo (Eds)

AREDS – Age-Related Eye Disease Study, a human clinical study for reducing the risk of developing age-related macular degeneration. The intervention agent was a mixture of 500 mg vitamin C, 400 IU vitamin E, 15 mg beta-carotene, 80 mg zinc oxide, and 2 mg cupric oxide.

AREDS-2 – Age-Related Eye Disease Study #2, a human clinical study designed to improve the formulation of AREDS [#1] and to further reduce the risk of age-related macular degeneration. The new formulation was a mixture of 500 mg vitamin C, 400 IU vitamin E, 80 mg zinc oxide, 2 mg cupric oxide, 10 mg lutein, 2 mg zeaxanthin, and omega-3 fatty acids.

ATBC – The Alpha-Tocopherol Beta-Carotene study, a human clinical trial in which alpha-tocopherol (vitamin E) and beta-carotene were the intervention agents for smokers.

Basal metabolic rate (BMR) - the energy necessary to allow normal function at the cellular, organ, and systemic levels, and to maintain homeostasis, body temperature, and heart and respiratory rate when the body is in a fasted state for 12 hours, awake and in a thermoneutral environment.

Beta-glucans-Polysaccharides made of glucose linked by β-glycosidic bonds. Beta-glucans are commonly found in fungi and bacteria, and they may enhance chemotherapeutic effects of conventional chemical cancer treatment.

Blocking agents-Chemical compounds that block the initiation phase of carcinogenesis by aiding in detoxification of carcinogens or by inducing DNA repair enzymes.

Body composition - The distribution and size of the components of total body weight

Body mass index (BMI)—a measure of weight in kilograms (kg) relative to height in meters (m) squared. It is also defined as a weight stature index used both as a measure of obesity and malnutrition. BMI is considered a reasonably reliable indicator of total body fat, which is related to the risk of disease and death. BMI status categories include underweight, healthy weight, overweight, and obese. Overweight and obese describe ranges of weight that are greater than what is considered healthy for a given height, while underweight describes a weight that is lower than what is considered healthy. Because children and adolescents are growing, their BMI is plotted on growth charts for sex and age. The percentile indicates the relative position of the child's BMI among children of the same sex and age.

Calorie - unit of (heat) energy available from the metabolism of food that is required to sustain the body's various functions, including metabolic processes and physical activity.

Cancer - a condition characterized by uncontrolled growth of abnormal cells.

Carcinogenesis-The three-stage process of the onset of cancer. Carcinogenic agents are those which cause cancer, or especially the initiation stage of carcinogenesis.

Cardiovascular disease—diseases of the heart and diseases of the blood vessel system (arteries, capillaries, veins) within a person's entire body.

CARET – the Carotene and Retinol Efficacy Trial, a human clinical trial in which beta-carotene and retinol (vitamin A) were the intervention agents for those at high-risk for lung cancer (smokers and those exposed to asbestos).

Carotenes – a sub-classification of carotenoids in which the chemical structures are hydrocarbon chains, such as beta-carotene.

Carotenoids – a class of phytochemicals that are fat-soluble molecules; many carotenoids are often natural colorants, such as lycopene in a red tomato.

Chemoprevention-A strategy for preventing the onset of a specific disease, through the use of chemical compounds. Chemoprevention requires the use of substances that are effective, but do not have as toxic qualities or do not possess as intolerable side effects as do chemotherapeutic substances.

Chemotherapy-Treating (halting or reversing) a specific disease with chemical compounds.

Cholesterol—a natural sterol present in all animal tissues. Free cholesterol is a component of cell membranes and serves as a precursor for steroid hormones (estrogen, testosterone, aldosterone), and for bile acids. Humans are able to synthesize sufficient cholesterol to meet biologic requirements, and there is no evidence for a dietary requirement for cholesterol.

Chromoplast – a plant organelle responsible for the production and storage of some pigments.

Cretinism – stunting of body growth and poor mental health development as a result of inadequate maternal intake of iodide during pregnancy.

Cruciferous vegetables – Vegetables from the Brassicaceae (also known as the Cruciferae) family: cabbage, mustard, broccoli, Brussels sprouts, bok choy, water cress, cauliflower, horseradish, *etc.*Cruciferous vegetables produce important phytochemicals called glucosinolates.

Culture – view and understanding of other people beliefs, customs, and knowledge to be grouped based on learned and shared behaviors in their lifestyle.

Cyclooxygenase-Enzymes that synthesize prostaglandins (lipophilic compounds that sensitize pain neurons and regulate inflammation) and that are inhibited by NSAIDs such as aspirin and ibuprofen.

Cytochrome P450 enzymes – A family of enzymes called cytochrome P450. There are several different isozymes within the family. Cytochrome P450 enzymes play a large role in metabolizing several prescription drugs (and other xenobiotics). Foods and phytochemicals that interact with cytochrome P450 isozymes are at high risk for food-drug interactions that may decrease the effectiveness of a pharmaceutical or even simulate an overdose, depending on which isozymes are interacting.

Daily value - recommended intakes of nutrients vary by age and gender and are known as Recommended Dietary Allowances (RDAs) and Adequate Intakes (AIs). However, one value for each nutrient, known as the Daily Value (DV), is selected for the labels of dietary supplements and foods.

Diabetes - a disorder of metabolism—the way the body uses digested food for growth and energy. In diabetes, the pancreas either produces little or no insulin (a hormone that helps glucose, the body's main source of fuel, get into cells), or the cells do not respond appropriately to the insulin that is produced. The three main types of diabetes are type 1, type 2, and gestational diabetes. About 90 to 95 percent of people with diabetes have type 2. This form of diabetes is most often associated with older age, obesity, family history of diabetes, previous his-tory of gestational diabetes, physical inactivity, and certain ethnicities. About 80 percent of people with type 2 diabetes are overweight. Pre-diabetes, also called impaired fasting glucose or impaired glucose tolerance, is a state in which blood glucose levels are higher than normal but not high enough to be called diabetes.

Dietary cholesterol - cholesterol found in foods of animal origin, including meat, seafood, poultry, eggs, and dairy products. Biologically, a liver is required to produce cholesterol, thus, plant foods, such as grains, vegetables and fruits, and oils contain no dietary cholesterol.

Dietary cholesterol—cholesterol found in foods of animal origin, including meat, seafood, poultry, eggs, and dairy products. Biologically, a liver is required to produce cholesterol, thus plant foods, such as grains, vegetables and fruits, and oils contain no dietary cholesterol.

Empty calories - solid fats and added sugars add calories to the food but few or no nutrients.

Energy balance – the state in which energy intake in the form of food and beverages, matches the energy expended, primarily through basal metabolism and physical activity.

Enriched - a food that is labeled as "enriched" with a nutrient must contain at least 10 percent more of the Daily Value of that nutrient than a food of the same type that is not enriched.

Essential nutrient - a vitamin, mineral, fatty acid, or amino acid required for normal body functioning that either cannot be synthesized by the body at all, or cannot be synthesized in amounts adequate for good health, and thus must be obtained from a dietary source. It must have at least one specific biologic function in the body; otherwise, the body leads to a decline in biologic function. Replacement of the deficient essential nutrient prior to permanent damage will restore normal biologic function.

Estimated Average Requirement (EAR) - the average daily nutrient intake level estimated to meet the requirement of half the healthy individuals in a particular life stage and gender group.

Ethnicity – group individuals based on nationality, shared language, social customs, and religion.

Fast food - foods designed for ready availability, use, or consumption and sold at eating establishments for quick availability or take-out.

Fats - a wide variety of compounds that are soluble in organic solvents and generally insoluble in water. The terms 'oils', 'fats' and 'lipids' are all used to refer to fats, 'oils' is usually used for fats that are liquids at room temperature, while 'fats' are solid at room temperature.

Fiber - a form of carbohydrate that is found in plant food. It's chief characteristic is that is is not digested by the processes in the human stomach or small intestine. It adds bulk to the stool – important to normal gastrointestinal tract function.

Flavonoids – a class of phytochemicals whose core structure consists of two phenyl rings and a heterocyclic ring (6 carbons in phenyl ring A, 3 carbons and 1 oxygen in ring C, and 6 carbons in phenyl ring B). Sub-classes of flavonoids include isoflavonoids, chalcones, flavones, and flavans, to name a few.

Fluid - often forgotten as an essential nutrient. It serves as a solvent, lubricant, and vehicle for transporting nutrients and waste.

Foodborne disease - disease caused by consuming foods or beverages contaminated with disease-causing bacteria or viruses.

Fortified foods - fortified means that vitamins or minerals have been added to the food.

Free radicals – an atom or molecule that has one extra electron or is missing an electron from having a full, stable valence. Free radicals often cause chain reactions of forming new radicals in an attempt to make itself electronically stable. Some free radicals play important roles in biological functions, but having too many causes cellular damage and increases the risk of developing certain diseases.

Functional foods – foods that contain important nutrients, allowing the food product to function as health-promoting agents within the human body.

Gluconeogenesis - production of glucose from non-glucose precursors.

Glucose load (GL) - the amount of carbohydrate in a serving of food multiplied by the glycemic index of the carbohydrate. The result is divided by 100.

Glucosinolates – Sulfur-containing compounds with sugar molecules attached. Several glucosinolates are possible chemopreventative agents often found in cruciferous vegetables.

Glutathione S-transferase-A phase II enzyme that conjugates a glutathione group (a molecule consisting of a cysteine, glutamic acid, and glycine unit) onto a xenobiotic substance to make the xenobiotic more polar, deactivated, and/or easier to excrete.

Glycemic index (GI) - the blood glucose response of a given food compared to a standard (typically glucose or white bread).

Glycoside – any molecule that has one or more sugar moieties attached. An anthocyanin would be a glycoside of an anthocyanidin. If all the attached sugars are glucose, the molecule could be called a glucoside or a glycoside (though glucoside is more specific).

Goiter – enlargement of the thyroid gland caused by insufficient iodide intake from the diet.

HDL – high-density lipoprotein.

Healthier-weight goal – the amount of weight loss that reduces disease risk rather than the amount necessary to achieve ideal body weight. A weight goal that is achievable and maintainable.

Healthy weight target – a reasonable upper limit for body weight that would offer a reduction in disease risk and be within reach for most healthy adults.

Hyperlipidemia - elevated lipid levels in the blood.

Hypertension - a condition, also known as high blood pressure, in which blood pressure remains elevated over time. Hypertension makes the heart work too hard, and the high force of the blood flow can harm arteries and organs, such as the heart, kidneys, brain, and eyes. Uncontrolled hypertension can lead to heart attacks, heart failure, kidney disease, stroke, and blindness.

Initiation-The first stage or carcinogenesis that involves encountering a carcinogenic agent for a few hours to days. In initiation, the carcinogenic agent damages DNA to an unrepairable state, or the DNA remains unrepaired after DNA repair attempts.

Isothiocyanates – Metabolites of glucosinolates that contain an isocyanate functional group (–N = C = S). Isothiocyanates are important cancer chemopreventative agents.

LDL – low-density lipoprotein.

Lean body mass - the combination of cell solids, extracellular and intracellular water, and mineral mass of the body.

Lipids - a broad group of naturally occurring molecules that include fats, waxes, sterols, fat-soluble vitamins, triglycerides, phospholipids and others. They function as energy source and storage, structural components of cells and physiologic processes related to stress response, immunity and coagulation. Lipid is often used as a synonym for fats which are a subgroup of lipids.

Macronutrient - a dietary component that provides energy. Macronutrients include protein, fats, carbohydrates, and alcohol.

Macular pigment – a region (called the macula) near thecenter of the retina that takes on a yellow color if there is enough lutein and zeaxanthin in the diet. The pigmentation absorbs blue and UV light, protecting the retina from those damaging wavelengths of light.

Minerals - inorganic substances which are either electrolytes or trace minerals. These are considered micronutrients since they are required in small amounts per day. Electrolytes serve several functions from fluid balance, to normal cardiac rhythms and gastrointestinal function. Trace minerals such as zinc, copper, chromium, manganese and selenium function as metalloenzymes facilitating the use of energy, cellular and organ functions.

Natural killer cells-A special type of cells, comparable to T-cells, that can detect stressed cells earlier than most immune cells. They acquired the name “natural killer” because they can detect the stressed cells and “kill” them before the cells are marked by antibodies that other immune cells detect.

Nitrogen balance - formula used to determine the adequacy of protein intake. Positive balance is considered to be supportive of lean body mass.

Nutraceuticals – Nutrients that are marketed as health-promoting agents with the idea of using food in a way similar to pharmaceutical drugs.

Nutrient – a substance obtained from food that is vital for growth and maintenance of a healthy body throughout life. Its function is to build and repair tissues, regulate body processes and to be converted to and used as energy.

Nutrients - may be divided into various classes: carbohydrate, lipids, proteins, vitamins, minerals and others (phytochemicals). A macronutrient is a nutrient that is required in large quantities (usually grams per day). A micronutrient is required in smaller amounts (milligrams or micrograms per day).

Nutrition (Miriam-Webster dictionary) - the sum of the processes by which an animal or plant takes in and utilizes food substances.

Obesity - a condition characterized by excess body fat.

Occupation - a person's usual or principal work or business, especially as a means of earning a living.

Organosulfur compounds – Any organic compounds that contain sulfur atoms. Important phytochemicals that are classified as organosulfur compounds are most commonly found in cruciferous vegetables or *Allium* species (such as garlic and onion).

Osteoporosis - decreased bone mass related to the effects of aging (including estrogen loss during menopause in women), genetic background and poor diet.

Phase I metabolism-Phase I enzymes (most commonly cytochrome P450 isozymes) metabolize xenobiotic substances, aiding oxidation, reduction, or hydrolysis reactions to reveal more polar products that are easily excreted from the body.

Phase II metabolism-Phase II enzymes (most famously glutathione S-transferase) metabolize xenobiotic substances, conjugating more polar functional groups such as glucoronate, acetate, or sulfate groups, onto the metabolite to deactivate it and excrete it from the body.

Pharmaconutrition - historically, refers to enteral diets enriched with nutrients and has been used to control inflammatory response and improve oxygenation in ICU patients on ventilators who have acute lung injury. It has also been seen as a great new word.

Phytochemical Index (PI) – The ratio of energy (calories) consumed from phytochemical-rich foods, to the total daily energy consumed; a comparative measure of phytochemicals consumed in one's daily diet.

Phytochemicals – Chemical compounds produced by a plant which may have important disease preventative properties, but that are not essential nutrients for the plant or for humans.

Phytoestrogens – Non-steroidal ompounds produced by plants that look and behave similarly to human endogenous estrogens. The most common examples are some of the soy isoflavones.

Phytosterols – Cyclic triterpenes that resemble the molecular structure of cholesterol. Phytosterols are well-known for their cholesterol-lowering abilities. Phytosterols differ from sapogenins in their substitution of the D ring.

Portion size - the amount of a food served or consumed in one eating occasion. A portion is not a standardized amount, and the amount considered to be a portion is subjective and varies.

Prehypertension - blood pressure that is higher than normal but not high enough to be defined as hypertension.

Proanthocyanidins – Polymers of anthocyanidins or flavonoids. Proanthocyanidins may also be called condensed tannins. Procyanidins are any proanthocyanidins with only catechin and epicatechin oligomers, wether the polymer has two units or 50.

Probiotics – Live bacteria administered *via* food with the intentions of depositing those bacteria in the human digestive system. The probiotics or healthy bacteria may aid in digestion, and are a major marketing campaign for yogurts.

Pro-carcinogen-A chemical substance that once modified or activated (usually by a phase I enzyme) becomes a carcinogen.

Progression-The third and final stage of carcinogenesis that involves replication of mutated cells that results in uncontrolled or misregulated proliferation, invasion, and/or metastasis of cells.

Promotion-The second stage of carcinogenesis where damaged cells are replicated to form a premalignant mass or population of cells over the course of 10-40 years.

Protective foods - from food guides (pyramids) are foods that contain adequate amounts of vitamins, minerals, and high quality proteins and that protect against development of a deficiency disease (as pellagra, beriberi, scurvy).

Race – group individuals based on physical characteristics such as skin color, facial features, and hair.

Recommended Dietary Allowance (RDA) - the average daily dietary nutrient intake level sufficient to meet the nutrient requirement of nearly all (97 to 98 percent) healthy individuals in a particular life stage and gender group.

Risk factor - a factor contributing to the development of a disease including heredity, lifestyle choices, and nutritional habits.

Salicylates-Anti-inflammatory agents that typically act through inhibition of prostaglandin synthesis, especially by inhibition of cyclooxygenase enzymes.

Sapogenins – Cyclic triterpenes that resemble the chemical structure of steroids. Their name comes from *Sapon*, which means soap because sapogenins look soapy or foamy when agitated in water. Sapogenins differ from phytosterols in their substitution of the D ring.

Saponins – Sapogenins with sugars attached.

Serum cholesterol - cholesterol that travels in the blood as part of distinct particles containing both lipids and proteins (lipoproteins). Three major classes of lipoproteins are found in the serum of a fasting individual - Low-density lipoproteins (LDL); High-density lipoproteins (HDL); Very-low density lipoprotein (VLDL). Another lipoprotein class; intermediate-density lipoprotein (IDL) resides between VLDL and LDL; in clinical practice IDL is included in the measurement.

Serving size - a standardized amount of a food, such as a cup or an ounce, used in providing information about a food within a food group, such as in dietary guidance.

Social class - people having the same social, economic, or educational status.

Socio-economic status - the combination or interactions of social and economic factors.

Suppressing agents-Chemical compounds that block the promotion or progression stages of carcinogenesis by inhibiting expression of mutated or malignant cells.

Terpenoids – A class of phytochemicals made up of one or more isoprene units. Common sub-classes of terpenoids include monoterpenoids (two isoprene units/10 carbons), diterpenoids (four isoprene units/20 carbons), triterpenoids (six isoprene units/30 carbons), and tetraterpenoids (eight isoprene units/40 carbons), among others. Terpenoids may either have linear or cyclic conformations, and sapogenins and phytosterols are triterpenoids.

The Estimated Energy Requirement (EER) - the average dietary energy intake that is predicted to maintain energy balance in a healthy, adult of a defined age, gender, weight, height, and level of physical activity consistent with good health.

Tolerable Upper Intake Level (UL) - the highest average daily nutrient intake level that is likely to pose no risk of adverse health effects to almost all individuals in the general population. As intake increases above the UL, the potential risk of adverse effects may increase.

Total energy expenditure – the sum of the energy components (BMR, thermogenesis, activity and growth).

Trans fats - rarely derived from dietary sources but are produced commercially for the purpose of converted 'oils' to 'fats' (solid is better for transport and easier to use in food preparation). It is an isomer with parts of the chain on opposite sides in contrast to being on the same side (cis-isomer) as occurs in nature. Therefore the isomer stacks easier, making it easier to freeze and remain solid rather than liquid.

Vitamins - defined by what they are not – carbohydrates, proteins nor fats. They serve vital (hence vita-) functions in the body. They act as coenzymes in the metabolism of energy yielding nutrients, coordinate growth and maintenance of tissues as well as assist in storage and utilization of energy.

Xanthophylls – A sub-classification of carotenoids in which the chemical structures are oxygenated hydrocarbon chains, where the oxygen atoms are typically located on both ends of the long molecules, as in zeaxanthin.

Xenobiotics-A chemical substance that is not produced by the body, but may be consumed. Typical xenobiotics include pharmaceutical drugs and phytochemicals, but also carcinogenic molecules.

Glossary includes definitions taken from original sources for educational purposes.

Subject Index

Esperanza J. Carcache de Blanco and Jay Mirtallo (Eds)

Printed in Germany
by Amazon Distribution
GmbH, Leipzig

16811500R00206